Nursing Policy Research

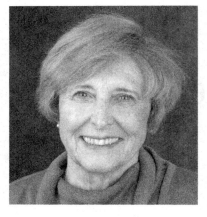

Geri L. Dickson, PhD, RN, is the founder and executive director of the New Jersey Collaborating Center for Nursing, in the College of Nursing, Rutgers University. The mission of the Center is to serve "as a future-oriented research and development organization," with a focus on developing data-based studies to take the pulse of the major issues confronting the discipline of nursing. The Center serves as a catalyst for change in New Jersey and makes evidence-based nursing recommendations to the state government. As a Wisconsin native, Dr. Dickson received a BSN from Alverno College, a MSN from Marquette University, and a PhD from the University of Wisconsin. She began her nursing career in psychiatric nursing, has taught nursing for 20 years, and engages in research, especially workforce issues and qualitative methods. In addition, she has been actively involved in guiding the development of the first university-based nursing program in post-Communist Romania.

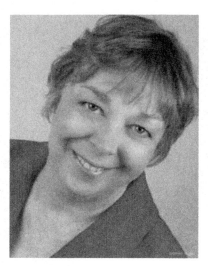

Linda Flynn, PhD, RN, earned her bachelor's degree from the University of Maryland, and her master's degree and doctorate from Rutgers University. She received postdoctoral education at the Center for Health Outcomes and Policy Research, University of Pennsylvania, under the direction of Dr. Linda Aiken. She is currently an associate professor at the University of Maryland School of Nursing and Research Director at the New Jersey Collaborating Center for Nursing, Rutgers College of Nursing. She has taught courses in research and policy to master's and doctoral students for many years.

Nursing Policy Research

*Turning Evidence-Based
Research Into Health Policy*

GERI L. DICKSON, PhD, RN
LINDA FLYNN, PhD, RN
Editors

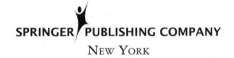
SPRINGER PUBLISHING COMPANY
NEW YORK

Springer Publishing Company, LLC
11 West 42nd Street
New York, NY 10036
www.springerpub.com

Acquisitions Editor: Allan Graubard
Production Editor: Julia Rosen
Cover design: Mimi Flow
Composition: Apex CoVantage

08 09 10 11/ 5 4 3 2 1

Library of Congress Cataloging-in-Publication Data

Nursing policy research : turning evidence-based research into health policy / [edited by] Geri L. Dickson, Linda Flynn.
   p. ; cm.
 Includes bibliographical references and index.
 ISBN 978-0-8261-3333-5 (alk. paper)
 1. Nursing—Research—United States—Methodology.   2. Evidence-based nursing—United States.   3. Medical policy—United States.   I. Dickson, Geri L.   II. Flynn, Linda.
 [DNLM: 1. Nursing Research—methods—United States.   2. Evidence-Based Medicine—methods—United States.   3. Health Policy—United States. WY 20.5 N97328 2008]
  RT81.5.N85   2008
  610.73072—dc22

                                    2008016042

Printed in Canada by Transcontinental.

This book is dedicated to all the nurses who make a positive difference in the lives of their patients, each and every day!

SECTION II: TOWARD EVIDENCE-BASED POLICY: COLLECTING AND MANAGING THE DATA   39

Introduction   39
Geri L. Dickson

3   Addressing the Complexities of Survey Research   43
Patricia Moulton, Linda M. Lacey, Linda Flynn, Christine Tassone Kovner, and Carol S. Brewer

It Is All About the Why: Determining Your Survey
   Research Topic   44
Do You Know What You Are Asking? Common Problems
   With Survey Questions   50
Mail Survey Method: Imperatives and Pitfalls   58
Collecting Data by Survey—The Best-Laid Plans
   Can Go Awry   62

4   Forecasting a State Supply and Demand of RNs Using the Revised 2005 HRSA Models   71
Lynn Unruh and Valerie Danesh

The HRSA Nursing Demand and Supply Models   73
Using the HRSA Models for Forecasting in Individual States:
   Three Approaches   81
FCN Experiences in Using the HRSA Models for Forecasting
   in Florida   85
Summary of FCN Experiences: Lessons Learned in Using
   the HRSA Models for Forecasting in Florida and
   Recommendations for Other States   98

5   Missing Data Effects on Nurse Workforce Analysis and Projections   103
Jennifer G. Nooney

Sources and Causes of Missing Data   104
Analyzing and Classifying Missingness: The Bias Analysis   107
Traditional Methods for Dealing with Missing Data   111
Recent Developments in Missing Data Techniques   115

Lessons Learned   121
Linda Flynn

SECTION III: RESEARCH AND WORKPLACE POLICY   125

Introduction   125
Geri L. Dickson

6   Work Satisfaction Among Staff Nurses in Acute Care Hospitals   127
Carol S. Brewer and Christine Tassone Kovner

Sample   128
Methods   129
Findings   130
Discussion   136
Policy Implications   138

7   Workload, Quality of Care, and Job Satisfaction
in Home Health Nurses   143
Linda Flynn

Background and Significance   144
Method   146
Findings   147
Policy Implications   150

8   The Emotional Demands of Nursing   155
Rebecca J. Erickson

A Crisis in Nurse Staffing   156
Why Nurses Leave Direct Patient Care   157
The Emotional Foundations of Burnout   158
Methods   162
Results   168
What Influences Burnout Among Registered Nurses?   170
Which Facets of the Emotional Context of Care Might Contribute to an
Understanding of Burnout Over and Above the Effect of Individual
and Occupational Characteristics?   172

Lessons Learned   179
Geri L. Dickson

SECTION IV: RESEARCH AND EDUCATIONAL POLICY   183

Introduction   183
Geri L. Dickson

9   Nursing's Long-Term Pipeline: A Study of High School Students Using a Unique Data Collection Approach   187

Rebecca Rudel and Patricia Moulton

North Dakota's Unique Nursing Education History   188
Tomorrow's Nursing Pipeline: A Literature Review   191
Nursing as a Specific Career Vision in High School   193
The High School Student Survey   194
Discussion   200

10   The Looming Crisis of an Inadequate Pipeline for Nursing Faculty   209

Brenda Cleary, James W. Bevill Jr., Linda M. Lacey, and Jennifer G. Nooney

Faculty Supply and Demand   210
The Pipeline for Faculty Roles   212
Discussion   214

11   Clinical Simulation and the Need for Evidence-Based Policy   219

Felissa R. Lashley and Wendy Nehring

Types of Simulation   221
Standardized Patients   225
Simulation and Policy   226

Lessons Learned   233

Geri L. Dickson

SECTION V: FUNDING THE RESEARCH TO POLICY CONNECTION   237

Introduction   237

Linda Flynn

12   Of Horses and Ponies: Taking Your Show to Washington   239

Claudia L. McDonald

Why Should I Learn to Dance?   239
The Dance: One Step at a Time   242
The Federal Budget Process   246

13   AHRQ Funding Opportunities for Nurse Researchers   253
Kathleen Kendrick, Gail S. Makulowich, and Mary L. Grady

AHRQ's Changing Mission   254
AHRQ's Research Priorities   255
Research Funding Opportunities   257
Training and Career Development Programs   263
Research Infrastructure Support Programs   265
Getting an AHRQ Research Grant   266
Overview of the Grant Application Submission, Review,
    and Award Process   267

14   From Issues to Action: How the Robert Wood Johnson
Foundation Influences Health Policy   271
Lori Melichar and Susan B. Hassmiller

Governmental Policy: RWJF's Role in Advancing the Nurse
    Practitioner Role   272
Organizational Policy: Transforming Care at the Bedside   273
The Process of Influencing Policy   275
Identifying Promising Solutions to Improve Health
    and Health Care   278
Creating the Evidence to Convince Policy Makers to Improve
    Health and Health Care Policy   279
Restrictions on Lobbying: A Delicate Balance   285
Building Capacity of Individuals and Institutions   288
Conclusion: How RWJF Influences Policy   289

15   A Metaphor for Addressing the Nurse Shortage
in Oregon   293
Judith L. Woodruff

Northwest Health Foundation   294
Farming and the Relationship to the Nursing
    Workforce Crisis   295
Cultivating the Environment for Nursing   296
Planning for Future Crops: Supporting a Nursing
    Policy Agenda   308
Conclusion and Key Findings   310

Lessons Learned   313
Linda Flynn

SECTION VI: MAKING THE RESEARCH TO POLICY CONNECTION   317

Introduction   317
Geri L. Dickson

16   Policy Development and Nursing   319
Lucille A. Joel

Citizenship in a Democracy   319
Nurses as Participants in a Democratic Community   320
The Power of Numbers   322
Politics for Policy   323
Beyond Baseline   327

17   State Funding for Nurse Faculty Loan Repayment:
The Vermont Experience   329
Mary Val Palumbo

Applying Kingdon's Framework   329
The Political Stream   333
The Policy Stream   333

18   Using Research to Influence Federal Policy:
The Nephrology Nurses' Experience   343
Linda Flynn, Charlotte Thomas-Hawkins,
and Sandra M. Bodin

The Research–Policy Connection   344
The Revised Model in Action   344

Lessons Learned   349
Linda Flynn

EPILOGUE   353

19   From Research to Policy—The Ultimate Translation   355
Linda Flynn and Geri L. Dickson

Index   359

List of Figures

CHAPTER 2

Figure 2.1   Nurse Practice Environments, Nurse Staffing, and Outcomes   25

CHAPTER 4

Figure 4.1   Overview of the NDM   75
Figure 4.2   NDM Operational Structure   78
Figure 4.3   Overview of the NSM   79
Figure 4.4   NSM Operational Structure   80

CHAPTER 5

Figure 5.1   Projected RN FTE Growth in NC Hospitals, 2004–2006   117

CHAPTER 8

Figure 8.1   Percentage Reporting Emotional Context-of-Care Experiences   169
Figure 8.2   Job Burnout Regressed on Emotional Experience   171
Figure 8.3   Job Burnout Regressed on Emotional Labor   171

CHAPTER 9

Figure 9.1   Reasons for Not Planning for a Nursing Career   197
Figure 9.2   Students' Agreement With Perception Statements   198

CHAPTER 10

Figure 10.1   Projected Faculty Supply and Demand Under Different
Retirement Thresholds and Student-to-Faculty Ratios   210

CHAPTER 12

Figure 12.1   Overview of the Federal Budget Process   248

Figure 12.2   Focus on the Congressional Budget Process   249

CHAPTER 13

Figure 13.1   Supply-side Research Paradigm   256

List of Tables

CHAPTER 4

Table 4.1   HRSA NDM Projections: Nurse Types and Health Care Utilization by Setting   76

Table 4.2   Summary of Data Sources and Corresponding Data Fields   87

Table 4.3   Baseline Comparisons of Employed Florida Nurse FTEs: HRSA Versus FCN Numbers   92

Table 4.4   Baseline Comparisons of Florida RN Populations: HRSA Versus FCN   93

Table 4.5   Baseline Comparisons of Florida RN New Graduates and Educational Upgrades: HRSA Versus FCN Values   94

CHAPTER 5

Table 5.1   Hospital Size and Response Status   109

CHAPTER 6

Table 6.1   Predictors of Job Satisfaction   135

CHAPTER 7

Table 7.1   Sample Characteristics ($n = 137$)   146

Table 7.2   Correlational Coefficients of Workload Variables and Quality Indicators ($n = 137$)   149

Table 7.3   Odds Ratios Associated With Unadjusted Effects of Workload and Quality Indicators on Home Health Nurses' Intentions to Leave their Jobs   149

CHAPTER 10

Table 10.1   Percentage of Cohort Members Achieving Master's and Doctoral Preparation   215

CHAPTER 17

Table 17.1   All Options Considered   335

Table 17.2   A Summary of all the Legislation that was Introduced for Nursing Faculty Loan Repayment in Vermont   340

Contributors

James W. Bevill, Jr., MSN, RN
Associate Director
Workforce Development
North Carolina Center for Nursing
Raleigh, North Carolina

Sandra M. Bodin, MA, RN, CNN
President 2007–2008
American Nephrology Nurses'
Association
Lead Clinical Informatics Analyst
St. Mary's Duluth Clinic Health System
Duluth, Minnesota

Carol S. Brewer, PhD, RN
Associate Professor
University at Buffalo School of
Nursing
Buffalo, New York
Director of Nursing
New York State System AHEC
Statewide Office
Department of Family Practice
Buffalo, New York

Sean P. Clarke, RN, PhD, CRNP, FAAN
Associate Director
Center for Health Outcomes and
Research Policy
Class of 1965 25th Reunion Term
Associate Professor of Nursing
University of Pennsylvania School
of Nursing
Philadelphia, Pennsylvania

Brenda Cleary, PhD, RN, FAAN
Executive Director
North Carolina Center for Nursing
Raleigh, North Carolina

Valerie Danesh, RN, BSN, MHSA
Doctoral Student
University of Central Florida
Orlando, Florida

Rebecca J. Erickson, PhD
Professor of Sociology
The University of Akron
Akron, Ohio

Mary L. Grady, BS
Health Communications Specialist
Agency for Healthcare Research
and Quality
Rockville, Maryland

Susan B. Hassmiller, PhD, RN, FAAN
Senior Program Officer
and Team Leader
Robert Wood Johnson Foundation
Princeton, New Jersey

Lucille Joel, EdD, RN, APN-C, FAAN
Professor
College of Nursing
Rutgers, the State University
of New Jersey
Newark, New Jersey

Kathleen Kendrick, MS, BS
Deputy Director
Agency for Healthcare Research
and Quality
Rockville, Maryland

Christine Tassone Kovner, RN, PhD, FAAN
Professor, College of Nursing
Senior Fellow at the Hartford Institute
for Geriatric Nursing
New York University
New York, New York

Linda M. Lacey, MA
Associate Director, Research
North Carolina Center for Nursing
Raleigh, North Carolina

Felissa R. Lashley, RN, PhD, ACRN, FACMG, FAAN
Dean and Professor
College of Nursing
Rutgers, the State University
of New Jersey
Newark, New Jersey

Gail S. Makulowich, BA
Health Communications Specialist
Agency for Healthcare Research
and Quality
Rockville, Maryland

Claudia L. McDonald, PhD
Associate Vice President for
Special Projects
Texas A&M University–Corpus Christi
Corpus Christi, Texas

Lori Melichar, PhD
Senior Program Officer
Robert Wood Johnson Foundation
Princeton, New Jersey

Patricia Moulton, PhD
Assistant Professor
Center for Rural Health
School of Medicine and Health Sciences
University of North Dakota
Grand Forks, North Dakota

Wendy Nehring, RN, PhD, FAAN, FAAIDD
Associate Dean for Academic Affairs
Director of the Graduate Program
and Associate Professor
College of Nursing
Rutgers, the State University
of New Jersey
Newark, New Jersey

Jennifer G. Nooney, PhD
Associate Director, Research
Florida Center for Nursing
Orlando, Florida

Mary Val Palumbo, FNP, GNP-BC
Director
Office of Nursing Workforce,
Research, Planning and Development
University of Vermont
Burlington, Vermont

Rebecca Rudel, PhD, RN, CNE
Assistant Professor
Minnesota State University
Mankato, Minnesota

Charlotte Thomas-Hawkins, PhD, RN
Assistant Professor
College of Nursing
Rutgers, the State University
of New Jersey
Newark, New Jersey

Lynn Unruh, PhD, RN, LHRM
Associate Professor
Department of Health Professions
University of Central Florida
Orlando, Florida

Judith L. Woodruff, JD
Program Director, Nursing
Northwest Health Foundation
Program Director
Partners Investing in Nursing's
Future
Portland, Oregon

Foreword

More than 150 years ago, Florence Nightingale inalterably influenced the evolution of the modern hospital and the establishment of the profession of nursing through outcomes research. Nightingale meticulously used statistics to demonstrate to British officials that more soldiers in the Crimean War died because of unsafe care environments in military hospitals than of wounds received in battle. She then demonstrated a dramatic reduction in deaths following the introduction of nurses whose roles included making the care environment safer (Cohen, 1984). Despite such an auspicious beginning, nursing policy research is still in its formative phases, having experienced little development between Nightingale's research and the late 20th century.

There are lessons from Nightingale's research that can guide the further development of policy-relevant research concerning nursing. First, her topic, preventable deaths in government institutions, was a problem that military and government representatives had already identified as needing attention. Policy research is more likely to have impact if framed in the context of a social problem that policymakers or health care leaders have already agreed is necessary to address. Policy research on problems that have not risen to visibility on the public's agenda is much less likely to have an impact on change, even if the research is carefully designed and implemented. Thus, the first step in successful policy research is the identification of a problem to which policy makers are seeking solutions. This requires nurse researchers to read the broad health policy literature including the mass media and to have collaborators from other disciplines whose knowledge base is different from nursing. Therefore, a fundamental requirement of successful policy research is an interdisciplinary team.

A second lesson from Nightingale's research is presentation of research findings so that they can be easily understood by an informed general audience. Nightingale's innovative charts created a form of communication that could be understood without knowing statistics. Of course, social statistics were just evolving in Nightingale's time; indeed she is credited with having a major role in the development of proportional statistics. Today we have often-conflicting requirements: the demands of peer reviewers and editors of scientific journals for the use of complex statistical presentations of findings versus the need for readability and simplicity of research design and presentation of results to communicate with those who can actually implement the findings by changing practice and policy.

Balancing the competing demands for complexity and simplicity is one of the great challenges of policy research. The challenge is made even more difficult by the power of stakeholders in political discourse who tend to refute inconvenient research findings by attempting to discredit the scientific legitimacy of the research rather than debating the practice and policy implications of research findings they do not like. This leads experienced policy researchers to "defensive practices" involving the use of complex research designs and methods that then become difficult to explain clearly. Stakeholders need only to confuse policy makers with research rhetoric, not necessarily disprove findings that run counter to their interests. Sometimes third-party neutral research organizations such as the Institute of Medicine or the New York Academy of Medicine can be helpful in interpreting evidence from competing points of view. In the end, however, nothing is as effective in influencing policy as clear answers to important questions gained through powerful but simple research designs.

In the chapters that follow, experienced policy researchers address how to manage multiple challenges to successfully make the transition from statistical significance to policy. Policy research shares with all forms of research the requirement for scientific rigor and clearly presented results. Usually the best research in any field is elegant in its simplicity and clarity. However, policy research often requires more front-end investment in the selection of the research question and its framing in a policy-relevant context than do disciplines where the primary audience is other researchers who together are trying to advance knowledge through cumulative research contributions. As well, significantly more investment is required in translating the findings of policy-relevant research to audiences who are not scientists.

Despite the difficulty of policy research, there is nothing as thrilling as seeing the results from rigorously designed research translated into public policies that benefit millions of people. Nursing has solutions to many of the most challenging issues in health care. Policy research is a vehicle to promote the widespread adoption of effective nursing solutions for the benefit of the public and for the continued advancement of the nursing profession.

Linda H. Aiken, PhD, RN, FAAN

REFERENCE

Cohen, I. B. (1984). Florence Nightingale. *Scientific American, 250,* 128–138.

Preface

A reoccurring theme among the chapters of this book centers on the powerful potential of nursing research to influence health policy decisions and initiatives. Additionally, the benefits of evidence-based policies, informed by findings from the scientific analyses of real-world observations compared to a "best guess," are similarly highlighted.

Throughout the book, contributors share their knowledge, skills, and experiences related to various aspects of the research enterprise and its impact on the research to policy connection. The foci of their respective research agendas frequently include nurse workforce issues, nurses' work environments, and the nature and outcomes of nurses' work. Consequently, these chapters may be of particular interest to leaders, researchers, and evaluators engaged in nursing workforce issues and nursing outcomes research.

Yet the principles and processes related to policy-influencing research, as shared throughout these chapters, transcend specific investigative agendas. Whether your interests are in maternal–child health, vulnerable populations, cardiac care, mental health disorders, or any population, health risk, or disease state, the use of research findings in the development of evidence-based policy decisions is, likewise, imperative. Toward that end, the chapters offered throughout the book have been designed to inform activities that may enhance your research to policy connection, regardless of your practice area or the nature of your research questions.

The book is divided into seven sections, and the editors have shared the responsibility of tying the chapters and sections together. Each section begins with an introduction and the theme of the section and concludes with a summary of the lessons learned from the studies in that section.

Section I is devoted to two introductory chapters: chapter 1 features a beginning of a dialogue of the research to policy connection, and chapter 2 presents an overview of nursing outcomes research and its relationship to policy decisions. These suggest that evidence does not just "happen." Instead, the production of trustworthy evidence requires a rigorous process and an ongoing refinement of research skills.

Toward that end, Section II offers "how to" chapters: three substantive chapters based on the experiences of seasoned researchers. The first, chapter 3, describes the processes and potential problems of collecting and managing data. A detailed description is found in chapter 4 of the procedures necessary to select, input, and analyze existing databases to project supply and demand for nurses on a state level, using the standardized national supply and demand models. Chapter 5 focuses on a problem that plagues most survey researchers—missing data. The author details methods of imputing data into survey research and describes the effects of missing data. All of these methods, however, are relevant to surveys of other topics.

Section III is devoted to research and workplace policy, with chapter 6 focusing on a study of work satisfaction among nurses in acute care hospitals. The findings from this regional study of RNs provide strong evidence for the authors' recommendations for policy changes.

The section continues in chapter 7 with the report of a national study of home health nurses and stresses the findings of the relationships of workload, quality of care, and job satisfaction for nurses in community settings. The author submits potential policy changes based on her findings. Chapter 8 concludes this section with a study based on statistics and the words of nurses about the emotional labor of nurses in hospitals. This author also puts forth evidence-based recommendations for policy changes aimed at retaining nurses in the workplace.

Section IV focuses on research and educational policy. In chapter 9, two North Dakota researchers report on their online survey of high school students in North Dakota and the students' perspectives on nursing as a career. Particularly interesting is the context of the study—the repeal of the North Dakota legislative mandate for two levels of licensure. North Dakota was the only state to implement that position, advocated by the 1965 American Nurses Association's position statement on nurse education.

In chapter 10, a team from the North Carolina Center for Nursing, the first state nursing workforce center, projects the future supply of faculty based on potential retirements of current North Carolina faculty. They present scenarios demonstrating reduction in the projected faculty shortage resulting from a staged increase in the student–to–clinical faculty ratios. Rounding out this section is chapter 11, in which experts in the field present discourse about the use of simulation models in nurse education. The authors, well known for their studies in this area, present the research suggesting pros and cons of simulation clinical education and the regulatory changes that may be necessary.

Section V presents critical information about securing funding for your research. In chapter 12, we find a description of how to seek funding through the U.S. Congress to obtain federal grants for your state research work. In chapter 13, colleagues from the Agency for Healthcare Research and Quality (AHRQ) describe their agency's mission and goals. They offer examples of funded nurse research, tips for writing proposals, and common problems to avoid in order to obtain AHRQ funding for your research.

In the succeeding chapter, officers from the Robert Wood Johnson Foundation delineate the impact of this national foundation and the grants they make to provide evidence that can influence policy in the United States. The foundation has devoted a good share of its philanthropic mission to nursing grants. In chapter 15, an officer in the Northwest Health Foundation takes a state perspective that outlines its role as a local foundation in funding grants to address workforce issues in Oregon. She views the nurse workforce as a living system and convincingly uses the metaphor of "farming" for the foundation's active role in sustaining state grants to address the local nurse shortage issues.

Last, but certainly not least, is the section on making the research to policy connection, offering suggestions and examples of how to make that policy connection. Chapter 16 lays out how *nurses as citizens* of health care can use their expertise in work settings, professional organizations, or public policy arenas to influence policy change. The following chapters offer examples of how nurse researchers have been able to make that research to policy connection. In chapter 17, the author carefully describes how nurse leaders in Vermont were able to make that connection, based on findings from the Vermont Office of Nursing Workforce. Collaborators in research in chapter 18 delineate the research, the political process, and the professional organization's strength they used to persuade the Centers for Medicare and Medicaid to adopt regulations mandating an RN be present during dialysis treatments.

The book concludes with an epilogue in which we address a means to carry out the ultimate research to policy connection—translation of research findings into policies. Thus, our research to policy journey concludes with an understandable framework from which to begin the process of connecting the research to the policy—an arduous and worthwhile venture!

Acknowledgments

Many of the chapters in this book began as presentations at the national conference for leaders in state workforce centers hosted by the New Jersey Collaborating Center for Nursing in 2006. Some of those presentations, together with additional authors, now provide a roadmap to identify how scientific, patient-oriented research is developed, administered, and presented and how it can drive many levels of policy change so that the health care system can achieve better, more cost-effective outcomes.

We gratefully acknowledge the philanthropy of the Robert Wood Johnson Foundation for their support of the conference and for continuing to fund the Jersey Collaborating Center (the Center). Making the Center a public/private venture, the state of New Jersey also has provided funding for the Center.

We extend an enthusiastic thanks to the authors who have shared their research, innovation, compassion, and talents with you, the readers of this book. Although most are nurse researchers, five of the authors are non-nurses, indicating the value of interdisciplinary collaboration.

We also want to acknowledge the fine technical assistance in the preparation of this book by Allison Creary and Mary Ellen Cook. Further, this book would not have been possible without the continuing support and love of our husbands: Carlisle Dickson and Roger Flynn.

A special thanks to the editors of Springer Publishing, whose helpful consultation has enabled us to achieve our goal to fill an educational void. They have helped us to put a useful resource into the hands of graduate students.

And finally, to the students who are studying how to ensure that nursing will be at the table when key health care policy decisions are made—we invite you to learn the skills and to build on the strong legacy of history's nursing leaders and researchers for the benefit of your patients.

Discovering the Research to Policy Connection

1

Back to the Future: From Evidence to Policy

GERI L. DICKSON

We who are nurses are inheritors of a great tradition. It is ours to guard, to strengthen, to enlarge where needed, and to equip ourselves worthily for so doing.

—M. Adelaide Nutting (1939)

As we embark on our journey of discovering the research to policy connection, this chapter provides an introduction for the ongoing journey. How far has nursing come in terms of providing evidence as the basis for policy change? Where are we today in that journey toward creating change through clinical, organizational, educational, professional, and public policy? As Aiken points out in this book's foreword, Florence Nightingale led the way in introducing the idea of quantifying and displaying data linking the work of nurses to the soldiers' survival during the Crimean War. This is part of the great tradition that we, as nurses, have inherited.

Nightingale developed and used her coxcomb diagrams, which are credited with having spawned the use of pie charts, to identify the differences nurses' care made in the lives of British soldiers during the 1854–1856 Crimean war. However, what was most unusual and unique was how she presented her data to demonstrate the number of *preventable* soldier deaths before and after the advent of nurses' care. Trained nurses, indeed, did make a quantifiable difference in the lives of the British soldiers.

Accordingly, the death rate of soldiers, resulting from disease and infections, decreased from 47% before the introduction of trained nurses to 2% after their arrival (Florence Nightingale Museum, 1854–1856). Nightingale used her evidence to support a sea change in nursing by identifying a problem—the lack of nursing care—around which the public, interest groups, media, and others could rally. She provided the evidence for a policy change in 1860 that has had an impact on health care ever since—the first organized program of training for nurses.

Over the last 150 years, and despite an increase in nursing research, policy questions have seldom been the major foci of research. As the twentieth century drew to a close, nurse researchers began to return to Nightingale's use of statistics to demonstrate with empiric evidence the differences nurses' care made in the lives of their patients. In time, clinical and patient outcomes research began the connection to policy-oriented change.

In this chapter, I provide a historical context for this book, citing select examples of how policy created by others has changed nursing and how some nurses, even without empirical evidence, were able to create policy changes. The policy changes are framed from a perspective of the merging of a policy agenda (Kingdon, 2003) and the support of others to fill a societal need, thereby creating a window of opportunity in which change can occur. From this perspective on the past and present of nursing policy development, an important question for the future is considered: how might we best move forward to translate our knowledge and evidence into policy changes that will improve the health of our nation's citizens?

SELECT EXAMPLES OF PAST POLICY CHANGES

The Formation of Nursing Schools

Because of the public's appreciation for Nightingale's work, a public trust was established that financed the Nightingale Training School for Nurses as an entirely independent educational institution. St. Thomas Hospital in London was chosen as the site of the school, but not without opposition from most physicians, who did not support the idea of any teaching for nurses beyond the "how to" of poultice-making (Donahue, 1985). Nevertheless, the public, the media, and the politicians of the day all supported Nightingale and her work. Consequently, the school thrived and became extremely important to nursing's future as a profession—a change made by virtue of evidence and social need.

Although there were no formal training programs in the United States, the Civil War, just like the Crimean War, brought the need for nursing care to others' attention. As the 19th century wore on, a growing sense of social responsibility for citizens' health in the United States contributed to the recognized need for formal training for nurses (Grippando, 1977). Accordingly, in 1873 three U.S. schools of nursing were started, based on the Nightingale system of nurse education. However, the schools in the United States, contrary to Nightingale's model, were not independent in financing or infrastructure; they were placed under the jurisdiction of the hospital and medical staff (Kalisch & Kalisch, 1986).

The Public Health Movement

As the 19th century drew to a close, social responsibility for health increased, and public health gained a new emphasis. Nurse leaders such as Lillian Wald rose to the occasion and demonstrated the value of nurses to provide care to the community and to advance public health. Although the nurse leaders did not employ the use of empirical evidence, nurses were recognized by the public as valuable and were the forerunners of the Visiting Nurse Associations and, later, public school nursing.

Based on business and the private sector's belief in the value of nurses and health, the Metropolitan Life Insurance Company provided free home nursing to policyholders, helping to keep them well during the early 20th century. Other community nurses worked in organized efforts to improve maternal and child care. The focus was on new immigrants and their families and involved assessment of social conditions as well as health needs. In this new role and before the development of vaccines or medications, nurses managed major infectious diseases, such as tuberculosis, in the community. Additionally, improving family health in the rural and country areas of our nation became a focus of nurses' care in the early 20th century.

By 1910, the nurses working in the various communities formed the National Organization for Public Health Nursing. Lillian Wald became the first president, and the founders of the organization declared that "the experience data available emphasized the urgency and practical necessity for the extension of public health nursing service to a much larger proportion of wage-earners and people of moderate means than now have the benefit of same" (Kalisch & Kalisch, 1986, p. 288). Indeed, infectious diseases had decreased, but so many societal changes (e.g., improved water supply, sewage disposal, cleaner streets, and regulation of food and dairy products) were made that nurses could not take credit for all of the changes. Rather, they cited what people experienced as the basis for change. Nevertheless, public health nurses had the support of the public and business and made an important difference in people's lives—they filled a social and health need.

Impact of Scientific Medicine on Nursing

In the following decade, nurses remained busy starting schools of nursing, educating teachers of nursing, advocating for regulation through licensure of nurses, and taking care of the sick in patients' homes. The superintendent of nursing supervised both the school of nursing and the hospital. She and supervisors oversaw the students' clinical practice, and, of course, physicians taught many of the classes. The superintendent and a supervisor were generally the only graduate nurses in the hospital as the student nurses provided the care for the patients. Their care included domestic work, cooking meals, and keeping the wards warm and spotless, as well as caring for the patients' comfort and physical needs.

At the same time, physicians were organizing their own schools, but neither regulations nor standards were in place. In 1910, with a grant from the Carnegie Foundation, Abraham Flexner conducted a review of all 155 medical schools in the United States and Canada, ranking their quality and value (Flexner, 1910). The outgrowth of the Flexner Report was that medicine became a university discipline with strict standards of admission and hospital affiliations to achieve quality medical education, based on the scientific model in place at Johns Hopkins University.

However, nursing education remained hospital based; the students cared for the patients and kept the hospitals running. As a result, the atmosphere in the hospital nursing schools remained one in which the doctors were in charge. A sense of what it was like to be a student at this time can be found in the first verse of this poem written by an early hospital nursing student:

Nurses moving quietly,
Voices hushed in awe.
All things silent waiting.
Obedient to the law
That we have heard so often.

But I'll repeat once more:
"All things must be in order
When doctor's on the floor." (Kalisch & Kalisch, 1986, p. 216)

Nevertheless, the nursing leaders of the day saw this movement of medical education into the university as an opportunity for a Flexner-like report to be conducted to revamp nursing education. Although the Carnegie Foundation funded other educational reports—for example, dental, legal, and teacher education—the nurses' pleas were passively ignored (Kalisch & Kalisch, 1986). An educational policy shift designated the medical school as the sole center for the production of physicians, and the apprenticeship programs passed into history. At the same time, the reform also was successful in creating medicine as a profession almost exclusively for white, male, upper-class Americans, leaving out women and Blacks (Reissman, 1983). Try as they might, nurse educators never were able to move nurse education from the hospitals into universities and colleges. Even today, the bulk of nurse education is found in 2-year community colleges or hospital schools, with a smaller percentage of the total new nurses graduating from 4-year colleges and universities.

The Start of Higher Education for Nurses

The U.S. Children's Bureau was established in 1912, and the welfare of America's children became a matter of national concern (Worcester, 1914). The passing of the federal Sheppard-Towner Act of 1921 provided the states with federal grants-in-aid for services for the welfare and hygiene of mothers and children. These services were most often free to the participants, with the costs borne by the federal funding or, in some cases, by charitable or private funding.

Although the majority of nurses remained private duty nurses, paid by their patients, public health nursing was growing, as hundreds of nurses were employed to make home visits and to supply health education and health screenings to mothers and infants. Under the leadership of M. Adelaide Nutting, the roles of nurses in the community led to the beginning of nursing education in a university: Teacher's College in Columbia University in New York City. The program, in 1910, was started with an endowment from wealthy female donors and was used to educate a small body of teacher-nurses to carry the theory and practice of physical welfare for children, as well as hygienic living practices, into private homes, schools, and communities (Christy, 1969).

Although this was a first for nursing, the reality of the situation led to a sense of divisiveness among nurses. Many of the nurse leaders and Columbia students were women who had private means of support and came from educated families, whereas the majority of nurses were women who were hospital trained, who had an opportunity to perform altruistic work, and who, at that same time, were able to be independent and self-supporting (Roberts, 1954). All things considered, it was the merger of support of the public citizens, private education, an endowment of financial support, and a societal need that created a window of opportunity for the beginning of higher education for nurses.

After the establishment of nursing education in one university, and licensure by all states in place by 1914, nurse leaders devoted their renewed efforts to the production of an educational report for nursing, comparable to the Flexner Report for medicine. Finally, the Rockefeller Foundation commissioned a national study of nursing education, which was published in 1923 and known as the Goldmark Report ("Nursing and Nursing Education in the U.S.," 1923). Although it was as critical of nursing schools as Flexner was of medical schools, the desired impact of moving the standard for nursing education into the university did not occur. The vision and efforts of the leaders, by themselves, were not sufficient to create their desired policy change for nursing education. Without the overwhelming support of the public, business, or government, the site of nursing education did not change—the window of opportunity was not open.

Nurses and Hospitals

By the mid-20th century, the world was involved in a major war, World War II. Patriotism was rampant, and women left their homes to take jobs helping the war effort while the men were off to war in the South Pacific, Europe, and Africa. At the same time, the Army Nurse Corps needed nurses, and President Roosevelt considered a nurse draft. Instead, Congress took action and established the Cadet Nurse Corps within the Public Health Service, which provided education for nurses through hospital schools. The Corps granted scholarships and stipends to qualified applicants in exchange for providing military or other essential nursing services for the duration of the war. State-accredited nursing schools also were provided certain funds for the nurses' education (Office of the Public Health Service Historian, n.d.), all in the name of patriotism.

Not only did the nurses serve when needed for the war effort, but also many of the nurses educated through the Cadet Nurse Corps went on to become the next generation of nurse leaders. There was strong support for these efforts. This was another example of how a societal need and public policy came together to change the face of nursing by recruiting and educating women who otherwise might not have become nurses—another window of opportunity was opened.

After World War II, research and scientific advances, such as the use of antibiotics, the control of many contagious diseases, and advanced diagnostic and surgical technology, became part of medical practice. With the nation's increased prosperity after the war, Americans had an opportunity to worry about their health and sought medical treatment to take advantage of the new resources available to physicians. At the same time, private foundations no longer invested large sums of money into universities and the creation of professional knowledge. However, the federal government was about to take up the slack with increased support for medicine and financially troubled hospitals.

The Hill-Burton Act of 1946 provided construction funds to community hospitals, which were gearing up to serve as the new workplace of physicians; the federal government also subsidized medical schools and medical education. However, the expansion of hospitals occurred at the same time the supply of nurses was dwindling. The Cadet Corps nurses left their positions and returned to the at-home life they had had before the war just as the demand for hospital nurses exploded.

With the government's help in building hospitals and third-party payment emerging for medical services, the hospitals were now in a position where they could hire nurses. However, registered nurses were in short supply. To meet this shortage, in 1951 a new kind of nursing education was designed for nurse "technicians." This associate degree from community or technical colleges was awarded to nurses in a 2-year program, with hospital nursing, not the community, as its focus. The intent of the designer of the associate degree program, Mildred Montag, was for a separate license for graduates from these programs (Montag, 1951). However, the state board examination for registered nurse licensure became the same for the associate's degree, the hospital diploma, and the university nurse with a bachelor's degree. Successful completion of this one examination allowed graduates to become a registered nurse (RN)—an example of the unintended consequences of a new educational policy.

Before long, the majority of all nurses, regardless of their education, were employed in hospitals. To foster medical care of the elderly, the Medicare Enactment of 1965 awarded funds to hospitals that provided medical education; however, that public policy also had a provision to support hospital schools of nursing through the same source of funds—Graduate Medical Education dollars (Thies & Harper, 2004). This mechanism of payment continues today, as long as the hospital owns or, in some cases, affiliates with the school of nursing.

Graduate programs were developed in nursing during the 1950s and 1960s, again with the prodding of a new generation of nurse leaders. With an increased emphasis and interest in research, the programs became focused on specialty areas of practice to allow nurses to become experts in one particular area of practice as well as a functional area such as education or administration. To assist in the education and development of the nursing profession, the U.S. Nurse Training Act of 1964 provided a comprehensive financial package for school construction, plus faculty development, student grants, and loans (Dickson, 1993). The increased funding for nursing resulted in many capital improvements, as well as the education and development of nurse faculty and high-level administrators. Many of today's seasoned nurse leaders were able to take advantage of this new public policy—an example of how public policy indirectly has shaped nursing.

As health care became more organized, and schools and the public gradually came to rely on the federal government and their policies, politics entered the picture and formed the intersection of politics and public policy. A more recent example of a public policy that has had a major impact on nurses and their practices is the Balanced Budget Act of 1997, which reduced payments to states for Medicare and Medicaid patients. This act, along with the implementation of managed care, has devastated hospital finances and increased the work demands on nurses as hospitals pared their staff to make ends meet. This, too, represents how public policy, not of its own making, has had a major influence on nursing, which many believe was the impetus for the current nurse shortage—another example of an unintended consequence of a public policy.

Moving Toward a Scientific Base for Nursing

Nationwide, about one-third of nurse graduates who enter the workforce are graduates from a 4-year college or university. Nurses educated at the entry level receive a generalist education covering both hospital and community nursing. Although the percentage of graduates holding a college degree in nursing has gradually increased over time, the bachelor's degree in nursing is required for entry into graduate school for the nurse who wants to practice as an advanced-practice nurse or a teacher of nurses.

About the same time as graduate schools expanded as a result of the Nurse Training Act of 1964, nursing theories and research were added to the curriculum. Numerous nurses developed theories of nursing, and the profession moved toward becoming scientific; indeed, even a beginning science of nursing was evolving. A milestone was reached when the first research journal, *Nursing Research,* began publication in 1952. The focus was on research about nursing students, and the reports were so sparse that one edition contained the entire dissertation of a recent graduate from Teachers College (personal communication with Harriet Werley, one of the first nurse researchers). Since then, other research-oriented journals have been published as opportunities increased for the dissemination of new knowledge.

In 1962 the federal government again came to the rescue by establishing the Nurse Scientist Training Grant programs, which continued into the 1970s and enabled the applicant to obtain a PhD in nursing and a cognate discipline. Nine universities implemented these programs, with the cognate disciplines of anthropology, biology, psychology, sociology, microbiology, anatomy, and physiology (Grace, 1978). Many of these graduates became scientific leaders and continue to mentor a new generation of nurses with PhDs in nursing. Nursing research, using ever more current scientific methods, has continued to grow, and some research has been able to create policy changes in clinical areas, particularly in the maternal child realm (e.g., see Brooten et al., 2005).

As an example of how nurses have been able to collaborate for change, to use their numbers and their knowledge, we turn to the policy example of the establishment of the National Institute of Nursing Research. Legislation was proposed in 1986 to establish a Center for Nursing Research. Initially, President Reagan vetoed the bill. However, the nursing profession managed to gain support by finding its voice, and the veto was overturned, creating the center within the National Institutes of Health. Later, in 1993, the center was awarded designation as an Institute of Nursing Research, a result of major action taken by the profession working together to create a window of opportunity.

In sum, over time we have identified some policy changes put forth by others that have affected nurses: the 1946 Hill-Burton Act expanding the U.S. hospital system and thereby increasing dramatically the demand for nurses or the Balanced Budget Act of 1997 reducing funds for health care that placed additional workplace stress on nurses. On the other hand, nurses, through public awareness, have created some policy changes: for example, Lillian Wald demonstrated the value of nurses to the people of the community, and advances were made in public health. However, it is only recently that policy changes have occurred based on scientific data-driven research in the tradition of Nightingale, linking nurse characteristics and organizational variables to patient outcomes. Now we do have the human capital—nurse scientists—to take advantage of large numbers and the tenacity of nurses and most importantly the knowledge of nurses' experiences from which to build our political expertise and network (Joel, this text, ch. 16).

WHERE DO WE GO FROM HERE? THE INTERSECTION OF POLITICS AND POLICY

With a context of how nurses came to this point in our scientific history, the question now turns to how we might better use the evidence we are developing to benefit our patients through policy changes for nurses and their work. This book is focused on the research to policy connection through all phases of the process: from the "how to" of gathering evidence to the "how to" of influencing policy.

Although this book is not designed for final answers, given that the policy courses of action are a work in progress, some useful insights can be gained from the expert contributions to this book. For example, Joel in chapter 16 cites the process of how a legislative bill becomes law and reminds us that three elements are necessary to create policy change at any level: numbers, tenacity, and knowledge. A good example of the use of these three concepts to collaborate and advocate for change can be found in the establishment of the National Institute for Nursing Research presented earlier. Clearly, our history has taught us that change can be made when policy change is fostered by a window of opportunity.

The concept of an open window of opportunity in this context was coined by John Kingdon (2003) and is used by Palumbo in chapter 17 as she describes the political policy efforts of Vermont nurses in obtaining funds to increase nurses and faculty in her state. In a similar vein, Gladwell (2002) emphasizes in his best-selling book, *The Tipping Point,* that it takes three things to make ideas "sticky" or spread among others to affect change: the context, the message, and the messenger.

Let us now look at the idea of a window of opportunity from Kingdon (2003), which can provide the background for Gladwell's theory. We can explore situations in which nurses may find a "window of opportunity" opening to present their evidence regarding the relationship of nurses' care processes to patients' safety and the quality of their health care outcomes. Further, one can then view the window of opportunity as the context and carefully investigate what is the message and who is the best messenger.

Kingdon's Agenda Setting

The policy agenda is described by Kingdon as "the list of subjects to which government officials and those around them are paying serious attention" (Kingdon, 2003, p. vii). With demands by interest groups, the public, and influential individuals, policy making has a dynamic nature in which problems rise and fall from the government's agenda in an unpredictable manner. Kingdon identifies three streams in policy making: the problem, policy alternatives, and political opportunities. Convergence or "coupling" of the three streams is often chaotic and unpredictable but allows the problem to move onto the policy agenda when the streams converge and a window of opportunity opens.

There are many reasons a problem stream converges with the policy stream to form public policy. Some proposals work better than others, and some rise and fall without any rhyme or reason and may never become a policy. Of the three streams, the political one is the most difficult to tame. As Kingdon stresses, experts generate an agenda, and politicians set the agenda. It is useful to analyze the windows and patterns of behavior in different policy arenas to determine which problems actually make it to the policy agenda. However, Kingdon also points out that the forces that drive the political stream may be different from those that drive the policy stream. Ideas float around and sometimes collide and become fused or go off in diffuse directions. Because there is no one right way to go, policy making can, indeed, be chaotic.

Kingdon (2003) also identifies the role of communities of specialists and the ideas they develop. Especially for our purposes here, communities of specialists can be the expert researchers who have the benefit of conversing with large numbers of other experts, the attribute of tenacity, and the knowledge of the problem. These attributes can apply to a community of researchers who are coalesced around a particular problem, such as the work of nurses. According to Kingdon, there is then a long period of "softening up, ideas are floated, bills introduced, speeches are made, proposals are drafted, then amended in response to reaction and floated again" (p. 115). Moreover, of course, although politicians like ideas, the budget is always a consideration, and attention must be given to funding the idea.

However, Kingdon (2003) does stress that ideas can be powerful as a basis for policy change, even more so than aggressive lobbying, but interest groups and what he calls political entrepreneurs connect ideas together to reach the policy agenda for consideration. These entrepreneurs highlight "indicators" of a problem by sending out press releases, presenting hearing testimony, speeches, and other devices, and bringing problems into the personal experiences of important people by giving them a firsthand look at the effects of the problem. Interest groups generating feedback in the form of letters, visits to decision makers, and protest activities all push for one kind of a problem definition rather than another one—a major conceptual and political accomplishment.

Given Kindgon's theoretical framework of policy making, is it possible that nurse researchers are communities of experts who can become political entrepreneurs? Can we build through collaboration "experts" who will share ideas, promote feedback, and excite interest groups as well as use their knowledge of health care, their large numbers, and their tenacity to work for health care change? Kingdon's ideas were based on interviews and analysis with participants in the health care and transportation sectors. On the other hand, Gladwell (2002) developed his ideas by observations of people and ideas as those ideas grew into general acceptance, seemingly without an apparent plan, to create "stickyness" or sustainability. To compare the two theories of how knowledge spreads and raises to the level of a policy agenda, let us turn to the ways provided by Gladwell to legitimate ideas.

Gladwell's Stickyness of Ideas

Since the first edition in 2000, *The Tipping Point* has spent years on the best-selling list, and it is no wonder. Gladwell clearly demonstrates how an idea can spread like a contagious disease, with the right message and the right messenger. Here, I would like to begin with his concluding remarks, which provide hope to us as to how we might use his concepts to enhance our goal of connecting research to policy, in order to improve health care through changing the work of nurses: "Look at the world around you. It may seem like an immovable, implacable place. It is not. With the slightest push—in just the right place—it can be tipped," concludes Gladwell (p. 259).

Using examples from the spread of Hush Puppies to Bernie Goetz and the reduction in crime in New York City, Gladwell informs the reader of how change comes about. He describes it in a similar way to Kingdon (2003), by stressing it is unpredictable and even chaotic. Moreover, similar to Kingdon's concept of political entrepreneur, Gladwell stresses that the right person (the messenger) with the right message in the right context can bring an idea to the "tipping point," when "little ideas can make a big difference."

An example from Gladwell that is likely to resonate with you, the reader, is the example of a nurse who began a program designed to increase knowledge and awareness of diabetes and breast cancer in the black community of San Diego. For her grassroots movement, she selected black churches as her focus, but the results were disappointing. A few interested persons showed up, but she could not get her message to "tip." She realized that she needed a different context in which to reach many more women.

She found the right context upon moving the program from the black churches to beauty salons, where women spent up to 8 hours having their hair braided—a perfect context in which to reach a tipping point. To make the effort as effective as possible, the nurse trained the stylists to present the information about breast cancer in a compelling manner, using conversational methods of communication. As Gladwell (2002) noted, "And how much easier is it to hang the hooks of knowledge on a story?" (p. 255). This is a keen example of how to do a lot with little and be successful in changing attitudes and, in this case, getting women to have mammograms and diabetes tests, by using the right context, the right message, and the right messenger.

We can learn and gain some hope from seriously considering Gladwell's elements of change—context, message, messenger—as we search for ways to bring a strong idea based on a program of evidence to the agenda setting of politicians. Even more positive is the possibility of using these ideas at the clinical or educational institutional level to have an idea reach the tipping point to create a policy change resulting in quality care to patients. Let us now apply some of Kingdon's concepts of the window of opportunity and Gladwell's tipping point to connect evidence and policy to nurses and their work.

APPLYING KINGDON AND GLADWELL'S THEORIES TO POLICY CHANGE BY NURSES

One has only to turn to CNN news to hear information about the need for reform in health care, where problems abound: safety, quality, access, cost, and disparities in outcomes, for example. Certainly, the major problems of our dysfunctional health care system are rising to, and moving onto, the policy-setting agenda. However, solutions are generated, but no one solution seems to be the choice. However, what often is missing from the dialogue of ideas is the leadership of nurses in defining the policies that are changing nursing practice at the point of origin—the clinical setting and the educational setting. Further, there is no consensus among communities of nurse experts as to the important issues to address with research. Evidence is growing to support change in the education and practice of RNs; however, the perennial issues of "turf-dom" prevent nurses from presenting a strong message with messengers solidified around an identifiable problem. Without this basic contextual issue resolved, it is unlikely that the window of opportunity will open or that an idea will tip.

However, now that we have some ideas about how policy changes occur, perhaps a critical mass of nurse researchers can come to agreement about a problem, the evidence needed to present a strong message, and who might be the best messenger. For example, we know the safety of patients in hospitals is a major concern; it came to the attention of the Institute of Medicine (2000), who reported that as many as 98,000 Americans each year lose their lives needlessly in hospitals because of medical errors. As a result, numerous safety measures have been put into place through national recommendations—the accrediting bodies' requirement regarding the use of the traditional abbreviations not be used, clear labeling of medications that look-alike or sound-alike, and the reconciliation of patient pre-admission medications with their discharge medications, to name a few. Also as a result, nurses became the "doers" in seeing that physicians abide by these changes in mandated policies. Especially now, when nurses are in short supply, could we not demonstrate with evidence that this is a poor use of nurses' time and may have an impact on the quality of patient care and outcomes?

Additionally, there is evidence to suggest that the educational preparation of nurses has a relationship to patient outcomes, including mortality of and failure to rescue surgical patients (Aiken, Clarke, Cheung, Sloane, & Silber, 2003). Could not the community of experts leading this research be brought together to expand the research in a systematic, logical way, across settings, so that strong evidence can be presented regarding the educational preparation of nurses and the impact on patient outcomes? Given the focus on health care safety, "Look at the world around you. It may seem like an immovable, implacable place. It is not. With the slightest push—in just the right place—it can be tipped" (Gladwell, 2002, p. 259). Is it not possible to develop a carefully orchestrated campaign to spread the idea and bring it to the attention of policy-makers?

CONCLUSION

Quality in health care is a major problem, and registered nurses are the largest professional health care workforce. Can we not use our large numbers, our tenacity, and our evidence to bring about health care policy changes for the betterment of our citizens? What would it take? How could we build on our auspicious research beginnings? These are all questions for you, for me, and for us, as we consider some of the ideas put forth here and develop answers. Let us consider the principles of taking action as the window of opportunity opens and the ideas reach their "tipping point." As we move toward our future, we can look back and remember Nightingale and her use of evidence to support policy change. As this chapter closes, consider that evidence suggests the current health care system is changing, and according to O'Neil (1998), the emerging health care system has an ongoing commitment to research and improvement. He suggests, "It might be more important for a profession to control and advance its research agenda than to control its scope of its practice in traditional ways. In fact, one could argue that the future control of scopes of practice will be a function of research in outcomes, not the actions of legislators" (p. 221). It is time to equip yourself for the challenge!

REFERENCES

Adelaide Nutting's Introduction. (1939). Retrieved February 15, 2008, from http://www. countryjoe.com/nightingale/nutting.htm

Aiken, L. H., Clarke, S. P., Cheung, R. B., Sloane, D. M., & Silber, J. H. (2003). Educational levels of hospital nurse and surgical patient mortality. *Journal of the American Medical Association, 290*(12), 1617–1623.

Brooten, D., Youngblut, J., Blais, K., Donahue, D., Cruz, I., & Lightbourne, M. (2005). APN-Physician collaboration in caring for women with high-risk pregnancies. *Journal of Nursing Scholarship, 37*(2), 178–184.

Christy, T. E. (1969). *Cornerstone for nursing education.* New York: Teachers College, Columbia University.

Dickson, G. L. (1993). The unintended consequences of a male professional ideology for the development of nursing education. *Advances in Nursing Science, 15*(3), 67–83.

Donahue, M. P. (1985). *Nursing: The finest art.* St. Louis: C. V. Mosby.

Flexner, A. (1910). *Medical education in the United States and Canada.* New York: Carnegie Foundation for the Advancement of Teaching.

The Florence Nightingale Museum. (1854–1856). *Florence Nightingale's Statistical Diagrams.* Retrieved February 20, 2008 from http://www.florence-nightingale.co.uk/small.htm

Gladwell, M. (2002). *The Tipping Point.* New York: Little, Brown.

Grace. H. K. (1978). The development of doctoral education in nursing: A historical perspective. In N. I. Chaska (Ed.), *The nursing perspective: Views through the mist* (pp. 112–123). New York: McGraw-Hill.

Grippando, G. M. (1977). *Nursing perspectives and issues.* Albany, NY: Delmar.

Institute of Medicine. (2000). *To err is human: Building a safer health system.* Washington, DC: National Academies Press.

Kalisch, P. A., & Kalisch, B. J. (1986). *The advance of American nursing* (2nd ed.). Boston: Little, Brown.

Kingdon, J. W. (2003). *Agendas, alternatives, and public policies* (2nd ed.). New York: Longman.

Montag, M. L. (1951). *The education of nursing technicians.* New York: Wiley.

Nursing and nursing education in the U.S. (1923). *Report of the committee for the study on nursing education.* New York: Macmillan.

The Office of the Public Health Service Historian. (n.d.). *The Cadet Nurse Corps, 1943–48.* Retrieved February 28, 2008, from http://lhncbc.nlm.nih.gov/apdb/phsHistory/resources/cadetnurse/nurse.html

O'Neil, E. (1998). Nursing in the next century. In E. O'Neil and J. Coffman (Eds.), *Strategies for the future of nursing* (pp. 211–224). San Francisco: Jossey-Bass.

Reissman, C. K. (1983). Women and medicalization: A new perspective. *Social Policy, 14*(1), 13–18.

Roberts, M. M. (1954). *American nursing: History and interpretation.* New York: Macmillan.

Thies, K. M., & Harper, D. (2004). Medicare funding for nursing education: Proposal for a coherent policy agenda. *Nursing Outlook, 52,* 297–303.

Worcester, A. D. (1914). *Nurses for our neighbors.* Boston: Houghton Mifflin.

2

Nursing Outcomes Research: Connections to Workforce Issues and Policy Decisions

SEAN P. CLARKE

The current national workforce crisis in U.S. health care has emerged at a time of unprecedented concern about the safety and quality of the services being provided. Because health care delivery is so dependent on skilled human resources, the work of workforce researchers and analysts addressing supply and demand issues in the nursing labor pool has come to complement that of outcomes researchers interested in systems-level determinants of quality (for instance, staffing and the organization of settings of care). Each field produces findings that make the work in the other all the more pressing and relevant. Research clarifying the nature and severity of current and future workforce shortages makes findings connecting staffing levels with outcomes more meaningful and compelling, and vice versa.

Over time, outcomes researchers have generated a base of findings that connect patient and nurse safety with organizational features of health care settings. Although the best-studied organizational element so far has been staffing levels, research also covers a broad range of other work environment factors. Key studies in the nursing outcomes research literature have had a clear impact on the way clinicians, managers, executives, and policy makers understand nursing work and the factors influencing it. Papers in the field have inspired leaders to measure staffing, practice environments, and outcomes in their own health care facilities, interpret them in the context of these studies, or benchmark them against outcomes from peer institutions. Nursing outcomes research findings are also frequently used to justify investments of various types in building a well-qualified nursing workforce and in establishing positive practice environments in practice settings at all levels in the health care system.

In this chapter some basic ideas about what outcomes research is and how it is conducted will be reviewed. The state of knowledge regarding the impacts of the structural elements and organization of nursing services on patient outcomes is discussed. The concluding section outlines the role of outcomes research in guiding health care and workforce policy more broadly and provides an argument for the ongoing involvement of nursing scholars in the field.

HEALTH SERVICES RESEARCH AND NURSING OUTCOMES RESEARCH

What exactly is nursing outcomes research? Perhaps the place to begin is an explanation of how health outcomes research relates to the broader field of health services research. Health services researchers apply social science perspectives and methods to the study of health care and the delivery of health care services (notably sociology and economics, but political science and other disciplines as well). Researchers with clinical training, experience in a health care profession, or background in fields such as epidemiology often contribute methods and perspectives from their knowledge of approaches for studying disease occurrence and outcomes, or their understanding of clinical care and its contexts. Health services researchers commonly study the flow of workers, patients, and money in health care facilities and systems. They focus much attention on variations in structures and outputs or outcomes across institutions and countries. Health services research encompasses many areas including health care labor studies (i.e., "workforce research"), studies dealing with patient and provider behavior, and analyses of health care financing, particularly in relation to the competitive success of some providers over others and issues of access to services, as well as more clinically oriented research on outcomes of care.

Outcomes research is a subfield within health services research that deals with variations in health status among treated patients or clients in relation to differences in the patient-level and systems-level contexts of their care. Specifically, outcomes researchers explore background demographic, psychosocial, and clinical characteristics of patients, as well as aspects of the institutions and the health care providers that are associated with which patients fare well and which ones fare poorly (Kane, 2005; Mitchell, Ferketich, & Jennings, 1988). On occasion, outcomes researchers also examine the interaction of client and provider characteristics—that is, whether specific types of patients experience better types of outcomes when cared for by certain kinds of providers.

The purpose of outcomes research is to generate data that will improve the appropriateness of clinical or administrative decisions and raise quality of care. Clinicians' awareness of contextual factors affecting their patients can influence their practice with vulnerable populations and spur reflection on and change in their facilities' policies and procedures.

Sound outcomes research data also can facilitate a broad range of decisions by managers and executives regarding the allocation of resources and the structures of care settings. One class of systems-level decisions relates to the types of facilities that are associated with optimal outcomes for high-risk patients, for instance, premature infants, patients undergoing specialized surgeries, or patients who experience traumatic injuries. Should these patient groups be cared for in organizations that handle high volumes of specific patient types or that have high technology facilities? A great deal of research analyzes differences in outcomes for various patient populations in relation to the volume of cases handled by treating physicians and hospitals—as well as many unanswered questions about why the effect occurs when it does. Should policy makers attempt to engineer delivery of health care systems to ensure that most or all such patients are treated in high-volume, high-tech institutions? If so, which conditions or procedures should be targeted? The answer will depend on the political philosophy of the individual questioned and by financial and economic considerations, but can be, and has been, informed by research findings.

Nursing outcomes research, a specialty within the broader field of health outcomes research, asks questions regarding the health status of patients treated in different contexts and conditions related specifically to nurses and nursing care. Nursing outcomes research studies may address the best structures or management strategies for nursing units or hospitals, as well as the mix of health care workers best equipped to care for various clinical populations. Studies may aim to inform managers' decisions to recruit specific types of workers, such as registered nurses (as opposed to other types of nursing workers) or nurses with specialized experience or training. At a state or national level, findings from outcomes research can be extrapolated and used to guide policies about subsidies for health care worker training or can influence the development of regulations for the operation of health care facilities.

CHALLENGES IN NURSING OUTCOMES RESEARCH

Nursing outcomes researchers face a number of challenges, some shared with the broader field of outcomes research and some fairly distinct. Data sources providing information about patients and providers that has been collected reliably and consistently across providers are a basic ingredient for outcomes research. If data collected for other purposes are not available, such as documentation in the course of providing care, meeting regulatory mandates or billing third-party payors, then other approaches are needed for gathering high-quality information in a cost-effective manner.

Nursing outcomes researchers must identify measurable outcomes plausibly related to nursing care that are of interest to multiple stakeholders. Working conditions that make it difficult to provide sound nursing care may lead to errors and accidents (especially accidents and errors causing injuries), complications, and ultimately, prolonged hospitalizations and increased costs and mortality rates, particularly death rates higher than those expected based on patients' clinical conditions. Such outcomes can be measured easily, albeit imperfectly, with existing data sets and are readily understood by many different groups inside and outside the profession.

Ideally, long-term outcomes of nursing care such as patient quality of life would also be studied. Unfortunately, with a few limited exceptions, quality of life data are rarely collected systematically, and even more rarely are they gathered in a manner that would allow formal analyses in research contexts. Although specific types of outcomes may be of great interest to clinicians, the public, and policy makers, there simply may be no validated measures available or no data sources from which appropriate measures can be drawn.

Studying the impact of nursing care on the organization of nursing services in the context of real-world care delivery is another challenge. A wide range of factors influences managerial decision making regarding staffing. Yet other factors affect the extent to which staffing coverage meets the needs of any given patient, as well as whether a particular patient will experience specific outcomes of care. These factors include aspects of health care outside of nursing.

Nurses are involved directly or indirectly in many different aspects of care delivery; however, so are many other health care workers and disciplines—so identifying readily measurable and consistently recorded variables that are closely tied to the delivery of nursing care can be quite difficult. Researchers also need to measure as many as possible of the different non-nursing background elements that may explain variation in outcomes.

The complexity of the systems in which nursing care is delivered (multiple nurses, within nursing teams, within institutions or facilities) poses yet more challenges. The nested structures involved raise questions about the best research designs as well as theoretical issues about which variables to measure and which associations to test and at what levels within organizations. Obtaining data on enough different patients and care settings to permit statistical analyses, taking both the layers of organizations and structures of care and most or all relevant non-nursing factors into account, is often very challenging. Even with data in hand, analyses are often complex and demand careful reflection on statistical and theoretical issues.

A final critical issue is making sense of how the outcomes of care occur because patients are never randomly allocated across facilities and providers. Many different factors influence the types of patients who seek care in particular facilities. Some of the same factors also affect the events that befall patients during their stays as well as the health status of patients as they leave care. Selection biases, whereby patients who are sicker, wealthier, better insured or who reside in different areas are cared for by different health professionals and in different institutions, are all but guaranteed. In order to understand differences in rates of adverse events across providers, including mortality, it is critical to carefully consider important differences in essential characteristics that may influence patients' outcomes independently of any care they may or may not receive. Fortunately, well-known statistical methods can help researchers handle this problem but require both high-quality data and methodological expertise to implement (Iezzoni, 1997, 2003).

Research on Staffing, Work Environments, and Hospital Outcomes

Researchers in nursing and related fields have at least partially overcome many of these obstacles in a number of areas of investigation. Among the largest bodies of findings that have accumulated in nursing outcomes research relate to nurse staffing levels in acute care settings and their impact on patients. Researchers have used administrative or survey data to gather information about staffing levels in hospitals and have found data regarding outcomes potentially sensitive to nursing care for hundreds of thousands, and sometimes millions, of patients in those discharge abstract databases.

Especially over the last 10 years, researchers have found a good deal of evidence for what frontline nurses and their managers have always known—that as staffing levels drop (sometimes in terms of personnel-to-patient ratios or hours per patient day, but often also in terms of credential and education mix), the risk of adverse patient outcomes rises. There is a critical mass of studies suggesting clearly that adverse outcomes are more common in institutions and in subunits within those institutions where staffing levels are lower. Many reviews of the literature on nurse staffing and patient and nurse outcomes reach very similar conclusions (Hickam et al., 2003; Kane, Shamliyan, Mueller, Duval, & Wilt, 2007; Lang, Hodge, Olson, Romano, & Kravitz, 2005; Seago, 2001). The body of findings is broadest in acute care hospitals, and much, but not all, of the work has been done in the United States. There is also a growing literature on long-term-care facility outcomes in relation to staffing levels (Bostick, Rantz, Flesner, & Riggs, 2006).

It is clear that staffing does not explain all variability in hospital outcomes—that even where staffing is found to have a significant effect on patient outcomes, there is usually much variation left unaccounted. Factors relating to the organization of nursing services other than staffing levels may be responsible, in addition to patient characteristics, structures, and processes relating to other health care disciplines. Many believe that high nurse staffing levels will produce optimal outcomes only when work environment conditions favor the high-quality nursing practice (see Figure 2.1 for a conceptual framework developed at the University of Pennsylvania that integrates a number of these concepts). The specific conditions of the nursing practice environment often cited include administrators' support of autonomous clinical decision-making by nurses, effective collaboration between members of different health disciplines, and resources for promoting quality, reinforcing competency, and continuing professional development. Nurse job outcomes, including satisfaction and physical and emotional well-being, are especially critical in nurse shortages but have clear potential impact on the quality of care. A critical mass of studies documents connections between the quality of nurses' work environments and job satisfaction and other self-reported job-related experiences (Lake, 2007). Not surprising, a growing

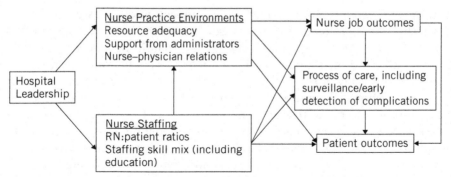

Figure 2.1 Nurse practice environments, nurse staffing, and outcomes
Source: Center for Health Outcomes and Policy Research, University of Pennsylvania School of Nursing.

literature also suggests that practice environment conditions also influence nurse occupational injuries (for recent examples, see Clarke, 2007, and Stone, Du, & Gershon, 2007).

There are still many questions regarding determinants of nurse and patient outcomes in hospitals and other settings that have not yet been addressed by researchers. Research exploring the impact of the practice environment features on patient and facility outcomes is still emerging, although research on Magnet hospitals and the Magnet Recognition Program has been a touchstone in this respect (Kramer & Schmalenberg, 2005; McClure & Hinshaw, 2002). Most research on the impact of practice conditions on outcomes has been conducted in adult medical-surgical inpatient settings. The literatures on community-based care, outpatient services, and mental health care are particularly sparse. The impact of staffing and other organizational factors on the delivery of direct care by frontline nurses also remains more or less unexplored (Clarke, 2006).

Health Care System and Workforce Trends That Make Outcomes Research Critical

The staffing outcomes literature has generated much discussion and has encouraged investments at the local, state, and national levels in interventions and programs to address long-standing and critical problems in the nurse workforce and its management. Well-conducted nursing outcomes research addressing related issues has also attracted attention and stimulated debate—for example, a high-impact outcomes study in nursing, this one on outcomes of care associated with nurse practitioners in primary care (Mundinger et al., 2000). Fortunately, researchers are also being attracted to the field, and resources are being committed to extending this body of research and to finding ways to apply it in practice.

A number of health care system trends are making understanding the impacts of human resources in outcomes vital. In brief, societal and health care forces are rapidly converging such that many, if not all, states, regions, and facilities, will face a shortage of registered nurses as well as a number of other types of health care workers within a decade.

The nurse shortage, first identified in the United States, has been evolving globally. Shortfalls of nurses have led to wage hikes that have helped to bring more nurses into the health care system working more hours. As of the middle of the century's first decade, enrollments and graduations from nursing schools have rebounded, foreign-born and foreign-educated nurses are filling a growing number of positions in the United States, and last, but not least, nurses work more hours and at older ages than ever before, presumably to take advantage of higher wages (Buerhaus, Auerbach, & Staiger, 2007). Currently, shortages remain confined primarily to areas where salaries are relatively low and for positions in hard-to-fill specialties that require specific education, training, or experience or a combination therein. However, much trouble is expected ahead, when the supply of new graduates from nursing education programs will be unable to compensate for retirements and an increased demand for health services in an aging American society (Health Resources and Services Administration, 2004). Fundamental rethinking of the way RN labor is used in American health care will be needed. This may be forced by financial considerations as well as labor supply. Human resources, including nursing personnel, are among the biggest drivers of exploding health care costs. Flat—and on occasion, falling—reimbursements are plaguing hospitals and health systems nationally (American Hospital Association, 2007). Interestingly, steep and steady capital expansions in many facilities that drive up demand for nurses are proceeding (for competitive reasons), even at a time when a supply cannot be guaranteed.

Of course, no discussion of the current shortage would be complete without reference to public and provider anxieties. Safety and outcomes researchers have raised public and professional consciousness about safety and quality issues in health care. Turn on a television news program or pick up a newspaper as of the last few years, and you are as likely as not to encounter a story that touches in some way on health care safety. The popular media have given a great deal of play to the nurse shortage, and stories including both anecdotes and research findings have alluded to suboptimal numbers and qualifications of nursing staff in some institutions. Policy makers and payors, responding to their constituents' concerns and frustrated by rising costs amid signs that health care is of inferior quality, are also making increasing moves to tie reimbursement to performance.

Outcomes research helps make the case for higher staffing levels and higher-cost professional workers. It helps stakeholders realize that connections between patient outcomes and workforce development, structural factors related to nursing, and the management of practice environments are based on empirical evidence as well as instinct. Downstream influences of nursing factors on patient satisfaction, institutional reputation, cost savings through efficient resource use, and lowered medicolegal liability are then easy to imagine. Should convincing data accumulate that nursing care or nurse staffing is also causally connected to process and outcomes measures that facilities have financial incentives to improve, such as in the case of the pay-for-performance reimbursement schemes, this may further influence executive-level decisions about investing resources in nursing care.

Overall, the deepening shortage and quality concerns amplified by research suggest how vital it is to understand how best to use limited human resources in health care. Sustaining high levels of nurse staffing may mean shifting budgets and investing in unit-level and institution-wide leadership and resources and community resources for educating nurses. Well-conducted research can help ground policy discussions about resource allocation at the local, state, and national levels in the coming years.

NURSING OUTCOMES RESEARCH AT THE UNIVERSITY OF PENNSYLVANIA'S CENTER FOR HEALTH OUTCOMES AND POLICY RESEARCH

Over the past two decades, an interdisciplinary team of researchers at the Center for Health Outcomes and Policy Research led by nurse sociologist Dr. Linda Aiken has been testing different aspects of a conceptual framework that proposes relationships between hospital outcomes and organizational characteristics that are affected by leadership decisions, as depicted in Figure 2.1. Some of the better-known studies have addressed the following:

- Models of specialty care, using AIDS inpatient care as a model (Aiken, Sloane, Lake, Sochalski, & Weber, 1999)
- Magnet hospitals (Aiken, Smith, & Lake, 1994; Aiken, Havens, & Sloane, 2000)
- The impacts of hospital restructuring on patients and nurses in the United States and in health systems worldwide (Aiken, Clarke, & Sloane, 2000; Aiken, Clarke, & Sloan, 2002; Aiken, Sochalski, & Lake, 1999; Aiken, Clarke, Sloane, Lake, & Cheney, in press)
- The association of nurse staffing (patient-to-nurse ratios; Aiken, Clarke, Sloane, Sochalski, & Silber, 2002; Rafferty et al., 2007) and nurse education (proportions of registered nurses holding bachelor's or higher degrees) on hospital patient outcomes (Aiken, Clarke, Cheung, Sochalski, & Silber, 2003)

Projects at the center have typically involved research designs combining organizational measures derived from surveys of nurses with information about hospital structures and patient outcomes from governmental and other data sources. International collaborations have been a consistent feature of the past decade's work. Across Western health care systems and, more recently, health systems in Asia, remarkably consistent findings have emerged: there has been similarity across countries in hospital nurses' reports of their experiences and concerns at work; within countries, striking variations are typically found in the staffing levels and work environments found in hospitals; and consistent associations have been identified between staffing levels, work environments, and patient outcomes in countries with very different health care systems.

The program of research at the center has stimulated a great deal of research activity elsewhere by providing some preliminary tools for investigating hospital nurses' work environments, notably survey measures of nurse staffing, the Nursing Work Index and Practice Environment Scales (Aiken & Patrician, 2000; Lake, 2002), and failure to rescue as an outcome potentially sensitive to nursing care (Clarke & Aiken, 2003). Results from the Magnet-related research have played a key role in the evolution of the Magnet movement and its evidence base. Survey findings and research on outcomes are cited frequently in discussions about nurse shortages, the shortages' causes and consequences, and potential policy decisions. The center's staffing research has stimulated a great deal of discussion and controversy in the United States, as well as internationally, and fueled a number of policy initiatives at state and national levels. Center researchers' findings relating nurse education levels to patient outcomes have injected empirical data into a long-standing and very emotional debate regarding educational standards for entry and continuing practice in American nursing. The entry-into-practice issue is one that was resolved in favor of a bachelor's degree as an entry standard in many other countries several decades ago. Overall, the center's research output, along with that of outcomes researchers in nursing nationally and internationally, has brought empirical findings about impacts on patients into complex policy decisions related to nursing that were previously made in a "data vacuum."

THE FUTURE AND THE ROLE OF NURSING OUTCOMES RESEARCH

More than ever, the consequences of resource allocation decisions in health care involving nursing services need to be documented. As nursing's workforce crisis deepens, the consequences of deploying various configurations of staff in different circumstances need to be quantified so that intelligent decisions regarding how and where to invest resources can be made. Nurses from all walks of the profession have an interest in this kind of information, but nurse managers and executives need these data most of all to assist them in effectively managing their workforces, in maintaining and improving operations in their facilities, in optimizing quality of care, and in "managing up" using evidence-based policies within their work systems. Again, understanding the determinants of nursing-related outcomes is vital for policy makers crafting workforce development strategies and reimbursement strategies for health care facilities and creating regulatory schemes to improve safety and quality.

For reasons discussed earlier in the chapter, carrying out sound outcomes research is challenging. A multidisciplinary perspective—bringing together methodological expertise with relevant social and clinical science expertise and integrating views in health policy from outside nursing—makes nursing outcomes research more rigorous and compelling. However, the perspectives of nurses who are practicing in clinical settings, educating nurses, and managing clinical facilities are also vital. Because the skills and resources needed to conduct such research are challenging to assemble, it can be tempting to leave the study of the outcomes of nursing services to other disciplines. However, not only is there a risk that important questions will not be asked in empirical research, but there are also serious consequences for the profession if poorly constructed research or incorrectly interpreted findings are applied. A critical mass of nurses must also be in a position to explain and critique this research, which brings about a need for the inclusion of outcomes research content in undergraduate and graduate research courses, to ensure that the profession keeps a hand in the application of these findings in local, state, and national policy contexts.

CONCLUSIONS

A remarkable amount of progress in nursing outcomes research has been made in a relatively short time, particularly in documenting connections between acute-care hospital nurse staffing and patient safety. However, this progress needs to be consolidated and built on with more funding; more cooperation between researchers; more exchanges between researchers, service providers, payors, and policy makers; and expansion of the scope of the questions asked and data sources being used to address them. As the workforce crisis deepens and expectations that the health care system improve its performance increase, nursing outcomes research has never been more critical. Leaders inside and outside the nursing profession must make crucial choices in the next years. They will need the best possible evidence about the consequences of their policy decisions so that the right choices about the nurse workforce and its management can be made, in the public's interest, in health care institutions and in facilities and at the state and national levels.

REFERENCES

Aiken, L. H., Clarke, S. P., Cheung, R. B., Sochalski, J., & Silber, J. H. (2003). Education levels of hospital nurses and surgical patient mortality. *Journal of the American Medical Association, 290,* 1617–1623.

Aiken, L. H., Clarke, S. P., & Sloane, D. M. (2000). Hospital restructuring: Does it adversely affect care and outcomes? *Journal of Nursing Administration, 30*(10), 457–465.

Aiken, L. H., Clarke, S. P., & Sloane, D. M. (2002). Hospital staffing, organization, and quality of care: Cross-national findings. *International Journal of Quality in Health Care, 14,* 5–13.

Aiken, L. H., Clarke, S. P., Sloane, D. M., Lake, E. T., & Cheney, T. (in press). Effects of hospital care environment on patient mortality and nurse outcomes. *Journal of Nursing Administration.*

Aiken, L. H. Clarke, S. P., Sloane, D. M., Sochalski, J., & Silber, J. H. (2002). Hospital nurse staffing and patient mortality, nurse burnout, and job dissatisfaction. *Journal of the American Medical Association, 288,* 1987–1993.

Aiken, L. H., Havens, D. S., & Sloane, D. M. (2000). The magnet nursing services recognition program: A comparison of two groups of magnet hospitals. *American Journal of Nursing, 100*(3), 26–35.

Aiken, L. & Patrician, P. (2000). Measuring organizational traits of hospitals: The revised nursing work index. *Nursing Research, 49,* 146–153.

Aiken, L. H., Sloane, D. M., Lake, E. T., Sochalski, J., & Weber, A. L. (1999). Organization and outcomes of inpatient AIDS care. *Medical Care, 37*(8), 760–772.

Aiken, L. H., Smith, H. L., & Lake, E. T. (1994). Lower Medicare mortality among a set of hospitals known for good nursing care. *Medical Care, 32*(8), 771–787.

Aiken, L. H., Sochalski, J., & Lake, E. T. (1999). Studying outcomes of organizational change in health services. *Medical Care, 35*(11 Suppl), NS6–NS18.

American Hospital Association. (2007). *2007 Health and hospital trends.* Retrieved July 9, 2007, from http://www.aha.org/aha/research-and-trends/health-and-hospital-trends/2007.html

Bostick, J. E., Rantz, M. J., Flesner, M. K., & Riggs, C. J. (2006). Systematic review of studies of staffing in nursing homes. *Journal of the American Medical Directors Association, 7,* 366–376.

Buerhaus, P. I., Auerbach, D. I., & Staiger, D.O. (2007). Recent trends in the registered nurse labor market in the U.S.: Short-run swings on top of long-term trends. *Nursing Economics, 25*(2), 59–66.

Clarke, S. P. (2006). Research on nurse staffing and its outcomes: The challenges and risks of grasping at shadows. In S. Nelson and S. Gordon (Eds.), *The complexities of care: Nursing reconsidered* (pp. 161–184). Ithaca, NY: Cornell University Press.

Clarke, S. P. (2007). Hospital work environments, nurse characteristics and sharps injuries. *American Journal of Infection Control, 35*(5), 302–309.

Clarke, S. P., & Aiken, L. H. (2003). Failure to rescue: Measuring nurses' contributions to hospital performance. *AJN: American Journal of Nursing, 103,* 42–47.

Health Resources and Services Administration, U.S. Department of Health and Human Services. (2004). *What is behind HRSA's projected supply, demand, and shortage of registered nurses?* Retrieved July 9, 2007, from ftp://ftp.hrsa.gov/bhpr/workforce/behindshortage.pdf

Hickam. D. H., Severance S., Feldstein, A., Ray, L., Gorman, P., Schuldheis, S., Hersh, W. R., Krages, K. P., & Helfand, M. (2003). *The effect of health care working conditions on patient safety* (Evidence Report/Technology Assessment Number 74, AHRQ Publication No. 03-E0204). Rockville, MD: Agency for Healthcare Research and Quality.

Iezzoni, L. I. (Ed.). (1997). *Risk adjustment for measuring healthcare outcomes* (2nd ed.). Chicago: Health Administration Press.

Iezzoni, L. I. (Ed.). (2003). *Risk adjustment for measuring healthcare outcomes* (3rd ed.). Chicago: Health Administration Press.

Kane, R. L. (Ed.). (2005). *Understanding health care outcomes research* (2nd ed.). Sudbury, MA: Jones and Bartlett.

Kane, R. L., Shamliyan, T., Mueller, C., Duval, S., & Wilt, T. (2007). *Nurse staffing & quality of patient care* (Evidence Report/Technology Assessment No. 151, prepared by the Minnesota Evidenced-Based Practice Center under Contract No. 290–02–0009,

AHRQ Publication No. 07-E005). Rockville, MD: Agency for Healthcare Research & Quality. Retrieved from http://www.ahrq.gov/downloads/pub/evidence/pdf/nursestaff/nursestaff.pdf

Kramer, M., & Schmalenberg, C. E. (2005). Best quality patient care: A historical perspective on Magnet hospitals. *Nursing Administration Quarterly, 29*(3), 275–287.

Lake, E. T. (2002). Development of the Practice Environment Scale of the Nursing Work Index. *Research in Nursing & Health, 25*, 176–188.

Lake, E. T. (2007). The nursing practice environment: Measurement and evidence. *Medical Care Research and Review, 64*, 104S-122S.

Lang, T. A., Hodge, M., Olson, V., Romano, P. S., & Kravitz, R. L. (2004). Nurse-patient ratios: A systematic review on the effects of nurse staffing on patient, nurse employee, and hospital outcomes. *Journal of Nursing Administration, 34*(7–8), 326–337.

McClure, M. L., & Hinshaw, A. S. (Eds.). (2002). *Magnet hospitals revisited: Attraction and retention of professional nurses.* Washington, DC: American Nurses Publishing.

Mitchell, P. H., Ferketich, S., & Jennings, B. M. (1998). Quality health outcomes model. *Image, 30*(1), 43–46.

Mundinger, M. O., Kane, R. L., Lenz, E. R., Totten, A. M., Tsai, W. Y., Cleary, P. D., Friedewald, W. T., Siu, A. L., & Shelanski, M. L. (2000). Primary care outcomes in patients treated by nurse practitioners or physicians: A randomized trial. *Journal of the American Medical Association, 283*(1), 59–68.

Rafferty, A. M., Clarke, S. P., Coles, J., Ball, J., James, P., McKee, M., et al. (2007). Outcomes of variation in hospital nurse staffing in English hospitals: Cross-sectional analysis of survey data and discharge records. *International Journal of Nursing Studies, 44*(2), 175–182.

Seago, J. A. (2001). *Nurse staffing, models of care delivery, and interventions* (Evidence Report/Technology Assessment No. 43, AHRQ Publication No. 01-E058). Rockville, MD: Agency for Healthcare Research and Quality.

Stone, P. W., Du, Y., & Gershon, R. R. M. (2007). Organizational climate and occupational health outcomes in hospital nurses. *Journal of Occupational and Environmental Medicine, 49*(1), 50–58.

SECTION I. DISCOVERING THE RESEARCH TO POLICY CONNECTION: LESSONS LEARNED

Geri L. Dickson

Suzanne Gordon, a journalist, has written several books highlighting the value of the caregiving work of nurses, most notably in *Nursing Against the Odds* (2005). In an earlier book, Buresh and Gordon (2000) had written a manifesto calling on nurses to speak out forcefully and effectively to the pubic and in the media about their research. They gave specific examples of how nurses may spread the word about the value of their work to the public and policy makers.

Most importantly, those authors describe a way whereby nurses may become, in Kingdon's (2003) terminology, "political entrepreneurs" or act in ways similar to Gladwell's (2002) "strong messengers," as previously described in chapter 1. Acting in this new role, as political entrepreneurs or strong messengers, nurses can provide the evidence to facilitate the opening of a window of opportunity for policy change. "The public will more readily understand the relevance of nursing to health and illness when nursing research becomes more visible" (Buresh & Gordon, 2000, p. 259).

In this section—indeed throughout this book—you may develop an understanding of the importance of research for and about nurses *and* the necessity of moving forward by presenting the science of nursing in all its different aspects. To help you, the reader, get a sense of the whole, each section has an introduction and an endnote of lessons learned. Section 1 is an introductory section, so, let us begin our journey discovering the research to policy connection by thinking about the lessons learned in this section.

LESSON 1. COMPLEMENT WORKFORCE RESEARCH WITH PATIENT OUTCOMES RESEARCH

Because the health care delivery system is so dependent on human resources, the studies by workforce researchers addressing issues related to supply and demand of the nurse workforce have come to complement the studies by outcomes researchers interested in systems-level determinants of quality (see Clarke in chapter 2). Together, the two types of knowledge can weave a powerful message to the public and to policy makers concerned about the safety and quality of their constituents' health care.

Outcomes research can make the case for increasing staffing levels and salaries for professional workers, according to Clarke. As a result, stakeholders come to realize the connection between patient outcomes and workforce development. The next task is causally connecting nursing care and nurse staffing to processes and outcome measures to demonstrate the financial impact. These studies, in turn, may influence executive-level decisions about investing resources in nursing care—a very important policy lesson to learn.

LESSON 2. IDENTIFY A PROBLEM OF GREAT CONCERN TO BOTH THE PUBLIC AND POLICY MAKERS

Chapters 1 and 2 have given some insight into the process of how policy is made. Using the concepts of Kingdon (2003), we can identify a problem—for example, a severe shortage of nurses—that can become of great concern to the public, associations, and academicians, thus creating a problem stream. The next stream, then, is the political one in which policy alternatives are considered.

As of this writing, a critical shortage of nurses has been experienced for approximately the past 8 years, and forecasts indicate that we have not hit the peak of the shortage. For example, the forecasting report of the Healthcare Research and Services Administration (Biviano, Fritz, Spencer, & Dall, 2004), which was based on 2000 RN data, forecasts a shortage of almost 1,000,000 FTE RN positions, or 36% of the workforce, by 2020. Buerhaus, Staiger, and Auerbach (2004), using census data, have revised the projections downward for a shortage of 340,000 RNs nationally, which would still be severe, at three times the shortage in 2001. In addition, according to the National League for Nursing (2006), a nursing faculty shortage is emerging that resulted in 137,000 qualified students being denied admission to nursing schools nationally, further increasing the shortage of nurses.

Many different aspects of the nurse shortage could be addressed by policy-generating research. For example, one could ask, "What are the consequences to patients and outcomes as a result of a nurse shortage?" An alternative question might be, "What are the economic and social costs of these shortage-related patient concerns?" Another question might consider, "How does the education of nurses impact patient outcomes in hospitals? In home health care? In long-term care?" Continuing on this journey of turning evidence-based research into health policy" can help the health care researcher firm up the questions for policy research and bring multidisciplinary teams together to collaborate on the evidence—a new direction to be taken seriously.

LESSON 3. PRESENT COMPLEX EVIDENCE TO THE PUBLIC IN SIMPLE, UNDERSTANDABLE TERMS

Clarke, in chapter 2, provides an overview of health services research that focuses on the impact of the work environment on nurses' satisfaction and patient outcomes. He provides the history and a framework outlining the complexity of variables crucial to the linking of nurse characteristics to patient health outcomes.

For our purposes here, the focus has been on workforce-related studies. However, health services research can be useful as well to describe the impact of nurses' care on the preventable deaths of Nightingale's time or the impact of home health visits by advanced practice nurses (Brooten et al., 2005) or the relationship between the presence of RNs in dialysis centers and a decrease in adverse patients outcomes (see chapter 18). In other words, any patient-related program of compelling original research has the potential to transform nursing and health care. The challenge, however, is translating the research into terms that the public can understand. As Aiken notes in the foreword, "balancing the competing demands for complexity and simplicity is one of the great challenges of policy research"—a lesson to consider as you continue on this journey of discovering the research to policy connection.

LESSON 4. NURSING HAS SOLUTIONS TO MANY OF TODAY'S MOST CHALLENGING ISSUES IN HEALTH CARE

Policy research holds the key to the "widespread adoption of effective nursing solutions for the benefit of the public" at many levels, but most notably for the safety and quality of care for patients across the continuum of health care (Aiken, this text, Foreword). However, what has been lacking is the ability of the profession to clearly and concisely blow its own horn. We must learn, after careful deliberations of the evidence on both sides of an issue, to take a reasoned and unified stance on the many complex and devastating issues in the U.S. health care system.

Hopefully, the journey outlined here will be taken as beginning steps to identify those evidence-based nurse solutions, which, in turn, can be introduced and adopted by the larger health care system to decrease the safety risks to patients. This is a very strong lesson to contemplate as you continue through this book.

LESSON 5. RECOGNIZE WHEN THE "WINDOW OF OPPORTUNITY" IS OPEN

In chapter 1, we learned of the convergence of three streams that are necessary to open a window of opportunity for policy change: the problem stream, the political stream, and the policy stream. Applying the concepts of Kingdon's (2003) theory can help us realize when the three streams are converging and when the time is ripe for the window of opportunity to open.

Health care, and lack thereof, continues to be an issue on both the national and the state level. Disparities in health care, the rising costs of health care, and the numbers of uninsured, underinsured, and undocumented people who are not able to afford health care are all issues of concern to the public. As the numbers of patients suffering medical errors increases, issues of safety, let alone quality, of hospital care are a major concern. With this increased concern, a problem stream can be identified and promoted. Action is then necessary for researchers to consolidate their evidence to prepare as the issue becomes a growing concern in the political stream and, hence, comes to the attention of the policy-making stream. The three steams converging result in an opening of the window of opportunity for nurses to influence the emerging health care system—a most important lesson to learn in creating change through policy.

In sum, this section introduces the reader to the development of policy in nursing and the use of patient outcomes research to complement research addressing issues of supply and demand for nurses. These lessons are especially useful for nurses who, like Aiken, want "to elevate nursing to a position where it can have greater influence because there is so much to offer" (Houser & Player, 2004, p. 247). For Aiken, influence *is* evidence!

REFERENCES

Biviano, M., Fritz, M., Spencer, W., & Dall, T. (2004). *What is behind HRSA's projected supply, demand, and shortage of registered nurses?* Retrieved September 10, 2005, from ftp.hrsa.gov/bhpr/workforce/behindshortage.pdf

Brooten, D., Youngblut, J., Blais, K., Donahue, D., Cruz, I., & Lightbourne, M. (2005). APN–physician collaboration in caring for women with high-risk pregnancies. *Journal of Nursing Scholarship, 37*(2), 178–184.

Buerhaus, P., Staiger, D., & Suerbach, D. (2004, November 17). New signs of a strengthening nurse labor market? *Health Affairs.* Web exclusive. Retrieved April 4, 2008, from http://content.healthaffairs.org/cgi/content/full/hlthaff.w4.526/DC1.

Buresh, B., & Gordon, S. (2002). *From silence to voice.* Ottawa, Ontario: Canadian Nurses Association.

Gladwell, M. (2002). *The tipping point.* New York: Little, Brown.

Gordon, S. (2005). *Nursing against the odds.* Ithaca, NY: Cornell University Press.

Houser, B. P., & Player, K. N. (2004). *Pivotal moments in nursing.* Indianapolis, IN: Sigma Theta Tau.

Kingdon, J. W. (2003). *Agendas, alternatives, and public policies* (2nd ed.). New York: Longman.

National League for Nursing. (2006, August). *Data reveal slowdown in nursing school admission growth.* Retrieved September 18, 2007, from http://www.nln.org/newsreleases/databook_08_06.pdf

Toward Evidence-Based Policy: Collecting and Managing the Data

INTRODUCTION

Geri L. Dickson

As we begin our journey in search of the research to policy connection, we pause to look at how to (a) begin the process of identifying research questions, (b) go about collecting data for a survey, (c) manage the data once we have collected them, and (d) identify some means to ensure reliable results. As this section continues, we delve into the value of using state and federal data in secondary analyses and learn how to use software to impute missing data. This section carries with it a "heavy lift" as we begin to explore these topics. However, all of these techniques are useful to researchers providing evidence for policy changes to stakeholders.

Surveys provide a means to collect data about a specialized topic from a targeted group of people who have knowledge about the topic. Researchers studying policy issues often use surveys to collect their data. These data, then, are analyzed and can be used to design evidence-based policy solutions at multiple levels—organizational, professional, and public.

In chapter 3, Patricia Moulton begins the research to policy quest by focusing on developing a research topic and questions. She describes a process that may involve a literature search and explains that you might find it necessary to collect data through interviews or focus groups. These latter methods are usually used when the research topics and questions are not clear-cut. Moulton gives specific examples of the process of guided focus groups with your targeted sample, which will provide direction as you form your research and survey questions. Alternatively, focus groups may sometimes be used to elicit information to clarify survey data that you have collected.

Linda M. Lacey continues, in this multiple-researcher chapter, to discuss some of the common problems with survey questions. She identifies ways to ask survey questions by limiting the answer choices and presenting clear and unambiguous questions. She gives multiple examples of questions most likely to bear fruit. She also describes some potential problems with scale items, question order, and knowing how to keep the survey at a reasonable length to obtain valid and reliable measures of your topic of interest.

Continuing in chapter 3, Linda Flynn identifies six imperatives to keep in mind when fielding a successful survey. Determining the sample is the first imperative, and how to obtain an effective response rate is the second of the six imperatives. Flynn also gives examples of ways to make a good impression and use the power of a stamp as means to ensure an effective response rate of 50% to 60%. Writing a powerful cover letter and, most importantly, scheduling multiple contacts with members of your sample to ensure that effective response rate are other imperatives presented by Flynn.

She provides an example of the implementation of these six imperatives in her recent study of New Jersey RNs. This survey yielded a response rate of 50.5%, producing data from 22,406 RNs who are actively licensed and who live in New Jersey. This was achieved by using the Dillman Tailored Design Method of survey methodology, partnering with the New Jersey Collaborating Center for Nursing, and the New Jersey Board of Nursing.

Chapter 3 ends with seasoned researchers Christine Tassone Kovner and Carol S. Brewer relating how their best-laid plans went awry in a recent mailed survey they completed of RNs in various states. To quote them, "The point of this litany of woes is not to discourage anyone from doing survey research, but only to say that things do and will go wrong, even when you try to anticipate everything you can."

Continuing on to chapter 4, we find the use of established national models of supply and demand of the nurse workforce adapted to calculate state projections by replacing model data with state-level data. Finding the existing state databases is an extremely arduous task because it revolves around finding the appropriate state-level data to serve as the variables in the models or having to rely on the default data, if unable to locate state-level data.

Nevertheless, the researchers conclude that the HRSA models work well enough to encourage other states to persevere or begin the process. The forecasts of supply and demand for the nursing workforce are invaluable for policy makers who are fostering state workforce planning and policy development.

The last chapter in this section is a technical report on the "how tos" of imputing missing data. Nooney describes missing sources of data and their implications for research findings and reviews correction strategies, as well as the pros and cons of various methods.

These chapters provide a gold mine of ideas for problems common to most researchers, be they novices or experts. In the following chapters, we continue in the research to policy journey. In keeping with our context of nurses and their work, we provide specific examples of evidence and policy in the workplace of nurses, the nursing educational system, available grant funding mechanisms, and exemplars of successful evidence-based policy strategies.

Addressing the Complexities of Survey Research

3

PATRICIA MOULTON, LINDA M. LACEY, LINDA FLYNN,
CHRISTINE TASSONE KOVNER, AND CAROL S. BREWER

Surveys are a useful and inexpensive approach to collect data from specialized groups of people. In contradistinction to the general public, "specialized groups of people" include aggregates such as members of a profession, employees within an institution, patients who have been admitted to a specific hospital, or members of just about any group of individuals for whom the investigator has a complete list of names and addresses. Survey data can be collected through multiple modalities such as through mailed surveys, through in-person interviews, over the phone, or through the Internet. It is also relatively easy to generate a large, representative sample, depending on your sampling parameters.

In recent years, mail surveys have been shown to be instrumental in collecting important research data that provide the evidences for the development of health care policy at the institutional, state, and national level. Nursing workforce centers, for example, have conducted mail surveys among licensed hospitals, skilled nursing facilities, and home health care agencies in their home states to determine current and future demand for nurses, nurse attrition rates, vacancy rates, and recruitment difficulties (Lacey & Nooney, 2005a, 2005b). These data have then been used to quantify and determine trends in workforce shortages, as well as to create evidence-based solutions to lessen the gaps between nurse supply and demand. Facility-level data from both North Carolina and North Dakota have also been used to explore models for nursing shortage designations at the national level. Likewise, mail surveys of nursing education programs have provided data on nursing faculty shortages; those data have informed the development of policies in the public and private sectors aimed at enhancing faculty supply and recruitment (Dickson & Flynn, 2005).

Regarding nursing workforce and patient care policies, Dr. Linda Aiken, director of the Center for Health Policy and Outcomes Research at the University of Pennsylvania, combined inpatient information with mail survey data from registered nurses employed at admitting hospitals to quantify the impact of nurse staffing and education levels on inpatient mortality. Findings from this pooling of survey and patient data influenced, among other policy initiatives, the decision by the Joint Commission on Accreditation of Healthcare Organizations (JCAHO) to add a staffing effectiveness standard to the accreditation criteria (Aiken, Clarke, Cheung, Sloane, & Silber, 2003; Aiken, Clarke, Sloane, Sochalski, & Siler, 2002; Rafferty et al., 2007).

According to the American Statistical Association (1995), the survey approach includes a clear research topic, and data are gathered by asking questions of individuals. Collecting these data is done in a systematic way, and the study produces aggregate results that can be generalized to the population studied. This chapter describes the steps necessary to collect data using a survey, including (a) determining the research topic, (b) writing survey questions, (c) collecting the data, and (d) avoiding pitfalls associated with surveys.

IT IS ALL ABOUT THE WHY: DETERMINING YOUR SURVEY RESEARCH TOPIC

It is important to design your survey with a clear and realistic research topic or question (Aday, 1996). You should be able to formulate discrete questions based on your topic, which will be used when designing your survey. An example of a research question follows:

Does my state have a nursing shortage?

This is a general topic and one that is difficult to answer. The definition of nursing shortage will change depending on whom you ask. A clearer question might be the following:

How many facilities in my state have vacant nurse positions?

When you frame your research question and your survey, you should first consult all available literature and sources for three reasons: (1) to determine whether the proposed study has already been done, (2) to find sample questions that might be utilized in the survey, and (3) to enable comparisons between the proposed study and other states or the national arena. Possible sources of information about nursing workforce include the 2002 AONE Acute Care Hospital Survey of RN Vacancy and Turnover Rates (HSM Group, 2002); the 2001 American Nurses Association staffing survey; the Colleagues in Caring minimum data set (2005); the 2002 NurseWeek and AONE National Survey of Registered Nurses; the National Sample Survey of Registered Nurses (Steiger, Bausch, Johnson, Peterson, & Arens, 2004); the National League for Nursing faculty census survey (2003); and other state-level surveys published in journal articles.

If you are unable to determine a discrete research question after consulting the literature, it might be prudent to collect information using qualitative methods. In contrast to quantitative survey research, qualitative research (i.e., focus groups, interviews) is useful when the research topic and the questions and options for a survey are not clear. In this case, many times qualitative data collection is used to develop a better survey (Sudman, Bradburn, & Schwarz, 1995). These methods can be useful not only for determining a research topic but also for designing survey questions on a topic that has not been explored.

Interviews with individuals from the group that you intend to survey can be very helpful in determining the best way to construct the survey (Bauman & Adair, 1992). Individual interviews are less helpful, however, with complex subjects such as nursing workforce issues. Consequently, instead of individual interviews, investigators frequently use focus groups to inform different stages during survey development (Morgan, 1993). Nassar-McMillan and Borders (1999) used a factor analysis to determine whether questions that were generated using focus groups were useful predictors in a national survey. They found that most of the focus group–tested questions loaded onto the factor analysis at .5 or greater, providing evidence that this process was useful in producing valid questions.

A focus group is a moderator-guided small group discussion with individuals from the same audience as your future survey (Krueger & Casey, 2000). In contrast to individual interviews, focus groups are especially useful for engaging in a dialogue about a particular topic for which group interaction is more valuable than individual input (Nassar-McMillan & Borders, 2002). Simply put, a focus group involves a series of open-ended questions on the topic of interest—the topic for which survey questions will be developed. These questions should also be formulated around survey topics. There are many excellent guides for putting together focus groups, such as Krueger and Casey, but this chapter does not go into this in detail.

The focus groups will be able to assist you in framing your overall research topic, as well as providing direction regarding the survey administration. For example, you might find through focus groups of the individuals that you intend to survey that your original sampling plan would not have produced enough, or the right kind of, information (O'Brien, 1993). Focus groups are particularly helpful, however, in developing questions for your survey. Consider the following example:

> Your survey is centered on whether nursing students in your state are planning to work in a rural area. After consulting the sources listed previously in this chapter and doing a literature search, you are unable to find suitable survey question, so you try to develop some potential questions.
>
> 1. *Do you plan to work in a rural area after graduation?*
> *Yes ___ No ___*

The primary problem with this survey question is that the concept of rurality is different for each individual. Is a rural area some place with 50,000 people or 1,000 people or both? You need to make sure that all of the words in your question are clear to your participants and are not open to varied interpretation.

Although this will be interesting information to report to policy makers, it does not really provide a complete picture. Often surveys are administered with questions such as this, and percentages are derived and presented to policy makers. Although they may be interested in what percentage of nursing students are planning to work in a rural area, policy makers are more interested in why students would or would not want to work in a rural area. This forms the basis for programs and policies. The easiest way to get this information is to ask a follow-up question about the students' reasons:

> *Why do you plan or not plan to work in a rural area?*

This open-ended question, however, would result in qualitative data with no real numbers. It might be difficult to determine a concrete answer because there could be hundreds of possible responses. Because this is a question where the information has to be written, you will not be able to collect information on this question using a scannable form and so would have to hand-enter this data, a daunting task if you are planning a large sample. You could also just make up possible answers and then leave an "other" option. But then you could end up with many "other" responses, making it difficult to provide the numbers that you want. There may also be problems with the understandability and validity of the survey question. In addition, depending on the nature of data collection, cultural differences might influence a respondent's understanding or interpretation of the survey question (Peterson, Schmidt, & Bullinger, 2004; Willgerodt, 2003). Asking a set of open-ended questions during a focus group could be invaluable in developing better response categories for your survey questions. You might start by asking the focus group a series of open-ended question, such as the following:

> *What benefits can you think of for working in a rural area?*

> *Prompts: Would the practice of nursing be different? Would the lifestyle be different? What might encourage you to work in a rural area?*

> *What barriers can you think of for working in a rural area?*

> *Prompts: Are there things that might deter you from wanting to work in a rural area? What would encourage you to work in an urban area instead?*

These focus group prompts will separate the issues into two sections—good things and bad things about working in rural areas. You will be able to use the responses to develop a survey question and response categories that have a better chance of including the potential responses and minimizing "other" responses. Following are questions that were derived from focus groups with students (Moulton, 2003). You will notice that there are many potential options that should encompass the majority of potential responses.

> *2. If you indicated yes to question 1, please indicate your reason(s) for seeking employment in a rural area. (You may indicate more than one answer.)*

> > *a. Better working conditions*
> > *b. Better pay and benefits*

    c. *Get to know patients*
    d. *Lower patient loads*
    e. *Low cost of living*
    f. *More likely to receive student loan reimbursement*
    g. *More autonomy*
    h. *Rural areas are a safe environment*
    i. *Will get a broad nursing experience*
    j. *Spouse/significant other has a job in a rural area*
    k. *Other (please indicate _____)*

3. If you indicated no on question 1, please indicate your reason (s) for not working in a rural area. (You may indicate more than one answer.)

    a. *Do not feel adequately prepared to practice in a rural area*
    b. *Few social activities*
    c. *Lack of new technology in rural areas*
    d. *Little cultural diversity in rural areas*
    e. *Not enough critical patients with complex health problems in rural areas*
    f. *Only want to work in a large city, no desire to work in a rural area*
    g. *Pay/benefits are not comparable to urban areas*
    h. *There aren't any jobs for my spouse/significant other in a rural area*
    i. *Unfamiliar with the rural environment*
    j. *Want to live close to family who are in an urban area*
    k. *Other (please indicate _____)*

You now have a series of more informed multiple-choice survey questions, but you are not done. It would be a really good idea to pilot test your entire survey instrument to see if it is understandable. In this case, pilot test it with nursing students. Depending on funding and time, you could also conduct another series of focus groups to pilot test the survey.

Sometimes after a survey has been administered, it is discovered that although a lot of information was collected, the "why" was not. This often results in a follow-up study or survey. Yet another possibility would be the use of a focus group as an economical way to augment the information from the survey by eliciting more details. After all, you may not have the funding to conduct another survey to discover the "why" of your findings. In addition, if you are collecting information from multiple groups, there is a possibility of conflicting findings. A focus group with a group of individuals close by would be a relatively inexpensive way to collect some additional information. You have the numbers that policy makers like, and through focus groups the numbers can come to life with personal stories. Now, you can paint a picture for policy makers. Here is another example:

On a survey of nursing program faculty in North Dakota, we asked the following:

1. Do you believe that your program with current resources could increase student capacity? Yes _____ No _____

If yes, how many more students do you think could be admitted each year?

_____ students

If no, what constraints exist that prevent expanding admissions?

Although this question resulted in some good quantitative data, when comparing the responses to this question with a separate survey of health care facilities, we found conflicting information. For example, nursing program faculty indicated that a major constraint to expanding admissions was the availability of clinical sites (Moulton, Christman, Dannewitz, & Wakefield, 2003). The health care facilities indicated that they could increase the number of students in clinical training (Moulton, Park, Muus, Wakefield, & Henderson, 2003). Rather than administering a second series of surveys, we conducted focus groups with several nursing programs (Moulton & Speaker, 2004). We concluded this would also be a great opportunity to tease out some details that could be useful when designing policy recommendations. The resulting focus group question follows:

A limitation in expanding admissions cited in last year's faculty survey was not having enough clinical facilities. However, our survey of employers indicated that they could increase the number of students. What actions could be taken to overcome those barriers and to increase the number of clinical sites, especially in rural areas? Have you attempted to set up new clinical sites? Did you encounter any problems?

This question resulted in a wealth of useful dialogue, and we were able to collect some information about the barriers of particular nursing programs. One program had several preestablished clinical sites and did not have the resources or time to expand its sites. Another program indicated that it had approached several facilities that were already overloaded with students.

Focus groups are a good beginning in designing survey questions, as well as for securing further information to clarify survey data. However, survey questions are not without their own set of issues in answering research questions, as Lacey identifies in the next section.

DO YOU KNOW WHAT YOU ARE ASKING? COMMON PROBLEMS WITH SURVEY QUESTIONS

Assume that all of the various factors that can affect a survey question—beyond the question itself—are all as they should be: the right sample has been drawn, the right respondents have been identified, your research questions have been clearly stated and agreed upon, and so on. This chapter covers many of those aspects of survey research. In this section, the focus is on the little things that can and do go wrong in crafting a survey question.

You have probably been asking questions all your life. Most of us start asking questions as soon as we can talk, and even earlier. Think of any small child you have known. Small children have mastered the art of asking questions using only body language, small gestures, and pointing. We have a lifelong association with asking questions, and it is often assumed that anyone can do it and do it well.

However, survey questions are not like other questions. They are actually data measurement devices like rulers or thermometers and, therefore, require a different approach. The test of a good survey question is not whether you—as the question author—think it is clear and direct, but whether each and every one of your respondents will understand what you are asking of them *and* be persuaded to share that information with you.

In this section, we quickly review some of the most common problems encountered by survey researchers as they struggle to develop accurate and reliable measures of the things in which they are interested.

Screening Your Respondents

The first common problem is the question that is not asked. Just because you have been able to identify your target population and locate a good sampling frame list for that population does not necessarily mean that your survey lands in the hands of the right person. It is a good idea to design a question that verifies that your respondent has the qualities you planned on when you designed your survey. If you are interested in learning the opinions of staff nurses, make sure that the person answering your questionnaire is actually in a staff nurse role or has been recently. People are mobile and ever-changing, but the lists that we use to draw samples are not. They may have been accurate when you identified them, but in most cases, they will already be at least somewhat out of date by the time you field your survey.

If you do use a screening question, be wary of instructing those who do not meet your criteria to "STOP NOW AND RETURN THIS SURVEY"—even if you are not particularly interested in their views. Chances are good that they will simply throw the survey away rather than make the effort to return it. That will have a negative effect on your response rate. It is better to simply identify them and then include those various identities in your analysis or subset them out of the analysis after you have received a completed questionnaire.

Language Barriers

The first rule of question development is *avoid jargon.* However, what exactly is jargon? Jargon refers to the specialized language that is used by a group of professionals. Jargon can also indicate nonsensical, incoherent, or meaningless talk and speech or writing having unusual or pretentious vocabulary, convoluted phrasing, and vague meaning.

It is often difficult for people to know when they are using jargon. The only way to know for certain is to have a wide range of people review your questions—especially people who are not nurses or workforce planners. The goal is to use words that have the widest shared meaning. Remember that it is the consistent interpretation of your question by the respondents that results in high-quality data.

Like jargon, abbreviations should also be avoided even though they save space. If you feel you must abbreviate a phrase or name you use more than three or four times in a questionnaire, be certain you define the abbreviation the first time you use it. FTE (full-time equivalent) is a common abbreviation in workforce planning. Because this is also a very common business term, you might expect that most nurses in a management position will be familiar with it. However, you would be wrong. That is because you and the nurse manager in the small home health agency you want to survey do not share the same knowledge base. You know about labor force and labor market issues. She knows about how to deliver services to the widest range of clients with a minimum of resources. There may be a fair bit of overlap, but no one knows the same combination of things that you do. Explain yourself and your terms if there is *any* chance of confusion or misunderstanding.

It is not enough that you think you have a clear question—your goal is also to have a consistent interpretation by your respondents. It is a point worth repeating.

Unanswerable Questions

Even if your question is clearly stated, you may be asking your respondent to make choices that are uncomfortable or not allowed by your answer format.

Double-barreled questions—those that combine two choices in one question—are a common mistake. Example:

> *Do you think the ANA and AACN are doing enough to combat the nursing shortage?*
>
> ___ Yes ___ No ___ Don't Know

What happens if you think the ANA is doing enough but the AACN is not? Or vice versa? Another common mistake is the use of vague references:

> *Do you think leaders in your organization understand the value of nursing?*
>
> ___ Yes ___ No ___ Don't Know

Who are the leaders in any given organization? It depends largely on who is answering the question. In the cognitive map of a chief nursing officer, the leaders might be the CEO and the chair of the hospital board of directors. A unit manager in that same organization might connect the word "leader" to the chief nursing officer and the chief of medicine. Unless you want that type of random association in your measure, be more specific.

What else is wrong with this question? It is also a double-barreled question. The words "leaders" indicates more than one, and maybe some do understand the value of nursing, and others do not. Rephrase the question (as follows) to ensure that all respondents use the same reference point and to make your meaning clear to your respondent. This will result in more completed questions and better reliability in your data.

Do you think the chief executive officer in your organization understands the value of nursing to the organization?

Vague and Ambiguous Questions

Vagueness and ambiguity are the primary enemies of good survey research questions. But they can be devilishly difficult to spot. The following example is the type of vague question that is often seen in questionnaires:

Employment Location _____

As the author of the question, you know exactly what you mean and how you intend respondents to interpret this question. Only a new set of eyes can—and will—read the words in a different way. This is why pretesting your questions is so important. However, even pretesting is no guarantee that the ambiguity in this question will be brought to light unless your readers and pretesters are aware of what you really want to know, which is the following:

Name the city or town where you worked the most hours last month
_____

It is important to develop "ambiguity radar." It will save you time and trouble down the road and improve the quality of your data. Some of the things that lead to ambiguity are using phrases rather than whole sentences; using words that can have multiple meanings, such as the word "location" in the example; and using negative statements—especially double negatives. An example of a double-negative question would be the following:

Are you against not having union representatives involved in quality-improvement initiatives?

The following would be a clearer statement:

Are you in favor of having union representatives involved in quality-improvement initiatives?

Inadequate Answer Categories

Another principle of question development is that answer categories must always be both comprehensive and exclusive of each other. That is, every possible answer must be available to the respondent, and none of those answer categories should overlap.

The first example here shows what can happen when answer categories are not exclusive of each other.

How long have you been a nurse?

____ *1–12 months* ____ *1 yr–3 yrs* ____ *3 yrs–10 yrs* ____ *11 yrs or more*

Imagine that your respondent is a person who has been a nurse for 3 years.

Which answer category should she choose on this first question? It is hard to say because the categories are not mutually exclusive. Now imagine your respondent identifies as a Native American Indian. How will she answer the second question about race?

Race: ____ White ____ Black ____ Asian

Chances are she will not. There is no category that accurately describes her race. She might write something in the margin, but more likely she will simply skip the question. She might decide at this point to throw the survey away. Why should she invest any more time and energy on it when those who sent it to her did not know that there are nurses whose racial background is something other than White, Black, or Asian? An "other" answer category will solve this problem, and it is always a good idea to provide respondents room to write in which race they identify with if different from the categories provided. This satisfies a respondent's need to be visible and also provides you with the information necessary to build a comprehensive set of answer categories for this question in your next study.

Common Problems With Scale Measures

Scale measures are extremely popular among survey researchers but may often be unnecessary. The first issue to address when considering the use of a scale measurement technique is whether it is the directionality of the respondent's opinion that matters most (e.g., good/bad, high/low, agree/disagree, etc.), or if you also need a measure of the intensity of their opinion. If directionality is all that is necessary, the best approach is to use a simple 2-point scale that leaves no doubt about how the respondents feel about an issue.

> *Do you agree or disagree with this statement? Please circle your response:*
>
> > *Short staffing has affected my patients in a negative way during the past month.*
> > *Agree   Disagree*

Depending on the question topic and your respondent group, the inclusion of a "no opinion" option may be a good idea. It can reduce the amount of respondent error because people who may not have a well-formed opinion on a certain topic thus will not be forced to choose an ill-fitting answer. It may also reduce item nonresponse if those with no strong opinion would otherwise choose to leave the question unanswered rather than accept an ill-fitting answer.

If it is intensity of opinion that you want to measure, then a multi-point scale will be necessary. In addition, the more points in the scale, the easier it will be to identify respondents with intense opinions. If you are interested in identifying those cases that fall at the very far ends, a longer scale of 7 or 9 points will help to differentiate those respondents. If, on the other hand, your interest is simply in putting people into two or three camps, a shorter scale of 3 or 5 points will work better.

There are some caveats to consider when using scales. The first is that, although it is very common, using the word "agree" in a survey question can introduce bias into your data. Research shows that scales using agree/disagree as the defining characteristic are subject to acquiescence bias—a tendency among respondents to place their answer in the "agree" area of the answer continuum. This happens because most people want to be agreeable. Furthermore, this type of bias toward agreement is strongest among those with less education and might introduce a non-random bias into your data (Czaja & Blair, 2005). If possible, craft

Exhibit 3.1 On a Scale of 1 to 5, Indicate How Important Each of These Factors is to You

Very Important	Somewhat Important	No Opinion	Not Very Important	Not At All Important
1	2	3	4	5

your question with other defining concepts that capture the opinion or feeling you want to measure—such as willingness to support an idea or perceived importance. (See Exhibit 3.1.)

Research that examines the effect of question format on the reliability of responses has found that scale measures such as the traditional 5-point Likert scale should be well labeled for *each* response point, leaving no doubt as to what you—the question developer—had in mind for the midpoint values on that scale. The alternative is to leave the interpretation of mid-scale values up to each and every respondent. Asking your respondent to intuit your intent is unlikely to lead to a shared and common interpretation.

The use of a middle alternative—a value of 3 in a 5-point scale, for example, that is neither positive nor negative—does not necessarily result in more reliability in your data than the use of a 4- or 6-point scale. A middle alternative may be most useful in longer response forms such as 7- or 9-point scales where they can serve as an anchor for an opinion (Czaja & Blair, 2005). Nevertheless, the opposing view also has merit: beware of forcing a choice onto a respondent—especially if your question topic is something that might not apply to your entire survey group. As noted earlier, forced choices are often biased in a positive direction and may substantially skew your results if more than a few fence sitters are forced to adopt an opinion in order to answer the question.

Creating a Shared Reference Point

It may seem obvious, but one of the ways to increase the likelihood that your respondents will interpret a question in a similar way is to use a qualifying phrase that grounds all of the respondents in the same time and place. Keep these short and simple, and make certain that they will apply to all of the respondents in your study. Ultimately, the purpose of a qualifier is to clarify the intended frame of reference for the measurement.

For example, to ground everyone in the same time frame, use phrases such as "in the past year," "as of October 1," and "during the last week you worked." To ground respondents in terms of place, use phrases such as "the last time you saw a patient," "in your system as a whole," and "among the staff RNs in your hospital."

Question Order

There are theories and schools of thought about the best way to order the questions in a questionnaire. Some suggest putting sensitive questions in the middle, with the assumption that it makes them easier to answer. Some recommend saving demographic questions about the respondents for the end of the questionnaire, and some put them at the beginning to help in the screening process. An in-depth review of questionnaire formatting is more than can be done here, but let me point out that the order of questions can be used to orient your respondents and improve their recall.

Here is one example of how that might work: The researcher's interest is in the most distant time point and how perceptions have changed over time. But asking someone to recall an opinion from two years past and expecting any kind of reliability in the person's recall is unrealistic. Instead, the question starts by grounding the respondent in the present and—using a relational thought process—moves them backward through time. Although not foolproof, giving respondents specific points in time for their assessments seems to reduce recall error (Converse & Presser, 1986).

On a scale of 1 to 5, with 1 being no shortage and 5 being a severe and persistent shortage, how would you rate the nursing shortage in your facility?

Today
6 months ago
1 year ago
2 years ago

Knowing When to Stop

For many researchers, the most difficult part of question development is knowing when to stop. Given the time, effort, and cost involved in primary data collection, there is always a temptation to ask just a few more questions while you have the attention of your respondent audience. However, response rates are undoubtedly affected by questionnaire length. In survey research, shorter is always better.

The challenges in survey research are in developing clear and concise questions that will produce valid and reliable measures of your topic of interest and doing it in the fewest questions possible. Now that you have your questions developed, what are you going to do to collect the data? The next section is devoted to the mail survey process.

MAIL SURVEY METHOD: IMPERATIVES AND PITFALLS

Despite the popularity, utility, and relatively low cost of mail surveys, this approach to data collection requires additional knowledge and skills in survey methods. Toward that end, in this section of the chapter, we review several essential elements, or imperatives, that will enhance the success of any survey process. Common mistakes during the survey process also are reviewed to help you avoid these survey pitfalls.

Imperative 1: Know Thy Targets...And Their Correct Addresses

Whether the survey is focused on nurses, patients, physicians, employers, or any other specialized collection of people, it is important to ensure that the sample selected to receive a mail survey actually represents the target population, or "survey population," defined as all of the individuals or units to which one wishes to generalize the survey results (Dillman, 2000, 2006). If the sample does not adequately represent the survey population, then obviously survey findings cannot be generalized to that population, and the entire survey process would have been fruitless.

For statewide surveys, a recommended sampling approach that enhances population representation is to simply obtain a mailing list of *all* members of the specialized survey population in the state, such as all registered nurses licensed by the state, and then randomly select a sizable sample from the list. This method of sample selection reduces the risk of coverage error by ensuring that all members of the survey or target population have an equal or known chance of being included in the sample. Consequently, there is an excellent chance that the sample will actually represent the survey population.

For nationwide surveys, however, a mailing list of all members of the survey population is not always available. In that case, one alternative approach to sample selection is to obtain a mailing list of members from a national organization that closely approximates the survey population.

If the survey population, for example, were registered nurses in the United States, the American Nurses Association might be a suitable source organization from which to obtain a member mailing list. Although this approach is relatively easy and inexpensive, it must be recognized that there is a higher risk of coverage error in that, most likely, not all members of the survey population have an equal chance of being included in the sample—because, most likely, not all members of the survey population would also be members of the selected organization.

In addition to the possibility of coverage error and its consequence of inadequately representing the survey population, another potential pitfall in choosing a mailing list from which to select randomly a survey sample involves inaccuracies in the contact information for persons on the list. Keep in mind that some organizations, journals, and even state agencies are more efficient than others in verifying and updating the names and addresses of their constituency. To avoid the pitfall of an inaccurate mailing list, the processes used by the source agency or organization to ensure the accuracy of contact information should be fully discussed and evaluated before the mailing list is requested or purchased.

Imperative 2: Response Rate Is the Name of the Game

Once the sample is selected, not every survey recipient, unfortunately, is going to take the time and effort to complete and return the survey. This can be problematic and lead to nonresponse error, which means that there is a chance that persons who do *not* participate are different from persons who *do* participate in ways that could affect study findings. Because of the risk of nonresponse error, it is a widely held belief among survey experts that when the response rate, or the percentage of the sample that completes and returns the survey, is low, the generalizability of findings to the survey population is seriously threatened. Consequently, the higher the response rate, the lower the risk of nonresponse error in survey research (Cui, 2003).

Fortunately for the survey process, Donald Dillman (1978, 2000, 2006) developed a comprehensive system currently labeled the Tailored Design Method (TDM), which research has demonstrated to be effective in ensuring survey response rates of 50% to 60%. Because an adequate response rate is vital to the success of the survey process, the remainder of the key imperatives discussed in the section focus on implementing important response enhancement strategies recommended by the TDM.

Imperative 3: Make a Good Impression

The first challenge faced in obtaining an adequate response rate is to ensure that survey recipients will actually *open* the survey envelope when it arrives in their mail. Consequently, the appearance of the outside envelope should never be such that it would be confused with junk mail or a mass mailing. Avoid bright colors, address windows, and stamped messages that state "important materials inside" because these tactics are hallmarks of the mass-mailing industry. Instead, the appearance of the outside envelope should represent a personal, yet professional, correspondence. When at all possible, hand-addressed envelopes are preferable because they convey to the recipient that the sender took the time to address the envelope personally. This simple act, when feasible, helps to establish a personal connection between the sender and the recipient that is vital to engaging the recipient in the survey process. When hand-addressed envelopes are not feasible because of a very large sample size, then according to the TDM, address labels are the next best choice.

If collaborating with a more influential sponsor or partner organization, it may be beneficial to use their mailing envelope as the outside envelope, so that their logo or information appears in the return address section on the upper left-hand side of the envelope. We at the New Jersey Collaborating Center for Nursing, for example, recently partnered with the New Jersey Board of Nursing (NJBON), among other stakeholders, in surveying 50% of all registered nurses licensed in the state. This partnership facilitated the use of NJBON stationery in the survey process. Anecdotal feedback from respondents indicated that when retrieving their mail, the NJBON stationary clearly distinguished that piece of mail from junk mail and hence influenced their decision to open the envelope.

Imperative 4: Tap the Power of a Stamp

The lower cost of bulk mail postage rates in comparison with first class may tempt survey planners to select the bulk mail approach, but generally, this has been found to decrease response rates. According to the TDM, postage stamps on the outside envelope personalize the attempted communication between the sender and the recipient and enhance response rates. Similarly, postage stamps affixed to the return envelope, which must be included in the survey packet, convey the sender's trust in the recipient, in that the sender has prepaid the return postage. Recognizing that individual stamps are not always feasible, the TDM indicates that metered postage is an acceptable alternative, but sending via bulk mail is a pitfall that should be avoided.

In addition to being impersonal, bulk mail will also not be forwarded to selected recipients who have had a recent change of address. Moreover, as the staff of the New Jersey Collaborating Center for Nursing discovered in our recent survey of nurses, delivery time can vary considerably with bulk mail and may take longer than with first class postage. Because the timing of multiple mailings is crucial to a successful survey process, as discussed in Imperative # 6, the use of bulk mail postage can easily hamper this imperative.

Imperative 5: Create a Personal Connection

The cover letter is one of the best opportunities to create a personal connection with the recipients and engage their interest and participation in the survey. It may be helpful to acknowledge, right up front, that the help of the recipients is needed because they have information that, if shared, could be useful in exploring a pressing problem or question. The purpose and importance of the survey should be explained early in the cover letter, as well as the reasons or methods by which the recipients were selected. Recipients will also want to know about the potential benefits of survey findings to the recipient, to the profession, or to society at large. Likewise, contact information for the survey director or principal investigator should be specified. Designate a time frame for responding, and highlight the inclusion of a self-addressed, postage-paid return envelope. Lastly, do not forget to say "thank you!"

Now for a real challenge—the TDM specifies that the typed cover letter should be no more than one page in length using a size 14 font and still contain lots of white space. Recipients can become overwhelmed with a cover letter that looks long or verbose or has print that is difficult to read. Consequently, they may simply discard the survey packet.

A final consideration is that although a signed consent form is usually not necessary in survey research, nonetheless, an explanation of the key elements of informed consent and recipients' rights as research participants should be outlined in the cover letter, on the back of the cover letter, or on a separate sheet within the survey packet. Elements of informed consent can be found through a local institutional review board or by visiting the following Web site: http://www.hhs.gov/ohrp/human subjects/guidance/45cfr46.htm#46.116

Imperative 6: Schedule Multiple Contacts

Last, according to Dillman (2000, 2006), multiple follow-up contacts increase the survey response rate by 20% to 40%! Therefore, multiple follow-up contacts are essential to the success of a mailed survey. The TDM recommends, generally, a total of five contacts, including (1) a pre-notice letter alerting recipients that an important survey is forthcoming, (2) the initial survey packet a few days to 1 week later, (3) a reminder or thank you postcard to all survey recipients approximately 1 week after receipt of the initial survey, (4) a second survey mailing to all nonrespondents approximately 3 weeks after the initial survey mailing, and (5) a final contact to all nonrespondents approximately 7 weeks after the initial survey mailing.

A key element of the TDM, however, is tailoring survey methods to the specialized needs and characteristics of the survey population. As an example of tailoring the method, the New Jersey Collaborating Center for Nursing, in its statewide survey of registered nurses, slightly modified the contact schedule by eliminating the pre-notice mailing and adding a third survey mailing to persistent nonresponders. To compensate for the lack of a pre-notice letter, the center's staff published notices and articles about the upcoming survey on the state nurses association's Web site, in the association's newsletters, and in local and regional news-papers. As a postscript to this example, the implementation of the slightly modified TDM was successful in that the statewide survey of registered nurses achieved a response rate of 50.5%, producing data from 22,406 New Jersey RNs (Flynn, 2007).

Although a highly useful method for collecting data, the conduction of surveys requires specialized knowledge and skills. The TDM (Dillman, 2000, 2006) provides a detailed and systematic guide for successful survey implementation and is a valuable resource to prospective survey researchers. However, even with careful planning, real-world problems can emerge for researchers, as pointed out in the next section.

COLLECTING DATA BY SURVEY—THE BEST-LAID PLANS CAN GO AWRY

> *A life spent making mistakes is not only more honorable, but more useful than a life spent doing nothing.*
> —George Bernard Shaw (1856–1950)

Collecting data using a mailed survey is a good way to obtain self-report data from nurses. Many excellent books describe how to develop survey questions, format surveys, and provide techniques to ensure high response rates. Rarely do these books describe the myriad of things that go wrong. The purpose of this section is to provide examples of what went wrong when two experienced survey researchers conducted mailed surveys of registered nurses (RNs) and what we did to correct those problems. The point of this litany of woes is not to discourage anyone from doing survey research, but only to say that things do and will go wrong, even when you try to anticipate everything you can. As Oscar Wilde wrote, "Experience is the name everyone gives to their mistakes" (*Lady Windermere's Fan,* 1892, Act III).

Among the necessary activities prior to mailing a survey is the development of the sampling frame (the list of the universe of people who are the target population for the survey) from which the sample who will receive the survey will be chosen. In some cases, everyone in the sampling frame receives the survey. Our goal was to invite first-time newly licensed RNs (new graduates who had passed the NCLEX) to participate in our survey. We planned to obtain the lists of contact information for new licensees from state boards of nursing. Our sample was limited to RNs from selected geographic areas in 35 states and the District of Columbia. Prior to requesting formally, we inquired about the availability and costs of mailing lists in the various jurisdictions. Just determining the actual person or unit responsible for providing the addresses in the format we needed in each state required some creative investigative work. Some state boards said they could sort based on our specified criteria, and for some states we knew we would have to do this ourselves. Eventually, all indicated that they could send us such lists with varying degrees of specificity. One state could not identify new licensees, and many states could not differentiate those who were first-time newly licensed from those who were first-time licensed in the state but who were also licensed in another state or country (e.g., were not new nurses). This meant that in some states we had to mail out many more surveys than actually were needed and sort out the usable respondents with a question in the survey. Jurisdictions required different formats for payment. Some required no payment. Others required a check, and others would accept a credit card. In many cases, we needed to pay for the lists and then be reimbursed by our universities.

Each state had lists in different file structures. The company mailing the surveys required that the name and address structure be identical for each state. We contracted with a research group to construct the final formatted name and address file. Among the difficulties encountered was that New York State (NYS) would provide the name and city of licensees but would not provide their addresses to researchers. Our mailing firm had to look up each address on an address database. What was particularly ironic was that if we had been providing continuing education programs (even if we were a for-profit company), NYS would have provided the actual addresses. Although we contacted various state officials, we could do nothing to change their minds. We briefly considered having one of our universities request the list for continuing education use and then "borrowing" the list, but our morals got the better of us, and we did not do that. Most nurses provide their home address to the state boards, but in Washington, DC, most nurses had provided work addresses, and we therefore could not get forwarding addresses. In another case, state zip codes were deleted when the lists were transcribed (electronically) from the state list to the lists that subcontractors created for the mailing house. Somehow, the zip codes of addresses from one state were missing. Therefore, we had to look up the zip code for each address, which delayed the mail process. One jurisdiction lost our check and thus did not provide the addresses; bureaucratic processes being what they are, this created enormous problems and slowed us down considerably. Overall, the process of constructing the lists took much more time than we anticipated.

We used a variation of the TDM (Dillman, 2000, 2006) to ensure a high response rate. We sent an alert letter and increasingly persuasive letters with each of the three survey mailings. A copy of each type of letter included in the survey was read by many people involved in the survey: the two investigators (twice), the project manager, New York University's human subject committee staff and review committee members, and the University of Buffalo's staff and human subject committee members. The survey firm included us in the survey mailing, so that we could participate in the process and make any necessary changes. When we read one of the letters we received, there was a spelling error: "its" instead of "it's"! An excellent approach to proofreading is for one person to read the text to another person as he or she reads along. We did not do that, but we will in the future.

In an earlier study, we had included a $1 incentive and a lottery for about $100, as well as a $2 incentive in the second wave of that survey. When we reread the literature on incentives, we were convinced that we should up the incentive to $5. Other options we considered were a gift card to a national chain, phone card for a long-distance phone company, or a check. We could see no advantage to a gift card and thought that so many people have cell phones with free long distance that respondents would not like that. The advantage of a check was that if the person did not cash it, we would not have to pay the $5, but we thought that a $5 check that needed to be cashed would annoy people and also create a huge bureaucratic and cost issue for the issuing university. We settled on cash, and our survey firm included a crisp new $5 bill in the first survey mailing. When we heard from potential respondents with various questions or comments, we found out that some people had not received the $5. Several said, "Oh, I threw out the envelope." We are confident that our survey firm put $5 in each package. Our advice is to make it very clear in the letter that there is a $5 bill and that people should look for it in the envelope. Second, use glue to attach the $5 bill to the top of the letter so that it is one of the first things the potential respondent sees upon opening the envelope. We did that in our second-year survey.

Fortunately (or not), we received many phone calls about the study. We had not budgeted time to handle the calls, and they became very burdensome. People will call. Be ready for the calls and develop a system for tracking and returning calls. Our calls fell into several categories. People returned the survey, but it crossed in the mail with the second survey mailing, and they wanted to be sure we had received the completed survey (and sometimes to let us know what terrible researchers we were for sending them a second mailing). People did not meet the inclusion criteria. We knew many people would not fit the criteria because of the lists that some states sent us. Many of these honest nurses wanted to return the $5. We urged them to keep the money.

We knew we would be sending two additional rounds of surveys at 1 and 2½ years after the first mailing was sent out, but we neglected to ask respondents for a change in address. Thus, if the original survey had been forwarded to a respondent, when we used that same address a year later, it would not be forwarded and would be returned to us. We actually considered asking for an address in the survey and rejected the idea because it would have been more difficult with our human subjects committee. We did two things to correct this error. First, we used a national change-of-address database to identify address changes and used those new addresses in year 2. Second, we asked for address change information in our year 2 survey to avoid a similar problem in the third survey. We also asked respondents to provide us with e-mail addresses if they wanted to be contacted by e-mail for future surveys. Although about one-third provided this information, we have decided to continue using mailed surveys because of the problems that multiple data collection methods can cause.

CONCLUSION

In this chapter, we have discussed the many steps involved in designing and collecting survey data and the potential problems that can occur. Topics included determining a research topic by using existing information or a mixture of research methods, writing clear and concise survey questions, taking steps to maximize the possibility that your survey will be completed and returned, and last, pitfalls associated with survey research.

Depending on funding levels for conducting research, a combination of approaches (quantitative and qualitative) could be combined into a rigorous research program that might be used, for example, when developing national surveys. A nine-step approach is detailed by Krause (2002) that includes focus groups, in-depth interviews, information gathering from other quantitative studies, preliminary survey development, expert panel review, cognitive interviews, pilot testing, nationwide survey administration, and psychometric testing.

Nurse researchers involved in gathering and interpreting evidence for policy makers to use in their policy decisions might find the experiences of these experienced nurse workforce researchers extremely helpful. Further, following are the classic texts designed to give you information regarding the tried and true methods of conducting a successful survey as an evidence-gathering tool. Carefully selecting the most appropriate method or methods to answer the questions you have with survey data from a specialized group of people is a skill well learned and respected in nursing workforce research and policy development.

SUGGESTED READING

Converse, J., & Presser, S. (1986). *Survey questions: Handcrafting the standardized questionnaire.* Quantitative Applications in the Social Science, No. 63. Thousand Oaks, CA: Sage.

Czaja, R., & Blair, J. (2005). *Designing surveys: A guide to decisions and procedures.* Sacramento, CA: Pine Forge Press.

Dillman, D. A. (2007). *Mail and Internet surveys: The tailored design method.* New York: Wiley.

Payne, S. (1951). *The art of asking questions.* Princeton, NJ: Princeton University Press.

REFERENCES

Aday, L. (1996). *Designing and conducting health surveys* (2nd ed.). San Francisco: Jossey-Bass.

Aiken, L. H., Clarke, S. P., Cheung, R. B., Sloane, D. M., & Silber, J. H. (2003). Educational level of hospital nurses and surgical patient mortality. *Journal of the American Medical Association, 290,* 1617–1623.

Aiken, L. H., Clarke, S. P., Sloane, D. M., Sochalski, J., & Siler, J. H. (2002). Hospital nurses staffing and patient mortality, nurse burnout, and job dissatisfaction. *Journal of the American Medical Association, 288,* 1987–1993.

American Nurses Association. (2001). *Analysis of American Nurses Association staffing survey.* Warwick, RI: Cornerstone Communications Group.

American Statistical Association. (1995). *What is a survey?* [Brochure]. Washington, DC: Author.

Bauman, L., & Adair, E. G. (1992). The use of ethnographic interviewing to inform questionnaire construction. *Health Education Quarterly 19*(1), 9–23.

Colleagues in Caring. (2005). Minimum supply-side data elements. In B. Cleary & R. Rice (Eds.), *Nursing workforce development: Strategic state initiatives* (pp. 214–217). New York: Springer Publishing.

Converse, J., & Presser, S. (1986). *Survey questions: Handcrafting the standardized questionnaire.* Quantitative Applications in the Social Science, No. 63. Thousand Oaks, CA: Sage.

Cui, W. W. (2003). Reducing error in mail surveys. *Practical Assessment, Research, & Evaluation, 8*(18). Retrieved September 9, 2007, from http://pareonline.net/getvn.asp?v=8&n=18

Czaja, R. F., & Blair, J. (2005). *Designing surveys: A guide to decisions and procedures* (2nd ed.). Sacramento, CA: Pine Forge Press.

Dictionary.com Unabridged. (2007). Jargon. Retrieved June 2007 from http://dictionary.reference.com/browse/jargon

Dickson, G. L., & Flynn, L. (2005). *New Jersey's educational capacity: Impact on the nursing supply.* Retrieved September 9, 2007, from http://www.njccn.org/pdf/RN%20Educational%20Capacity%202005%20data.pdf

Dillman, D. A. (1978). *Mail and telephone surveys. The total design method.* New York: Wiley-Interscience.

Dillman, D. A. (2000). *Mail and Internet surveys: The tailored design method.* New York: Wiley.

Dillman, D. A. (2006). *Mail and Internet surveys: The tailored design method* (2nd ed.). New York: Wiley.

Flynn, L. (2007). *The state of the nursing workforce in New Jersey: Findings from a statewide survey of registered nurses.* Newark: New Jersey Collaborating Center for Nursing.

HSM Group. (2002). *Acute care hospital survey of RN vacancy and turnover rates.* American Association of Nurse Executives, Washington, DC. Retrieved November 7, 2007, from http://www.wha.org/workForce/pdf/aone-surveyrnvacancy.pdf

Krause, N. (2002). A comprehensive strategy for developing closed-ended survey items for use in studies of older adults. *Journal of Gerontology: Social Sciences, 57B,* S263–274.

Krueger, R., & Casey, M. (2000). *Focus groups: A practical guide for applied research* (3rd ed.). Thousand Oaks, CA: Sage.

Lacey, L. M., & Nooney, J. G. *Nursing vacancy rates in North Carolina hospitals.* Raleigh: North Carolina Center for Nursing. Retrieved June 2005 from http://www.nursenc.org/research/empsurv2004/vacancy%20rates%20-%20Hospitals.pdf

Lacey, L. M., & Nooney, J. G. *Evidence of increasing demand for nursing personnel in North Carolina.* Raleigh: North Carolina Center for Nursing. Retrieved July 2005 from http://www.nursenc.org/research/empsurv2004/demand%20expect%20statewide.pdf

Morgan, D. L. (Ed.). (1993). *Successful focus groups: Advancing the state of the art.* Newbury Park, CA: Sage.

Moulton, P. (2003). *North Dakota nursing needs study: Student focus group results.* Grand Forks: University of North Dakota, School of Medicine and Health Sciences, Center for Rural Health. Retrieved May 28, 2007, from http://ruralhealth.und.edu/projects/nursing/pdf/studentfocusresults.pdf

Moulton, P., Christman, S., Dannewitz, H., & Wakefield, M. (2003). *North Dakota nursing needs study: Faculty survey results.* Grand Forks: University of North Dakota, School of Medicine and Health Sciences, Center for Rural Health. Retrieved May 28, 2007, from http://ruralhealth.und.edu/projects/nursing/pdf/FacultySurvey Results.pdf

Moulton, P., Park, R., Muus, K., Wakefield, M., & Henderson, T. (2003). *North Dakota nursing needs study: Facility survey results.* Grand Forks: University of North Dakota, School of Medicine and Health Sciences, Center for Rural Health. Retrieved May 28, 2007, from http://ruralhealth.und.edu/projects/nursing/pdf/facilities report.pdf

Moulton, P., & Speaker, K. (2004). *Nursing faculty focus group results.* Grand Forks: University of North Dakota, School of Medicine and Health Sciences, Center for Rural Health. Retrieved May 28, 2007, from http://ruralhealth.und.edu/projects/nursing/pdf/year2facultyfocusgroupresults.pdfNassar-McMillan, S., & Borders, L. (1999). Work behaviors of volunteers in social service agencies. *Journal of Social Service Research, 24*(3–4), 39–66.

Nassar-McMillan, S., & Borders, D. (2002). Use of focus groups in survey item development. *The Qualitative Report, 7*(1). Retrieved May 11, 2007, from http://www.nova.edu/ssss/QR/QR7-1/nassar.html

National League for Nursing (2003). *Nurse educators 2002: Report of the faculty census survey of RN and graduate programs.* New York: Author.

NurseWeek & AONE. (2002). *National Survey of Registered Nurses.* Retrieved November 2, 2007, from Harris Interactive, at http://www.nurseweek.com/survey

O'Brien, K. (1993). Using focus groups to develop health surveys: An example from research on social relationships and AIDS-Preventive behavior. *Health Education Quarterly 20*(3), 361–372.

Peterson, C., Schmidt, S., & Bullinger, M. (2004). Brief report: Development and pilot testing of a coping questionnaire for children and adolescents with chronic health conditions. *Journal of Pediatric Psychology, 29*(8), 635–640.

Rafferty, A. M., Clarke, S. P., Coles, J., Ball, J., James, P., McKee, M., & Aiken, L. (2007). Outcomes of variation in hospital nurse staffing in English hospitals: Cross-sectional analysis of survey data and discharge records. *International Journal of Nursing Studies, 44*(2), 175–182.

Steiger, D. M., Bausch, S., Johnson, B., Peterson, A., & Arens, Z. (2004). *The registered nurse population: Findings from the national sample survey of registered nurses.* Washington, DC: U.S. Department of Health and Human Services, Health Resources and Services Administration, Bureau of Health Professions, Division of Nursing.

Sudman, S., Bradburn, N., & Schwarz, N. (1995). *Thinking about answers: The application of cognitive processes to survey methodology.* San Francisco: Jossey-Bass.

Willgerodt, M. (2003). Using focus groups to develop culturally relevant instruments. *Western Journal of Nursing Research* 25(7), 798–814.

4

Forecasting a State Supply and Demand of RNs Using the Revised 2005 HRSA Models

LYNN UNRUH AND VALERIE DANESH

A reliable forecast of the supply and demand of nurses is essential for nursing workforce planning and policy at the federal and state levels. In this era of nursing shortages, it is especially important to be able to evaluate the current situation and anticipate the future in order to demonstrate the need for governmental expenditures, policies, and regulations that could ease actual current or predicted gaps.

Important federal policies that require nursing workforce information include nursing education, nursing immigration legislation, hospital and nursing home regulation and reimbursement, and other regulations and policies that promote the growth or contraction of nursing supply or demand. However, it is incumbent upon the states to initiate independent policies aimed at balancing supply and demand, rather than wait for the federal government to make changes. States must make decisions regarding funding and regulation of nursing education, professional licensure, workforce development programs, and other programs (Salsberg, 2003). These targeted decisions require assessments and forecasts of the supply and demand of nurses at the state and county levels.

Thanks to Manisha Agrawal, MPH, Rutgers Center for State Health Policy, Rutgers University, for assistance with the chapter.

71

National estimates of the present and future supply and demand of registered nurses (RNs) are conducted by the National Center for Health Workforce Analysis, Bureau of Health Professions, Health Resources and Services Administration (HRSA), of the U.S. Department of Health and Human Services (2000, 2002). The forecasts are obtained using two models, the nursing supply model (NSM) and the nursing demand model (NDM), with data from the quadrennial National Sample Survey of RNs (NSSRN), the Area Resource File (ARF), Bureau of Labor Statistics (BLS), Occupational Employment Statistics (OES), and national surveys such as the American Hospital Association (AHA) survey, National Home and Hospice Care Survey (NHHCS), and others (Dall & the Lewin Group, 2004a). Wherever state-level data are available, they are incorporated into the database, but many data fields rely on national values. The last national forecast was published in 2002, using these models; NSSRN data from 1992, 1996, and 2000; and other data from around that time period (U.S. Department of Health and Human Services, 2002).

State-level forecasts can be conducted using the two HRSA models and the databases that come with the models, but the accuracy of the predictions, given the older data and sparse state-level data, is a concern. Substituting more recent and more accurate state-level data when using the models should improve the accuracy. Several state nursing workforce agencies have forecasted the nursing workforce in their state using the NDM and NSM. North Carolina, Hawaii, Virginia, Washington, and Texas, for example, have used one or both of these models with updated data (Kishi, Douglas, Gunn, Ponder, & Menon, 2006; Lacey, Nooney, & Cleary, 2006; LeVasseur, 2007; State Council of Higher Education in Virginia, 2004; Skillman, Andrilla, & Hart, 2007).

Until 2005, the NSM and NDM used an MS-DOS operating platform. The models were essentially "black boxes." Data substitution required a significant time and skill investment. These formidable characteristics discouraged potential state-level use until 2005, when revised versions of the models were released. The 2005 models use a Windows® operating system, incorporate menu screens with pull-down bars, and offer data substitution in Excel® and Access® file formats. Furthermore, the models are redesigned to project nurse supply and demand at the state level and then aggregate the projections to the national level, and the user can set many model assumptions. In short, the 2005 revision made the models much friendlier for use at the state level.

This favorable change in the HRSA models influenced the decision of the Florida Center for Nursing (FCN) to use the models for state-level forecasting. Established by the state of Florida in 2002 to engage in research and policy analysis that supports state decision making on the nursing workforce, one of FCN's mandates is to forecast RN supply and demand. The FCN weighed several options for forecasting, including building a "simple" model with basic, available data; developing a more complicated econometric model; and using the NSM and NDM if revised models were made public. When HRSA released the revised models in 2005, FCN jumped at the chance to conduct a state forecast using the models with updated data.

This chapter discusses the FCN's experience in using the revised 2005 HRSA NDM and NSM. It begins with a review of the HRSA models' structure, function, capabilities, and output and discusses the steps and interventions needed to use the HRSA models at the state level. The FCN's experiences in data procurement, data replacement for both models, and model testing are reported. The chapter closes with recommendations for future state-level analyses. We conclude by identifying implications for other state-level nurse workforce researchers and planners.

THE HRSA NURSING DEMAND AND SUPPLY MODELS

Overview of Nursing Workforce Forecasting and the HRSA Models

The HRSA NSM determines RN supply, and the NDM determines RN, licensed practical nurse (LPN), and nursing assistant (NA) demand using a forecasting approach that can be classified as "nursing personnel-to-population utilization" (or nursing supply/utilization). This is one of three major approaches, the other two being "nursing needs-based," which projects the need for nursing personnel unconstrained by current or future resource limitations, and "econometric," which simultaneously determines future demand and supply (Benham, 1971; Deane & Yett, 1979; Dumpe, Herman, & Young, 1998; Hall & Mejia, 1978; Heckman, 1993; Markham & Birch, 1997; O'Brien-Pallas et al., 2001; Prescott, 1991). The nursing personnel-to-population utilization approach forecasts the demand for future nursing personnel given expected population and service-delivery changes (O'Brien-Pallas et al.; Prescott). Nursing supply is forecasted independently given projected demographics and participation rates and is then compared to the demand forecast.

The nursing personnel-to-population utilization approach uses known stocks and flows of nursing workforce supply and known utilization of the nursing workforce, along with estimated future changes in the population and responses of supply and demand to these changes, in its projections. The approach incorporates many assumptions regarding population growth, health care consumption patterns, workforce participation rates, workforce entry and exit rates, and other factors. Many of these assumptions are linked to population demographics, including, for example, health care utilization rates, which are assumed to be higher in the older population. Whether these factors are entered into the model as fixed or varying over time depends on each of the factors and the particular model.

The demand for nurses is derived from the demand for health care services. Therefore, forecasts of the demand for nurses are based on both the rates of health care utilization and the rates of the utilization of nurses in the delivery of those services. Two important assumptions are whether current rates of health care utilization will continue into the future and whether the current demand for nurses given the demand for health care should be projected into the future. Although the personnel-to-population models allow for overall changes in utilization over time given changes in population demographics, they characteristically tend to keep the rate of health care utilization fixed given the population characteristic. This assumes that cohorts of the population will use health care in the same way across time. The models also characteristically keep fixed the existing rates of nursing personnel to health care utilization. This assumes that the existing personnel-to-population ratios provide the desired quantity and quality of care (O'Brien-Pallas et al., 2001; Prescott, 1991).

The HRSA Nursing Demand Model and Its Operation

The HRSA NDM forecasts the demand for full-time-equivalent (FTE) RNs, LPNs, and NAs through 2020. Components of the NDM are baseline and projected data elements, equations that incorporate assumptions regarding health care utilization, and nursing intensity rates. The baseline data for the model are current per capita health care utilization and the current number of employed RN, LPN, and NA FTEs in several health care settings (Dall & the Lewin Group, 2004a). In addition, data for factors determining this health care utilization are also placed in the system as exogenous variables (values determined a priori outside of the model), with baseline values and estimates for all of the projected years (1996–2020). The factors that are considered to be exogenous determinants of health care utilization are population demographics and health status, the health care operating environment (e.g., payment systems, nurses' wages), and the economic environment (per capita income, percent uninsured, percent on Medicaid) (Dall & the Lewin Group).

The model equations describe the relationship between demand for health care services and its determinants and the relationship between nurse staffing intensity and its determinants. Equations assumptions can be modified. Based on these data and equations, the future demand for health care services and the demand for FTE nurses given the demand for health care services can be projected by geographic location, employment setting, and the three main nursing occupations (i.e., RNs, LPNs, and NAs) (Dall & the Lewin Group, 2004a). Figure 4.1, taken from HRSA manuals and reports on the NDM, illustrates the main structure of the model. The top three parallelograms correspond to the

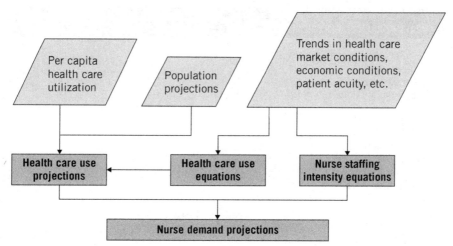

Figure 4.1 Overview of the NDM
Source: What Is Behind HRSA's Projected Supply, Demand, and Shortage of Registered Nurses? by M. Biviano, S. Tise, M. S. Fritz, & W. Spencer, 2004, report prepared for the National Center for Health Workforce Analysis, Bureau of Health Professions, Health Resources and Services by the Lewin Group: Falls Church, VA. Retrieved November 5, 2007, from ftp://ftp.hrsa.gov/bhpr/workforce/behindshortage.pdf; and *The Nursing Demand Model: Development and Baseline Projections,* by T. M. Dall & the Lewin Group, 2004a, report prepared for the National Center for Health Workforce Analysis, Bureau of Health Professions, Health Resources and Services Administration by the Lewin Group: Falls Church, VA. Available with demand model CD. Contact the Lewin Group at http://www.lewin.com/Spotlights/WorkforceMgmt/NurseWorkforce.htm

exogenous variables, whereas the next three rectangles relate to baseline data and model equations.

The NDM provides demand projections for health care utilization in short-term and long-term hospitals, nursing facilities, and home health. Projections for LPN and NA FTEs are available within the inpatient setting in hospitals, long-term hospitals, nursing facilities, and home health. Projections for RN FTEs include these settings, plus several types of short-term hospital settings, doctors' offices, occupational health, schools, public health, and nurse education (Dall & the Lewin Group, 2004a). Table 4.1 indicates these settings.

The 2005 NDM allows the user to adapt the model to use at the regional, state, or sub-state level. Adapting to the regional or state level

Table 4.1

HRSA NDM PROJECTIONS: NURSE TYPES AND HEALTH CARE UTILIZATION BY SETTING

HEALTH CARE DELIVERY SETTING	NURSE DEMAND RNs	LPNs	NAs	HEALTH CARE UTILIZATION
General, short-term (ST) hospitals				
Inpatient	X	X	X	X
Outpatient	X			X
Emergency department	X			X
Non-general and long-term (LT) hospitals	X	X	X	X
Nursing facilities	X	X	X	X
Home health	X	X	X	X
Doctors' offices	X			
Occupational health	X			
Schools	X			
Public health	X			
Nurse education	X			
All other settings	X	X	X	

Source: What Is Behind HRSA's Projected Supply, Demand, and Shortage of Registered Nurses? by M. Biviano, S. Tise, M. S. Fritz, & W. Spencer, 2004, report prepared for the National Center for Health Workforce Analysis, Bureau of Health Professions, Health Resources and Services by the Lewin Group: Falls Church, VA. Retrieved November 5, 2007, from ftp://ftp. hrsa.gov/bhpr/workforce/behindshortage.pdf; and *The Nursing Demand Model User Guide,* by T. M. Dall & the Lewin Group, 2004b, Manual prepared for the National Center for Health Workforce Analysis, Bureau of Health Professions, Health Resources and Services Administration by the Lewin Group: Falls Church, VA. Available with demand model CD. Contact the Lewin Group at http://www.lewin.com/Spotlights/WorkforceMgmt/NurseWorkforce.htm

requires updating the data for that region or state and running the model for projections isolated for that one region or state. Adapting to the sub-state level requires substituting sub-state data for state data and running projections as if the sub-state data were state data, in other words "tricking" the model.

One can also add to the input variables used to project nurse demand or to model demand under different assumptions regarding the future health care system. To make these changes requires systematic changes to the data tables and equations and may require additional empirical research to revise the projection equations (Dall & the Lewin Group, 2004b).

The 2005 NDM is operated through a Windows-based system. The program can be saved on the user's computer hard drive. When the program is opened, a main menu page pops up with the following links to new pages: scenario, reports, import, edit, and exit. Each of these pages is further divided into more pages. Figure 4.2 provides a flowchart of the operational structure of the model.

Data can be replaced via manual changes either through the "edit" menu screen and then the "data tables" screen or by changing the entire tables and replacing them through the "import" menu screen. In the 2005 NDM version, only tables in Access® can be imported into the system (Dall & the Lewin Group, 2004b). Equations can be changed from the "edit" screen, as well values for the policy variables such as wage growth. The initial reporting year is also changed from the "edit" menu (Dall & the Lewin Group). The model comes with a default scenario for equations and policy variables. New scenarios can be created and saved by opening a new scenario from the "scenario" screen and then making the changes to the equations and variables. The model saves those changes for that scenario. If the user wishes to return to the default scenario, he or she needs only to go to "existing scenarios" in the "scenario" menu and click on the default tab.

Once the data and equations are changed, when the user is ready to run the model, he or she opens the "report," page and the model runs with a few prompts. Output reports are produced that can be copied and pasted or printed.

The HRSA Nursing Supply Model and Its Operation

The HRSA NSM forecasts the supply of RNs through 2020 by year, state, educational level, and age. Components of the NSM are baseline data elements and equations that project the changes in supply

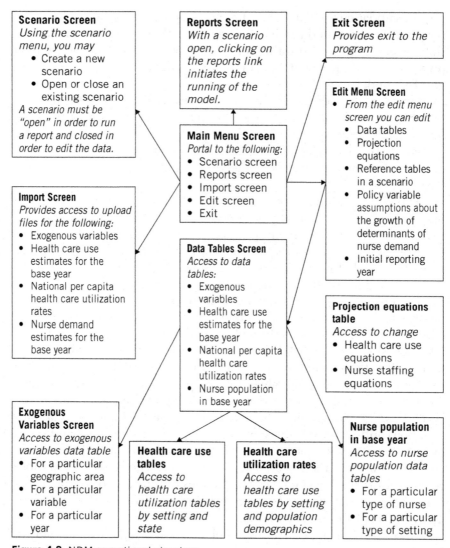

Scenario Screen
Using the scenario menu, you may
- Create a new scenario
- Open or close an existing scenario

A scenario must be "open" in order to run a report and closed in order to edit the data.

Reports Screen
With a scenario open, clicking on the reports link initiates the running of the model.

Exit Screen
Provides exit to the program

Main Menu Screen
Portal to the following:
- Scenario screen
- Reports screen
- Import screen
- Edit screen
- Exit

Edit Menu Screen
- *From the edit menu screen you can edit*
- Data tables
- Projection equations
- Reference tables in a scenario
- Policy variable assumptions about the growth of determinants of nurse demand
- Initial reporting year

Import Screen
Provides access to upload files for the following:
- Exogenous variables
- Health care use estimates for the base year
- National per capita health care utilization rates
- Nurse demand estimates for the base year

Data Tables Screen
Access to data tables:
- Exogenous variables
- Health care use estimates for the base year
- National per capita health care utilization rates
- Nurse population in base year

Projection equations table
Access to change
- Health care use equations
- Nurse staffing equations

Exogenous Variables Screen
Access to exogenous variables data table
- For a particular geographic area
- For a particular variable
- For a particular year

Health care use tables
Access to health care utilization tables by setting and state

Health care utilization rates
Access to health care use tables by setting and population demographics

Nurse population in base year
Access to nurse population data tables
- For a particular type of nurse
- For a particular type of setting

Figure 4.2 NDM operational structure

with each successive forecasted year. The NSM is an annual snapshot of licensed RNs in a particular cohort based on the RNs' age, educational level, and state. The number of RNs in each group is extrapolated over time by aging the RN population each year, determining subtractions and additions to the cell based on accessions and attrition (retirement, death, and disability), determining movement across states, and determining changes in highest level of nursing education (Dall & the Lewin Group, 2004c).

The NSM operates by making a series of calculations for each forecasted year. Starting in the first year (Y) with the beginning inventory, the NSM extrapolates the nurse population from year Y to year Y+1 by making the following calculations: adjusts state inventories for cross-state migration; adjusts cells for educational upgrades; subtracts for attrition; adjusts for the aging of the RN population; adds the net immigration of foreign-trained nurses; and adds the new graduates from U.S. nursing programs. After completing these steps going from year Y to year Y+1, the NSM repeats them for each year in the projection (Dall & the Lewin Group, 2004c). Figure 4.3 shows the process (Dall & the Lewin Group, 2004b).

The NSM forecasts three measures of RN supply by age and educational status: the number of licensed RNs, the number of RNs active in nursing, and the number of FTE RNs in nursing. In addition, the number

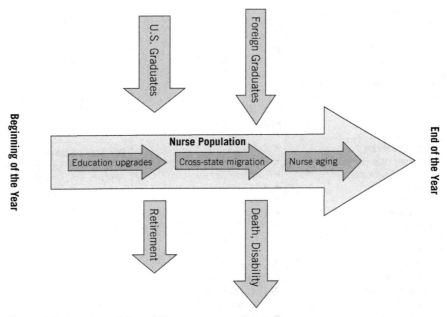

Figure 4.3 Overview of the NSM
Source: What Is Behind HRSA's Projected Supply, Demand, and Shortage of Registered Nurses? by M. Biviano, S. Tise, M. S. Fritz, & W. Spencer, 2004, report prepared for the National Center for Health Workforce Analysis, Bureau of Health Professions, Health Resources and Services by the Lewin Group: Falls Church, VA. Retrieved November 5, 2007, from ftp://ftp.hrsa.gov/bhpr/work force/behindshortage.pdf

of emigrants, immigrants, and new graduates can be forecasted by age and educational status. These figures can be reported for each state in the United States or in aggregate (Dall & the Lewin Group, 2004c).

As with the NDM, the 2005 NSM is operated through a Windows®-based system and can be saved on the computer's hard drive. Also, as with the NDM, when the program is opened, a main menu page appears with the following links to new pages: settings, reports, import, edit, calculate, and exit. Some of these are further divided into more pages, whereas others open directly into an active page that allows access to settings, editing, and so on. Figure 4.4 provides a flowchart of the operational structure of the model.

Data can be replaced either by making manual changes through the "edit" menu screen, which opens up to a choice of 17 tables to edit, or by changing the five main Excel® data worksheets in the NSM application folder (Dall & the Lewin Group, 2004c). In order to replace

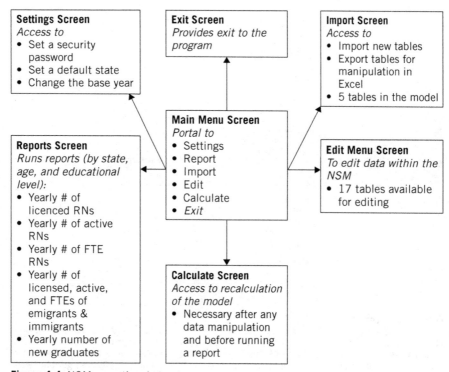

Figure 4.4 NSM operational structure

entire data worksheets, the user constructs a matching worksheet with the desired data changes and saves the file with the same name as the default worksheet in the same application folder as the original worksheet (this writes over the original worksheet, so the original should be saved in another folder). Replacing the Excel® worksheets requires that you keep the same column and row headings and sequence that are in the original Excel® file. Once the data files are replaced in the application folder, the "import" function must be used to transfer the revised files into the model.

In the NSM, rates of change in accession, attrition, and participation in the RN workforce are part of the data tables, not the equations. Therefore, these are changed not through an equation screen, as in the NDM, but through editing the data tables. By going to the "edit" screen and selecting one of these functions (e.g., "attrition rates"), the user can change the rates listed in the table. Through the edit screen, the user also can change policy variables that affect RN supply, such as wages, the number of nurse educators, costs of tuition, and other factors. For example, wages can be raised or lowered, or the number of nursing faculty can be increased or decreased. Finally, the elasticities for policy variables (the amount of the RN supply response to the policy variables) can be altered in the edit screen (Dall & the Lewin Group, 2004c).

Once the data are changed, the user must go to the "calculation" screen and perform a recalculation of the model. Finally, to receive the forecasts, the user opens the "report" page and chooses to run a report for the nation or for a single state and specifies one of the types of RN reports described earlier (projections of RN graduates, immigration and emigration, or RN participation or general RN population projections). Reports can be copied and pasted and printed.

USING THE HRSA MODELS FOR FORECASTING IN INDIVIDUAL STATES: THREE APPROACHES

There are three approaches to using the HRSA models for forecasting in individual states. The models can be used to forecast aggregate, state-level supply and demand with the default data; forecast aggregate, state-level supply and demand with replacement data from the state; or forecast supply and demand at a disaggregated sub-state level (county, metropolitan statistical area (MSA), or workforce region) with replacement data at the disaggregated level.

The simplest statewide forecasting is the first approach—to use the models with the default data contained in them. In this case, the user merely needs to access the report menus and run the various reports. However, state workforce organizations have compared forecasts using this method to actual numbers and report that the forecasts using the models with default data can be inaccurate (Nooney & Lacey, 2007). One reason for this bias is the older default data used to project into the future. The data in the 2005 models date back to 1996–2000. When data from those years become the baseline, future figures will be less accurate than updated data with a baseline closer to the current year. Another reason is that the default data may be estimated at the state level or may contain national values applied to each state. Default data in the NSM, for example, are largely taken from the NSSRN, in which specific state survey responses are applied to total licensees in the state to produce estimated values for responses. Moreover, fields such as attrition and workforce participation rates are estimated at the national level and applied uniformly to each state. Likewise, the NDM uses some national data uniformly across states and estimates other state-level data based on state survey data. NSSRN survey responses in each state are used to extrapolate the number of nurses employed in various health care settings.

The North Carolina Center for Nursing (NCCN) recently compared the default data in the NSM and NDM models to its own state-level data and tested the model predictions with its own data. Researchers found that many data points in the NSM, such as the number of licensed RNs, were similar. However, the default data significantly underestimated participation rates, the number of FTEs, and accessions while overestimating attritions. The overall effect of these differences was a consistent undercount of RN FTE supply that grew over the projection period. In their testing of the NDM, researchers found that the estimates of demand using their own data were close to 10% higher than estimates using the default data. Combining supply and demand, researchers found that whereas the HRSA models with default data underestimated both supply and demand, the estimates of the *gap* were similar between models run with default data and models with replacement data (Nooney & Lacey, 2007).

The good news from the North Carolina report is that for the NSM, "given adjusted inputs to the model derived from state-specific data sources, the model performs amazingly well" (Nooney & Lacey, 2007), indicating that the structure of the model is sound. The NCCN was less able to assess the validity of the NDM, but it was thought to perform well enough to be used by states with little or no replacement data. Therefore, the second approach to using the models for state forecasting—forecasting at the aggregate state level using replacement data from the state—is a viable option. The NCCN encourages other state nursing workforce organizations to use the models with whatever updated replacement data they have available, even if they have very little (Nooney & Lacey).

For states taking the second approach of using the HRSA models to forecast aggregate state-level supply and demand with replacement data, the first step of locating replacement data is one of the most difficult parts. For supply, state licensing bureaus may be able to provide numbers of licensed RNs, and perhaps LPNs, along with information about their age and educational level. Finding information about numbers of NAs can be much more difficult given that state certification is not necessarily required. The numbers of licensed nurses can form the base of many other data points for both supply and demand. For example, if the information about percentages of nurses in various health care settings can be obtained (e.g., through nurse surveys), these percentages can be multiplied by the number of nurses to provide estimates of numbers of nurses employed in various health care settings.

The U.S. Census Bureau, BLS, and ARF are sources of state-level population demographics, employment figures, and employment policies such as wages. Data sources listed by Nooney and Lacey (2007) include nursing education programs in the state, health services research departments or research centers within the state university system, and state workforce information and planning organizations.

Once data have been obtained, the default data for that state are replaced with the new data in those cells. Because this involves changing the data for only that state, it may be easiest to use the "edit" functions within the program to accomplish this, rather than exporting, changing, and importing revised files. Data replacement for the NDM is more complicated than for the NSM, especially given that the files are in Access® formats.

In the third approach to state forecasting using the HRSA models, the forecasts are performed at the workforce region, MSA, county, or zip-code levels within the state. This requires data gathering at the substate level and replacement of default statewide data points in the models with the sub-state data points. We warn you, however, that this is a very complicated undertaking. First, one has to find the data. Second, one has to find a way to replace the default data with the sub-state-level data in models that do not have much flexibility in allowing alterations of column or row entries. In the experience of the FCN, which is detailed in the next section of this chapter, both models must be essentially tricked into using the sub-state data.

Sub-state data may come from many of the same sources as state-level data, including state nurse licensure data, the U.S. Census Bureau, nurse surveys, the ARF, and workforce agency statistics. What is needed to make the sub-state-level data available is an identifier for that level or smaller, or individual data points at that level or smaller. We mention "at that level or smaller" because different data fields may present to forecasters at various levels (county, zip code, regional), and all of the data can be used if the smaller levels are aggregated to the largest available level. For example, licensure data typically have zip codes or county codes, whereas the ARF has county-level data points.

Because of the more granular nature of this approach, it is highly doubtful that sub-state data will be located for all data fields within the models. When sub-state data cannot be obtained, state-level data may need to be substituted. As is seen in the discussion of Florida in the next section of the chapter, at times even national data may need to be used.

In data replacement, because the models cannot merely be expanded to accommodate one state's disaggregated data, the approach must be to replace all the existing default data in the models with sub-state data and run the models as if the universe of each model is the individual state under study. This produces the following dilemma: technically, how does one keep existing column and row placements and headings when the number of sub-state observations may be different from the number of state observations present in the models? In addition, how does one use Access® for this type of data entry anyway?

The answer to the first question is that no column or row headings within the tables can be renamed, added, or deleted. Sub-state IDs must be proxied by the state names present in the tables. If there are fewer sub-state observations than the number of states, the remaining state headings must remain in the table, but the data cells can be left blank. If there are more sub-state observations than the number of states, it does not appear to be possible to enter additional observations. The answer to the second question (as to how to use Access®) is "with difficulty." In the next version of the NDM an Excel® option may be available.

One additional set of manipulations that can be performed with all three approaches to state forecasting is to change model assumptions by changing policy equations within the NDM and likewise changing policy, elasticities, and other data tables in the NSM. State forecasters, for example, can change participation rates, wages, and elasticities to match available data or assumptions. Although these changes will be more effective when other data have been updated and when the changes are evidence-based, forecasts with alternative assumptions regarding policy and workforce participation can be interesting to compare even in states where no or little data are available.

The advantage of the second approach to forecasting in individual states in comparison with the last is that there is less data replacement, a greater chance of data availability, and a much less complicated data replacement process. The disadvantage of the second approach in comparison with the last is that the forecasts apply to the state as a whole. Issues and trends pertaining to particular regions cannot be assessed.

FCN EXPERIENCES IN USING THE HRSA MODELS FOR FORECASTING IN FLORIDA

In the fall of 2005, the FCN made the ambitious decision to replace the data in both the NDM and the NSM with sub-state Florida workforce-region data in order to forecast RN supply and demand in each of these areas. The 24 workforce regions in Florida are designated by the state workforce planning agency, Workforce Florida. Each region comprises several distinct counties. Workforce regions were used in lieu of counties for several reasons. First, the use of workforce regions strengthens the accuracy of the analysis, given that the data for some surveys at the county level is sparse. RNs may or may not work in their county of residence, or patients may live in one county but receive health care services in another, so the use of workforce regions may capture the workforce distribution and the population demand for health care more accurately. Second, because Florida has 67 counties, and the HRSA models have input areas for the 50 U.S. states plus the District of Columbia, we would need to add new input areas to the model setup, which would be difficult, if not impossible.

The steps we have taken in forecasting so far are obtaining data for replacement, replacing the HRSA default input data in the NSM, comparing Florida baseline data to HRSA default data in both models, and running a supply forecast with the new NSM data. The following sections provide details.

Data Collection

Data collection and preparation consumed most of the first year of the project. Once the required data fields for the models were identified, possible data sources were sought. This entailed Web searches, phone calls, and networking. The partnership between FCN and Workforce Florida was strengthened, and new partnerships were formed as Workforce Florida assisted FCN with data source contacts, such as the Florida Agency for Workforce Innovation, which provided data on median wages for NAs, home health aides, LPNs, and RNs by regions within Florida. We obtained data from a total of ten different sources, including the ARF, the U.S. Census Bureau (2004), the Florida Board of Nursing (BON), a 2004 Florida Licensure Renewal Survey, the Florida Agency for Workforce Innovation, and other sources identified in Table 4.2.

We found that most of the needed data were not *directly* available but that we could combine data, with some manipulations, to produce the data fields we needed. Sometimes this entailed three data sources and four manipulations to produce one data field for the model. In fields where we could not produce data by any means, we kept the default HRSA data. Sometimes the default data that we had to use were state-level, and sometimes they were national. For example, to produce the number of part-time RN FTEs working in ambulatory care and physician offices, the number of RNs from the 2002 Florida Board of Nursing Licensure Database was aggregated from zip code to workforce region. That number was multiplied by the participation rates by workforce region and then by the percentage of RNs working part-time in ambulatory care and physician offices according to the ARF and converted to part-time (0.5 FTE) and full-time FTEs according to the ARF.

Data Replacement

In the replacement phase of the forecasting project, we had four NDM tables to replace in an Access® database and five NSM tables in an Excel® workbook. The data fields in the tables are either national percentages identically applied to all states or state values for each states. To make the models work at the state level, we replaced the default national and state data with state and workforce-region data. Data that had national-level values in the original HRSA model became state-level values in the new model. Data that were state-level values in the original model

Table 4.2

SUMMARY OF DATA SOURCES AND CORRESPONDING DATA FIELDS

DATA SOURCE	DESCRIPTION	SUPPLIER	DATA FIELDS IN MODELS
Area Resource File (ARF)	(2004) A database of more than 6,000 variables for county-level information on health facilities, health professions, health care resource scarcity, health status, economic activity, health training programs, and socioeconomic and environmental characteristics.	Purchased from http://www.arfsys.com/	Mean age of population; % of population without medical insurance; per capita personal income; HMO enrollment rate, 1996–2020;
Bureau of Labor Statistics (BLS)	(November 2004) national, state, and metropolitan area occupational employment and wage estimates, Employment: the estimated total occupational employment (not including self-employed) according to the Standard Occupational Classification (SOC) system. (Excel® file)	http://www.bls.gov/oes/oes_2004_n.htm	The number of LPNs and NAs; NAs by setting
Florida Agency for Workforce Innovation (FAWI)	(2004) Data on workforce employment and wages in Florida by county or workforce region.	AWI provided data in Excel® files upon request from FCN.	Wage for home health aides, LPNs, nurse aides, RNs by state average, 1996–2020;

(Continued)

Table 4.2

SUMMARY OF DATA SOURCES AND CORRESPONDING DATA FIELDS (Continued)

DATA SOURCE	DESCRIPTION	SUPPLIER	DATA FIELDS IN MODELS
Florida Board of Nursing-Licensure Database and NCLEX-RN Pass Rates	(2002) RN demographic data collected at the time of relicensure with the state of Florida.	Data obtained from the Florida Board of Nursing upon request.	The number of RNs by age by county; The number of new AND and BSN graduates.
Florida Center for Nursing-License Renewal Survey	(2004) Voluntary survey of Florida RNs conducted with the 2004–2005 license renewal regarding RN demographics, population numbers, activity numbers, and workplace settings. Due to Board of Nursing omission, only $\frac{1}{2}$ of the licensees were offered the survey. $N = 4,425$, a response rate of 4.1% for one-half of the RN licensees.	FCN	FTE participation rates for RNs in nurse education, occupational health care, doctor's offices, public health, school health care, and other health care settings; Educational upgrades; RN FTEs by educational level.
Florida Department of Health, Licensure Look-Up	(2006) Florida Department of Health search for health care provider information. Indicates whether the license is clear and free from restrictions, null and void, or deleted or has disciplinary action. Data are available by profession and by county.	https://ww2.doh.state.fl.us/IRM00PRAES/PRASLIST.ASP	The number of LPNs and certified nursing assistants (aides, orderlies, surgical technicians) in Florida.

(Continued)

Table 4.2

SUMMARY OF DATA SOURCES AND CORRESPONDING DATA FIELDS (*Continued*)

DATA SOURCE	DESCRIPTION	SUPPLIER	DATA FIELDS IN MODELS
National Council of State Boards of Nursing, Inc. (NCSBN)	(2002) Licensure and examination statistics. Research brief.	http://www.ncsbn.org/pdfs/2002LicExamStats.pdf	National nurse graduates by educational level; foreign nurse graduates
Office of Economic and Demographic Research (OEDR)	(2004) The Florida Legislature (Excel® file)	http://edr.state.fl.us/population.htm	General population demographics
National Sample Survey of Registered Nurses (NSSRN)	(2000) Survey conducted by the National Center for Health Workforce Analysis, Bureau of Health Professions, Health Resources and Services Administration, U.S. DHHS.	HRSA NSM default program data available upon request from BHPr: http://bhpr.hrsa.gov/	Default data built into HRSA NSM and NDM
U.S. Census Bureau Quick Facts	General population numbers and population numbers by specific demographics (age, sex, etc.) by county.	http://quickfacts.census.gov/qfd/states/12000.html	Total population by state, total population by age 5–17 and by age 18–64 by state; % of population non-White by state, 1996–2020; % of population Hispanic by state, 1996–2020.

became workforce-region values. Cross-state migration in the NSM was translated to workforce-region migration. International migration in the default NSM represented migration to and from all outside states.

A base year of 2004 was used for both models. This contrasts with the original HRSA model base years of 1996 for demand and 2000 for supply. We chose 2004 in order to update the baseline to a more recent year, while at the same time allowing for a test of forecasting of 2006 supply and demand against actual numbers.

Replacing the data in the models was, shall we say, challenging. Starting with the NDM, which uses Microsoft Access® (.mdb) files rather than Excel® files, we found that we could not export the original Access® file to make changes or even to see what the tables in the file looked like. Instead, we had to study the tables in the "edit" mode and fill out the tables accordingly. Complicating this was the fact that the exogenous table is three-dimensional, and we were able to view only two-dimensional pieces of it at a time. At this juncture, we had to contact Timothy Dall of the Lewin Group, who sent us the proper layout. We built new data tables in Excel® for import into an Access® file, with the expectation of replacing the existing default Access® files.

With the NSM, the input data file is an Excel® workbook with five worksheets. This file can be opened for viewing and editing. The default Excel® file was saved in an alternate folder and removed from the model folder. Tables in a new Excel® file were created using the shell of a copy of the default file. The new file was given the same name as the default file and was resaved in the model folder.

We found that the number of cells could not be changed through editing of the original Excel® workbook, and only substitutions or blank spaces were accepted. Cells representing labels or categories could not be modified, added to, or deleted. None of the column headings in any of the worksheets could be renamed. The listed ages, years, and state abbreviations could not be modified, eliminated, or otherwise changed. Even the worksheet names and filename "NSM Input Database.xls" could not be modified. The contents of the data cells could be changed, and data cells that were not needed could be cleared and left blank.

There are 51 state categories (50 states and the District of Columbia) in the HRSA NSM, so without changing any headings, we converted this to 24 workforce regions for Florida. The cell contents of all states after the 24th state (Minnesota) were cleared and left blank.

Comparing Baseline Data

To test the similarity between the HRSA default baseline year data and our updated Florida baseline year data, we selected important data fields to compare. In the NSM, the data field we selected was RN population, and in the NDM the data were RN, LPN, and NA FTEs demanded. For the Florida data, we aggregated these from the workforce-region level to the state level so that the numbers could be compared to the state-level numbers in the default HRSA data. Although the HRSA baseline years are 1996–2000, and ours was 2004, we reasoned that whatever natural differences there were should be reflected in a slight increase in both demand and supply between 1996–2000 (HRSA model baseline years) and 2004 (our baseline year). We also compared the numbers of new graduates and education upgrades between the HRSA and FCN baselines.

We found significant discrepancies between HRSA and FCN values for both demand and supply baselines. Demand-side comparisons are reviewed in Table 4.3. The FTEs employed by setting are significantly different when our data for 2004 are compared with the default NDM. Our numbers for the RN population are less than the HRSA numbers across several settings even though our baseline year is more recent and should not have reflected a large drop in demand. In contrast, our numbers for LPNs and NAs are greater.

For RN FTEs demanded, the FCN count of total demand was around 1,500 less than the HRSA count. There were differences by setting as well. RN FTEs in short- and long-term hospitals, home health, public health, and educational settings were lower in the FCN data, whereas the numbers in nursing facilities, ambulatory care, occupational health, school health, and "other" were higher in the FCN data. In the hospital setting, if RN FTEs in all types of hospitals were combined, FCN numbers were lower than those of HRSA by approximately 26,000.

For LPN FTEs, FCN estimates of total demand were nearly double that of HRSA. Demand was higher in all settings in the FCN data. For NA FTEs, FCN total demand was also nearly double that of HRSA, with demand higher in all settings.

Supply-side comparisons between FCN and HRSA data are reviewed in Table 4.4. The total RN population in the FCN baseline data is 13,390 less than the RN population in HRSA's baseline. However, the differences vary with education and age group. HRSA counts over 25,000 *more* RNs in the diploma/associate degree (AD) category than FCN, around

Table 4.3

BASELINE COMPARISONS OF EMPLOYED FLORIDA NURSE FTEs: HRSA VERSUS FCN NUMBERS

	HRSA DEFAULT (1996) FL	FCN (2004)
RNs		
Short-term hospitals (outpatient)	2,710	1,839
Short-term hospitals (inpatient)	45,569	30,929
Short-term hospitals (emergency)	5,323	3,612
Long-term hospitals	11,400	2,586
Nursing facilities	7,139	12,395
Ambulatory care	8,502	13,824
Home health	12,692	8,051
Occupational health care	654	993
School health care	1,018	5,909
Public health	5,775	5,284
Nursing education	1,749	867
Other health care	4,737	19,334
Total	**107,268**	**105,630**
LPNs		
Short-term hospitals	7,570	10,545
Long-term hospitals	574	800
Nursing homes	11,993	16,706
Home health	3,424	4,770
Other	11,794	16,429
Total	**24,555**	**49,250**
Nursing assistants		
Short-term hospitals	11,075	26,638
Long-term hospitals	1,794	3,460
Nursing homes	29,315	56,533
Home health	28,099	27,300
Other	9,294	31,200
Total	**79,577**	**145,130**

10,000 *less* in the bachelor's degree (BSN) category, and around 1,500 *less* in the "master's +" category.

Age counts vary the most in the ages 43–45, 48, and 62. The most important age differences are in the 65-year-old group. HRSA numbers are very large for 65-year-olds in comparison with FCN numbers. The difference between FCN and HRSA data in the 65-year-old bracket is 10,815, which accounts for all but 2,575 of the 13,390 overall differences in RN population.

Table 4.4

BASELINE COMPARISONS OF FLORIDA RN POPULATIONS: HRSA VERSUS FCN

AGE	HRSA (2000) DIPLOMA/ADN	FCN (2004) DIPLOMA/ADN	HRSA (2000) BSN	FCN (2004) BSN	HRSA (2000) MASTERS +	FCN (2004) MASTERS +	HRSA (2000) TOTAL	FCN (2004) TOTAL
22	0	140	0	140	0	0	0	280
23	296	323	813	323	0	0	1,109	645
24	323	377	810	453	53	0	1,186	830
25	470	420	837	630	88	0	1,396	1,050
26	505	442	874	589	88	147	1,467	1,178
27	544	699	794	629	70	210	1,409	1,537
28	460	715	971	1,021	35	0	1,466	1,736
29	904	624	1,134	1,382	123	45	2,162	2,050
30	1,198	724	1,387	1,058	195	613	2,780	2,395
31	1,401	931	1,103	1,372	248	441	2,752	2,744
32	1,158	716	1,108	1,829	160	477	2,426	3,021
33	1,510	1,096	1,182	1,461	53	417	2,745	2,974
34	1,817	1,312	1,292	1,274	53	375	3,162	2,961
35	1,925	1,095	1,313	1,729	195	231	3,433	3,055
36	1,683	1,360	1,070	1,410	299	403	3,051	3,173
37	2,078	1,673	1,219	1,619	490	216	3,788	3,507
38	2,553	1,632	1,230	1,695	402	753	4,185	4,080
39	2,835	1,913	1,515	1,971	351	290	4,702	4,173
40	2,818	2,234	1,597	1,596	213	365	4,628	4,194
41	3,102	1,971	1,563	1,757	443	600	5,108	4,328
42	2,938	2,151	1,698	1,861	674	698	5,310	4,710
43	3,135	2,808	1,840	1,809	869	286	5,844	4,902
44	3,477	2,441	1,651	2,062	787	589	5,915	5,092
45	4,236	2,743	1,845	2,286	688	457	6,769	5,486
46	4,084	2,946	1,765	1,878	452	854	6,302	5,678
47	3,876	3,095	1,627	1,835	368	792	5,871	5,722
48	3,587	3,388	1,045	1,838	342	685	4,974	5,911
49	3,373	2,988	820	1,559	576	1,007	4,769	5,553
50	2,983	2,700	934	1,908	596	734	4,512	5,341
51	2,640	2,889	898	1,642	652	456	4,190	4,988
52	2,677	2,407	607	1,376	628	661	3,912	4,444
53	2,566	2,373	455	1,625	652	438	3,673	4,436
54	2,478	2,300	392	1,348	621	555	3,491	4,204
55	2,462	2,569	601	1,297	559	467	3,622	4,333
56	2,217	2,629	852	704	452	435	3,521	3,768
57	2,164	1,848	768	666	431	400	3,363	2,914
58	1,839	1,937	568	768	250	314	2,657	3,019
59	1,852	1,885	302	671	231	362	2,385	2,918
60	1,966	1,780	290	770	173	266	2,429	2,816
61	1,837	1,382	262	635	267	243	2,366	2,259
62	2,164	1,412	309	511	320	122	2,793	2,045
63	1,884	1,250	471	383	214	182	2,569	1,815
64	1,591	1,143	771	343	0	229	2,362	1,715
65	9,438	771	1,915	534	945	178	12,297	1,482
Total	99,042	74,229	44,502	54,245	15,307	16,988	158,852	145,462

Total difference = 13,390

FCN and HRSA data also differ throughout all age groups for BSN RNs. Aside from the 22-year-old age group, the HRSA data show greater numbers of young RNs, whereas FCN data show greater number of older RNs.

A curiosity with both the FCN and HRSA supply data is the low numbers for 22- to 24-year-olds. These numbers are significantly lower than those for the 25-year-old bracket, even for RNs graduating from the three-year (diploma) and two-year (AD) educational programs. Within this similarity, FCN differs from HRSA in that FCN counts more diploma and AD RNs and fewer BSN RNs. FCN counts no master's-level RNs in the 22- to 25-year-old age bracket.

An important difference between HRSA and FCN baseline numbers for the RN NSM is in the distribution of new RN graduates and education upgrades. FCN counts 751 fewer new graduates at the diploma/AD level and 173 fewer new graduates at the BSN level than does HRSA. On the other hand, the FCN number for educational upgrades from diploma/AD to BSN is higher by 2,487, and the number for upgrades from BSN to master's or higher is greater by 1,775. Table 4.5 reviews these results.

Table 4.5

BASELINE COMPARISONS OF FLORIDA RN NEW GRADUATES AND EDUCATIONAL UPGRADES: HRSA VERSUS FCN VALUES

NSM WORKSHEET: VARIABLE SUPPLY	HRSA (2000)	FCN (2004)	FCN DIFFERENCE
Base year number of new RN graduates at diploma or ADN level	2,760	2,009	−751
Base year number of new RN graduates at BSN level	881	708	−173
Base year number of RNs upgradings from diploma or ADN to baccalaureate level	549	3,036	+2,487
Base year number of RNs upgrading from baccalaureate to master's or higher level	419	2,194	+1,775

Why Do We See Baseline Data Differences?

The differences between HRSA and FCN baseline values in both models could be due to a number of factors. On one hand, in some cases the FCN data could be more accurate. In some of the supply areas, especially those involving the actual numbers of RN licensees supplied by the Florida BON, this could be true. However, much of the time the number of Florida licensees obtained from the BON was manipulated with other data sets, such as the 2004 FCN License Renewal Survey, a data set that had a low response rate. The data resulting from these manipulations were therefore not necessarily more valid than the HRSA data.

A questionable area for the HRSA data is the high RN population in the 65-year-old bracket. It is possible that the 65-year-old age group was large because the data included all RNs 65 *and older,* although this is not stated in the HRSA manuals. The FCN numbers did not include RNs older than 65. Even so, the numbers appear high. Are there really 12,297 nurses age 65 and older who maintain their RN license in Florida? Further data analysis with Florida data will investigate this further. Finally, is it valid to include RNs older than 65 in the RN population just because they maintain an active license? The RN population should represent the pool from which RN participants can be drawn. Is it realistic to include nurses at a retirement age?

One problem area for both the HRSA and FCN data is the low RN population in the young age groups for diploma/AD and BSN RNs. We checked the validity of these numbers by using data from the Florida BON and the University of Central Florida (UCF) School of Nursing (2004). The Florida BON reports that there were 34 associate degree and 19 BSN degree nursing programs in the state of Florida in 2004 (Florida Board of Nursing, 2004). Fifty-two students ages 22–24 graduated in 2004 from the UCF nonaccelerated BSN program alone. Seventeen of these were age 22. Roughly, then, the number of 22-year-olds graduating from Florida BSN programs should be in the 100s. For some of the 22-year-olds graduating from the BSN programs, there may be a lag between graduation and licensing that puts them at 23 years of age upon licensing. That may explain why the number in the 23-year-old bracket is high, but it does not explain why the number is 0 for 22-year-olds. The number graduating from AD programs at age 22 or younger should be even higher, given that these programs are shorter and graduate roughly 60% of the RN graduates.

We note the following problems affecting the validity of our data:

- We frequently lacked direct data, so the numbers often were a result of multiple data sources and involved several manipulations of that data.
  - There were 10 different data sources used throughout the two models
  - Example: The numbers for RN FTE employment in public health, occupational health, and nurse education were a result of three data sets and four successive manipulations.
- The accuracy of the original data was questionable.
  - The Florida Center for Nursing License Renewal Survey did not always provide accurate estimates because the number of nurses responding to the survey was low (see Table 4.2). This, compounded by the specificity of the input data demanded by the HRSA models, resulted in very low response rates in some workforce regions.
- Missing data within a given data source forced estimation of some values or the use of HRSA default data.
  - This relates to the example of the FCN License Renewal Survey data noted previously. When very specific data were needed, such as the number of RNs by age, by education, and by workforce region, some cells had no data, requiring extrapolation of the survey data or the use of HRSA default data at the state level.
- We were often forced to use generalizing assumptions.
  - For example, data were not available for health care utilization rates by age, by gender, or by rural or urban setting in six health care settings by workforce region. In order to use the HRSA default data, we assumed that health care utilization rates in Florida by these demographics were close to those at the national level.
- We often had to use state- or national-level data for the Florida workforce regions.
  - For example, data were not available for health care utilization rates by age, sex, or gender at the state or workforce-region level, so national rates from the HRSA default data were used.
- The ARF data did not compare well to other data sources such as the Florida BON Licensure database and the NCLEX-RN

National Council of State Boards of Nursing. After these significant discrepancies were realized, the ARF was used only for portions of the Exogenous Variables table in the NDM.
■ Migration is particularly difficult to track.
   ■ Nurses may hold licensure in more than one state.
   ■ New entries are captured by licensure, whereas exits are not realized until the licensure expires within the state.

In sum, in some cases, discrepancies between HRSA default baseline values and FCN baseline values raised concerns regarding the accuracy of the HRSA default data; in other cases, concerns were raised with the accuracy of the FCN data; and finally, in some cases, it could have been that neither baseline was accurate. On the side of FCN baseline values, inadequate access to accurate, specific data is an enormous problem that impedes accurate forecasting. In the future, as the FCN collects increasingly valid supply data (such as through a full licensee survey with an adequate response rate), we will be better able to compare FCN's baseline supply data with default HRSA data.

Further Testing: Running the Models

After the NSM was set up with the replacement Florida data, the model was run by clicking the "calculate" button on the main menu screen. On the screen offering a choice of years, we entered the years 2004–2020. Once calculations were finished, a report of the RN population was generated. In the future, other forecasts can be reported, such as the number of RNs participating in the nursing workforce or the number of participating RN FTEs, among other reports. Our initial runs have been unsuccessful in producing credible forecasts. We obtained negative numbers for RNs 42 and older in the diploma/AD educational category and occasional negative numbers in age categories greater than 50 in other educational categories. We will troubleshoot this problem in the months to come. Steps to investigate the problem are as follows:

■ Make sure the data were replaced correctly.
■ Contact other state workforce centers working with the models.
■ Contact the Lewin Group representative if unable to correct the problem.

SUMMARY OF FCN EXPERIENCES: LESSONS LEARNED IN USING THE HRSA MODELS FOR FORECASTING IN FLORIDA AND RECOMMENDATIONS FOR OTHER STATES

The FCN experience of using the HRSA models to forecast supply and demand of RNs in Florida workforce regions has been a challenging journey that is not yet complete. Yet we have already learned many important lessons regarding data issues and operation of the models that we can share with others. Many states are similar to Florida in that there are few data sources related to nursing supply and demand, especially at the regional level. The HRSA models require very specific data, making complete data substitution difficult for state-level analysis, let alone sub-state analysis. At the sub-state level, forecasters can be guaranteed that many of the data fields will not be replaced with actual sub-state data but will instead be estimates of state or national numbers or trends. Therefore, our first recommendation is to begin forecasting with state-level analysis. If state-level data are obtained and replaced in the models, and models are successfully run at the state level, forecasters may then attempt the sub-state forecasts if so desired.

In our experience we found that keys to obtaining data include cooperation and collaboration among public and private agencies within the state, as well as funding and support to conduct large surveys of the RN population. Because RN licensure information is so critical, the cooperation and support of the state board of nursing is especially important. A survey of RNs that is completed with licensure renewal information or that is funded for a large sampling of the RN population is important for obtaining more detailed information about RN demographics, educational levels, employment settings, and other data used in both models. Employer surveys of non-hospital settings regarding the number of RN, LPN, and NA FTEs they employ are also needed, at least in the long run.

Another reason to avoid sub-state forecasting initially is the complicated method of loading data into the models at the sub-state level. In forecasting at the sub-state level, all of the data elements in all of the tables must be carefully replaced with the sub-state data. Aside from the difficulty of removing and replacing default tables, the chances of unintentional changes with the data substitution are high. In contrast, in state-level forecasting, only data elements for that state are changed, which can be done in editing modes rather than table replacements.

The data substitution is simpler, and the chances of problems with data substitution are lower.

In using the 2005 NDN and NSM, we found that the models are more user-friendly than prior models but that they continue to be challenging. Replacing data in tables is difficult, and user guides do not have detailed instruction. Running the models and troubleshooting are not straightforward, and user guides do not have any troubleshooting sections. That being said, it must be kept in mind that we were using the models in an unusual way—in essence, tricking them into running our workforce-region data as if they were running data for the 50 states, which was probably not the intent of the models' designers. When we contacted the staff at the Lewin Group with questions, we found them to be very accessible and helpful.

A final observation and recommendation is that it is helpful to share experiences with other states engaged in forecasting. Exchange of experiences and information from other state centers using the HRSA models helps with questions regarding data procurement and replacement and operation of the models. It has been beneficial for the FCN to have communication with the North Carolina Center for Nursing and others engaged in forecasting the nurse workforce.

Several state nursing workforce agencies are attempting to use the HRSA NDM and NSM models to forecast nursing supply and demand in their states. New Jersey, Iowa, Texas, Virginia, Washington, Hawaii, and North Carolina have published nurse forecasting reports using the models (Dickson, 2004; Hansen, 2004; Kishi et al., 2006; Skillman et al., 2007; LeVasseur, 2007; Nooney & Lacey, 2007). North Carolina, in particular, has successfully run the supply model and arrived at credible forecasts (Nooney & Lacey). The issues that the FCN is encountering with the HRSA NDM and NSM are similar to those being addressed by these other state workforce groups. The discrepancies are part of data problems and learning curves associated with using these complex and not-well-documented systems. Nursing workforce centers undergoing this process tend to agree that the models have improved from prior years and that support from HRSA's technical staff is good.

Supply and demand projections provide evidence to state and national policy makers that is needed to conduct workforce planning and policy. Legislators, in particular, are interested in these data so that they can provide adequate funds for state-supported schools of nursing, to ensure an adequate nurse workforce. The hope at this time is that the process will lead to more accurate knowledge of the supply and demand of nurses on which to base workforce planning. Our Florida experience leads us to encourage other states to continue on their journey or to begin one.

REFERENCES

Benham, L. (1971). The labor market for registered nurses: A three-equation model. *The Review of Economics and Statistics, 53*(3), 246–252.

Biviano, M., Tise, S., Fritz, M. S., & Spencer, W. (2004). *What is behind HRSA's projected supply, demand, and shortage of registered nurses?* Report prepared for the National Center for Health Workforce Analysis, Bureau of Health Professions, Health Resources and Services by the Lewin Group: Falls Church, VA. Retrieved November 5, 2007, from ftp://ftp.hrsa.gov/bhpr/workforce/behindshortage.pdf

Dall, T. M., & the Lewin Group. (2004a). *The nursing demand model: Development and baseline projections.* Report prepared for the National Center for Health Workforce Analysis, Bureau of Health Professions, Health Resources and Services Administration by the Lewin Group: Falls Church, VA. (Available with demand model CD. Contact the Lewin Group at http://www.lewin.com/Spotlights/WorkforceMgmt/NurseWorkforce.htm)

Dall, T. M., & the Lewin Group. (2004b). *The nursing demand model user guide.* Manual prepared for the National Center for Health Workforce Analysis, Bureau of Health Professions, Health Resources and Services Administration by the Lewin Group: Falls Church, VA. (Available with demand model CD. Contact the Lewin Group at http://www.lewin.com/Spotlights/WorkforceMgmt/NurseWorkforce.htm)

Dall, T. M., & the Lewin Group. (2004c). *Nursing supply model: Technical report and user guide.* Report prepared for the National Center for Health Workforce Analysis, Bureau of Health Professions, Health Resources and Services Administration. Falls Church, VA: Bureau of Health Professions. (Available with supply model CD. Contact the Lewin Group at http://www.lewin.com/Spotlights/WorkforceMgmt/NurseWorkforce.htm)

Deane, R. T., & Yett, D. E. (1979). Nurse market policy simulations using an econometric model. In R. M. Scheffler (Ed.), *Research in health economics* (Vol. 1, pp. 255–300). Greenwich, CT: JAI Press.

Dickson, G. L. (2004). *Issue brief: Projections of supply and demand of registered nurses in New Jersey, review of "What is behind HRSA's projected supply, demand, and shortage of registered nurses?"* Retrieved October 17, 2007, from http://njccn.org/pdf/HRSA_NJ_Review.pdf

Dumpe, M. L., Herman, J., & Young, S. W. (1998). Forecasting the nursing workforce in a dynamic health care market. *Nursing Economics, 16*(4), 170–179, 188.

Florida Board of Nursing. (2006, September 30). *NCLEX Pass Rates 2003.* Retrieved November 5, 2007, from http://www.doh.state.fl.us/mqa/nursing/NCLEX-Results_fl-nat.pdf.

Hall, T. L., & Mejia, A. (Eds.). (1978). *Health manpower planning: Principles, methods, issues.* Geneva, Switzerland: World Health Organization.

Hansen, M. M. (2004). *Issue brief: Registered nurse supply, demand and shortage projections in Iowa.* Des Moines: Iowa Department of Health, Center for Workforce Planning.

Heckman, J. J. (1993, May). What has been learned about labor supply in the past twenty years? *The American Economic Review, 83*(2), 116–121.

Kishi, A., Douglas, N., Gunn, B., Ponder, A., & Menon, R. (2006). *The supply and demand for registered nurses and nurse graduates in Texas: Report to the Texas legislature.* Austin: Texas Center for Nursing Workforce Studies.

Lacey, L. M., Nooney, J. G., & Cleary, B. L. (2006). *The next nursing shortage in North Carolina: Causes, projections and solutions.* Raleigh: North Carolina Center for Nursing.

LeVasseur, S. A. (2007, January). Projected registered nurse workforce in Hawai'i 2005–2020. Report for the Hawaii State Center for Nursing. Retrieved September 15, 2007, from http://www.hinursing.org/rp_rn_workforce.htm

Markham, B., & Birch, S. (1997). Back to the future: A framework for estimating healthcare human resource requirements. *Canadian Journal of Nursing Administration, 10,* 6–23.

Nooney, J. G., & Lacey, L. M. (2007, October). Validating HRSA's nurse supply and demand models: A state-level perspective. *Nursing Economics, 25*(5), 270–278.

O'Brien-Pallas, L., Baumann, A., Donner, G., Murphy, G. T., Lochhaas-Gerlach, J., & Luba, M. (2001). Forecasting models for human resources in health care. *Journal of Advanced Nursing, 33*(1), 120–129.

Prescott, P. A. (1991). Forecasting requirements for health care personnel. *Nursing Economics, 9*(1), 18–24.

Salsberg, E. (2003). Making sense of the system: How states can use health workforce policies to increase access and improve quality of care. New York: Milbank Memorial Fund and Reforming States Group. Retrieved June 26, 2007, from http://www.milbank.org/reports/2003salsberg/2003salsberg.html

State Council of Higher Education in Virginia. (2004). *Condition of nursing and nursing education in the commonwealth.* Richmond: Author. Retrieved November 1, 2007, from http://healthresearch.gmu.edu/ConditionOfNursingReport-Jan2004.pdf

Skillman, S. M., Andrilla, C. H. A., & Hart, L. G. (2007). *Washington state registered nurse supply and demand projections: 2006–2025.* Seattle: Washington Center for Nursing.

U.S. Census Bureau. (2004). *U.S. interim projections by age, sex, race, and Hispanic origin.* Retrieved November 5, 2007, from http://www.census.gov/ipc/www/usinterimproj

U.S. Department of Health and Human Services. (2000). *The registered nurse population: Findings from the national sample survey of registered nurses.* Washington, DC: Author. Retrieved November 5, 2007, from http://bhpr.hrsa.gov/healthworkforce/reports/nursing/samplesurvey00/default.htm

U.S. Department of Health and Human Services. (2002). *Projected supply, demand and shortages of registered nurses, 2000–2020.* Washington, DC: Author. Retrieved November 5, 2007, from http://www.ahcancal.org/research_data/staffing/Documents/Registered_Nurse_Supply_Demand.pdf

University of Central Florida School of Nursing. (2004). *Graduating class of 2004 basic BSN by birth year.* Orlando: Author. [Excel® file transmitted to Dr. Lynn Unruh from the School of Nursing.]

5

Missing Data Effects on Nurse Workforce Analysis and Projections

JENNIFER G. NOONEY

Missing data are an everyday problem for the researcher. They are encountered when analyzing data collected by someone else—a respondent did not answer the item on income, and a convenient placeholder (typically a "dot" or period) appears in the electronic data file you received. Missing data are even more obvious during analysis of data you collect yourself—you painfully record who responded and who did not, and you begrudgingly place your own dot in the electronic data file when you find that a respondent left an item blank. Luckily, the modern researcher has a number of options for dealing with missing data that were all but unavailable to researchers in the past. With the advanced data-processing capabilities offered by today's computers and statistical software, the modern researcher can accomplish in seconds the necessary computations that previously would have taken weeks to do by hand.

These capabilities also mean, however, that the modern researcher is increasingly obliged to consider missing data in cases where it might have been acceptable to ignore in the past. Studies of missing data effects on statistical models and resulting interpretations have revealed how damaging it can be to ignore the phenomenon (Horton & Kleinman, 2007; Penn, 2007; Pigott, 2001). For the nurse workforce researcher, missing data can bias conclusions about characteristics of the workforce, the number of licensed nurses working in nursing, the number of nurses demanded by employers, and forecasts of nurse labor supply and demand. These inaccuracies may yield inappropriate policy and funding recommendations. Clearly, missing data are of more than academic concern for the nurse workforce researcher—they may be of critical importance to workforce planning efforts.

This chapter provides a crash course on missing data for the nurse workforce researcher. The techniques described here can be used in any quantitative or survey research study, but the examples underscore the benefits to nurse workforce research of correcting for missing data. I begin by describing sources of missing data and their implications for research findings. I then describe how researchers can assess the impact of missing data in a particular study. Finally, I review correction strategies and discuss their pros and cons.

Throughout the chapter, I provide examples from a study of North Carolina nurse employers conducted in 2005. The survey was conducted by the North Carolina Center for Nursing (NCCN), and it included all hospitals, long-term care facilities, home health agencies, and public health departments in the state. The study's purpose was to understand the current and future nurse workforce needs of the state's employers, as well as their difficulty in recruiting nursing personnel and adverse experiences related to the nursing shortage. My examples use data from the hospital portion of the survey. For more detail on the study design and response rates for all industry groups, see NCCN (2005a). Employment projections for other industry groups—after correction for missing data—can be found in NCCN (2005b).

SOURCES AND CAUSES OF MISSING DATA

There are two possible sources of missing data in research. The first we might call "the missing record." In survey research, this is called *survey nonresponse,* and it occurs when a sample member—whether an individual or a facility—fails to return a questionnaire. Other types of data, including data collected for administrative or regulatory purposes, can also suffer from missing records. In survey research, the omission is usually a known quantity because the researcher typically knows how many questionnaires are expected (the sample size) and how many are returned. In work with administrative or regulatory databases, the missing record is often an unknown. It may be a facility whose operating license, for whatever reason, is absent from the database of regulated health care facilities. The fact of an omission and its content are unknown both to the researcher and to the regulatory body maintaining the database. Because there is little that can be done to assess or correct for unknown missing records, this chapter focuses on known missingness that is common when a researcher fields a survey and analyzes the resulting data.

The second source of missing data occurs when a record identifying a sample member is present in the data file, but the record is incomplete in some way. We might call this "the missing item." In survey research, this occurs when a respondent skips over an item of interest while completing a questionnaire. Again, other types of data may also suffer from item missingness. For example, a facility record from a database of licensed health care facilities might be missing information on the number of licensed beds if someone entering the data inadvertently skipped over the field or if the facility did not provide updated information to the regulatory agency as scheduled. In either case, the fact of missing data is a known commodity, and corrections for the omission might be possible.

In many survey research projects, both types of missing data are present. Combined, they can present the researcher with a serious obstacle. Suppose you are interested in computing nursing staff turnover rates for hospitals in your state. You survey each of the 100 hospitals in your state, but only 50 respond to your survey. Further, suppose that only 30 of the respondents provide the data elements you need to compute a turnover rate. You will report that you achieved a 50% response rate for your survey of hospitals, but for the purpose of understanding nursing staff turnover, you effectively have a 30% response rate.

To understand the consequences of missing data, it is important to understand what might cause each type to occur. There is one case in which the amount of missing data has little bearing on the accuracy of your results, and that is when the responses of the people who *did not* respond to your survey or to a specific item are, in the aggregate, no different from the people who *did* respond. That is, your data are missing more or less randomly. Suppose the average nursing staff turnover rate is identical within hospitals that did and did not provide data for your survey. You could compute an average turnover rate for the responders and confidently apply that to the entire sample selected for participation in your survey. Unfortunately, it is not possible to know precisely how different the nonresponders are if they do not respond.[1] And there is very good reason to suspect that there *are* important differences. Survey respondents skip items or fail to return surveys for reasons, and those reasons are often linked with the responses they would have provided.

Take, for example, the case of missing staff turnover rates in a nurse employer survey. A hospital chief nursing officer, noticing how prominent the items related to turnover are on the questionnaire, considers her nursing turnover rates to be unacceptably high. She is not confident that the information she provides will be kept confidential, and she is concerned that her hospital may be subject to bad publicity as a result of survey participation. She decides to throw away the survey, and as a result, the researcher's results are biased downward, toward the lower turnover rates reported by remaining hospitals. Another chief nursing officer at a small hospital completes the survey but fails to answer the items on turnover because his hospital's staffing records are insufficient. He judges his turnover rates to be admirable, but because they are not included in the study, the researcher's results are biased toward higher turnover rates.

There are some usual suspects among the reasons for missing data that apply to survey research on any topic. Interested readers can find a very thorough description of motivations for response (or nonresponse) in Dillman (2007).

1 Respondent burden. If your survey or item requires too much effort from the respondent, some sample members will refuse the survey or skip the item. This problem is not likely to plague opinion pollsters to the same degree it does the nurse workforce researcher. Employer surveys, in particular, often require respondents to consult records for staffing information. If the information is not easily accessible, which may be likely in very small facilities using less complex record-keeping systems, the probability of nonresponse increases.

2 Lack of necessary information. If your respondent does not know or cannot obtain the answer to your question, the item will be skipped. If the respondent cannot answer most of the items on your questionnaire, he or she is likely to discard the questionnaire entirely. In employer surveys, facility size is again a consideration given that more complex organizations tend to keep more sophisticated records.

3 Sensitivity. If your survey or item solicits sensitive information that respondents consider proprietary, you may not get a response. This is particularly likely when the honest response is embarrassing to the respondent.

4   Relevance to the respondent. When the subject of a survey or an item is interesting to respondents, or when it addresses an issue of importance to them, they are more likely to respond. Conversely, the probability of nonresponse increases if a survey is boring or irrelevant to respondents.

5   Design factors. Survey researchers must not overlook the visual and other ancillary elements of the survey research process. When too many questions are squeezed into a small space, for example, the effect is a questionnaire that looks busy and daunting. The cover letter accompanying the questionnaire is also an important element of the survey because it is typically used to convey the importance of the study and other information that may encourage response.

If the researcher can identify the likely cause of missing data, the appropriate corrections may be more obvious. Although most data sets—and indeed single items—contain missing data for multiple reasons, researchers can often use information that they *do* have to learn more about missing data and ultimately adjust for it.

ANALYZING AND CLASSIFYING MISSINGNESS: THE BIAS ANALYSIS

A bias analysis can be used to understand how your respondents and nonrespondents differ. Ultimately, the purpose of a bias analysis is to gain knowledge of how biased your data may be as a result of survey nonresponse. Of course, in order to do any analysis including nonresponders, you need at least a little information about them. The good news is that you probably *do* know something useful about your nonresponding nurse employers. If you have sent out a mail survey, somewhere in your electronic records you have the mailing address of every facility in your sample. If you know the zip code of a facility, you have access to a wealth of geographic information that may help you understand how nonresponders differ.

A number of software packages can transform zip codes into other, more meaningful bits of information. For example, ZipList5 CBSA (available for purchase from http://www.zipinfo.com) can convert zip codes to metropolitan statistical areas and Federal Information Processing Standards (FIPS) codes. For researchers who use SAS statistical software, free zip code data sets can be downloaded from http://support. sas.com. These data sets can be merged by zip code into the file containing address information for each facility you surveyed. In the process, information on county, FIPS codes, metropolitan statistical areas, and geographic coordinates is attached to each facility's record.

FIPS codes uniquely identify U.S. counties, so they enable users to link survey records to county-level data. For the health services researcher, one important county-level data set is the Area Resource File (ARF). It contains many variables describing the health of a county's population as well as the prevalence of health professionals and levels of health care utilization. Your state demographer or other data-driven agencies in the state may have additional county-level information useful for understanding the context in which your sample members live and work.

Finally, the regulatory agency that licenses health care facilities in your state may have other publicly available information on the facilities in your sample. In North Carolina, the Division of Facility Services (DFS) publishes the number of licensed beds at each hospital and long-term care facility in the state. Though not a perfect measure of facility size, the number of beds is a good proxy for the volume of services provided and is strongly related to the size of the nursing staff a facility employs.

Once you have assembled a data set containing records with all information you can get on your nonrespondents, plus the information provided by those who responded to the survey, you are ready to analyze differences. A cross-tabulation of response status (responded = 1; did not respond = 0) by facility attributes such as size and location is a good place to start. In our survey of North Carolina nurse employers, we analyzed response status by facility size, region of the state, metropolitan (or rural) status, and the Health Professional Shortage Area (HPSA) status of the county in which the facility was located.

We sent 125 surveys to acute-care general hospitals in North Carolina, and 84 were returned, for a response rate of 67.2%. As Table 5.1 shows, however, the probability of responding to the survey was not random with respect to hospital size. Little more than half of small hospitals responded (55.9%), whereas nearly 90% of large hospitals responded (87.8%). No other facility or geographic variables were strongly associated with response status. Clearly, hospital size is a factor we needed to consider when correcting for missing data.[2]

A look back at the factors contributing to survey nonresponse helps to make sense of our findings with regard to response status and hospital

Table 5.1

HOSPITAL SIZE AND RESPONSE STATUS				
RESPONSE STATUS	**ALL HOSPITALS**	**SMALL HOSPITALS (LESS THAN 100 BEDS)**	**MEDIUM HOSPITALS (100–199 BEDS)**	**LARGE HOSPITALS (200 OR MORE BEDS)**
Responded	84 67.2%	19 55.9%	29 60.4%	36 87.8%
Did not respond	41 32.8%	15 44.1%	19 39.6%	5 12.2%
Totals	125 100.0%	34 100.0%	48 100.0%	41 100.0%

size. We know, for example, that respondent burden and lack of information needed to complete the questionnaire are prominent reasons for survey nonresponse. Larger hospitals may have more thorough record-keeping systems and a larger human resources staff to update them. As a result, it may be easier for chief nursing officers at large hospitals to pull up the staffing information necessary to complete our survey. Does survey nonresponse among smaller hospitals lead to bias? Not necessarily. If the smaller hospitals would have provided information similar to that provided by larger hospitals, our results are not biased by their lower probability of response. But we will never know for sure because the nonresponding hospitals did not complete surveys. However, we *can* see if there are differences between the small and large hospitals that *did* respond to the survey, and we can use this difference as a kind of proxy for bias resulting from nonresponse.

We analyzed vacancy rates, turnover rates, and projected growth in employment over the next 2 years (demand expectations) by hospital size in order to determine whether any differences exist that provide clues regarding response bias. We found that among small, medium, and large hospitals, vacancy and turnover rates were very similar. We inferred from this that our report of average rates across the responding hospitals is not biased with respect to hospital size. However, we did find a difference in the number of full-time equivalent (FTE) RN positions the hospitals planned to add over the next 2 years. Small hospitals, on average, expected to grow their staff sizes by about 3 RN

FTEs. Large hospitals, in contract, expected to grow by an average of 19 FTEs.

Employment projections are an important reason for conducting an employer survey. When aggregated across all hospitals in our study, the expectations of growth tell us how many new nursing positions will be created in North Carolina hospitals. However, because only 67.2% of hospitals responded to the survey, our total count of new positions based on respondents likely underestimated substantially the number of new nurses North Carolina hospitals would demand over the next 2 years. We clearly needed to address this missing data in order to provide more accurate projections. The first question we needed to answer, given the need for some correction, is what *type* of missing data we had.

Statisticians classify "ignorable" missing data as missing completely at random (MCAR) or missing at random (MAR) (Allison, 2002). The selection of a strategy for dealing with missing data often depends on assumptions a researcher makes regarding the causes and correlates of missing data. MCAR means that none of the variables in your analysis (which may be one or more, depending on the analytic model used) have missingness that is related to the values of the variables. Another, less precise way of putting it is to say nonrespondents would have provided answers similar to the ones provided by respondents—in this case, the mean of the variable for nonrespondents would equal the mean of the variable for respondents. MCAR means that this condition is satisfied for all variables to be included in a given model or analysis. Note that this is a very strong assumption that is not likely to be true very often. As noted previously, there are usually reasons for missingness related to the value a respondent would have provided for a variable.

MAR, on the other hand, is much less strict. It means that missingness is not related to a variable's value *after* the researcher has controlled for other variables in the analysis. Suppose a researcher wanted to estimate a regression model that predicted a nurse's income, but nearly 20% of cases in her data set were missing data on income. Suppose further that those respondents whose income information was missing were much older than those who provided the information, a common finding related to suspicion about sharing this information among older individuals. If the researcher includes age in her regression model, and if age is the only thing explaining missingness, the researcher has data that are MAR for this regression analysis. Although not as strict as MCAR, MAR is also hard to satisfy from a conceptual standpoint. It seems unlikely, for example, that age is the only thing that explains missingness on income.

Luckily, many strategies for dealing with missing data are considered robust to violations of the MAR assumption (Allison, 2002), which means they tolerate some unexplainable missingness if at least a portion of it can be explained by variables in the analysis.

If missing data do not meet either of these assumptions, they are said to be "nonignorable." In this case, the missing data mechanism must be modeled explicitly for results of an analysis to be unbiased. This type of modeling is beyond the scope of the present chapter. Here, we review some traditional and more recent methods for dealing with missing data that are MCAR or MAR and ignorable.

TRADITIONAL METHODS FOR DEALING WITH MISSING DATA

Listwise or Casewise Deletion

The closest thing to actually ignoring the ignorable MCAR or MAR data is to exclude cases with missing data on the variables in your analysis. This is called listwise or casewise deletion because it involves excluding records (observations) from your analysis if they contain missing data on any of the variables in your analysis. Most statistical software programs use listwise deletion by default. When estimating a regression model, for example, most programs use only those cases with complete data.

One problem to consider with this method is the number of cases that remain for analysis after listwise deletion. Suppose you begin an analysis with a random sample of 1,000 nurses in your state, and your goal is to estimate a regression model to predict the income of those nurses. If 20% (200) cases are missing data on income, 20% of the remaining cases are missing data on age (160), another 15% are missing data on setting of employment (96), and another 10% are missing data on education (54), you would only use 490 cases in your regression model—less than *half* of the full sample. Although your data set will hopefully contain more complete cases than this, the example illustrates the cumulative effect of missing data in a multivariate analysis.

Listwise deletion has become less popular as more sophisticated methods have become easier to implement, but as Allison (2002) points out, there *are* cases where listwise deletion may still be the best strategy for dealing with missing data. If your data are MCAR, your results after listwise deletion will be unbiased (though your standard errors will be larger and statistical significance harder to find given a smaller sample size). If your data are MAR, but you have no missing data on your dependent variable, your regression analyses will be unbiased; missing data on the independent variables will operate like a stratified sample, but the relationship to your dependent variable is unchanged.

When nurse workforce research is directed toward legislators and other stakeholders with little knowledge of statistics, it is more typical to present univariate and bivariate (rather than multivariate) analyses in reports. In particular, legislators may desire a count of some sort, such as the number of new nurses that will be needed over the next 2 years. Stakeholders may want averages or other measures of a variable's central tendency, such as the mean vacancy rate or the median turnover rate of nursing personnel within the state's health care facilities.

When data are missing in univariate analyses, the problems (and solutions) are similar to those encountered in multivariate analyses, at least where averages are concerned. Take, for example, the case of vacancy rates within North Carolina hospitals. Our bias analysis demonstrated that these rates are uncorrelated with facility size, region of the state, metropolitan status, or HPSA. In addition, nonrespondents are similar to respondents on each of these characteristics with the exception of facility size. Because facility size is unrelated to vacancy rates among respondents, we may conclude that our measured vacancy rates are likely to represent all hospitals fairly well. In effect, we think that vacancy rates are MCAR. We might report the average vacancy rate for respondents and generalize that to all hospitals with confidence. However, if we had found that vacancy rates were much higher in larger hospitals, our data would be MAR because we *could* control for hospital size. If we used listwise deletion and reported the average for responding hospitals only, our average would be biased toward the higher vacancy rates reported by the overrepresented large hospitals.

If you are interested in counts, however, missing data must be considered whether your data are MCAR or not. Say we are interested in the number of new RN positions that North Carolina hospitals will budget. If we simply sum up the number of new positions reported by our responding hospitals, we will underestimate the true number of new positions because some hospitals did not respond, and others did not provide information on that variable. Clearly, listwise deletion is inappropriate in this case even if your data on staff expansions are missing completely at random.

Simple Mean Imputation and Conditional Mean Imputation

An alternative to deleting cases with missing data is to assign or impute a value for missing variables in those cases. An imputation is essentially a guess about what value might be reasonable for a given case. To make this guess, a researcher can use one or more variables that are not missing for that case. Note that each of the imputation strategies covered in this section involves *single* imputations. In other words, the researcher assigns one (and only one) value for a variable to each case.

The most commonly used imputation, and the easiest to implement, is the simple mean (or marginal mean) imputation. The researcher simply imputes the mean of a variable among all respondents to each of the nonrespondents. In this case, the guess is that nonrespondents are similar to the average respondent on the variable. If there is little response bias associated with your variable, this sort of guess is not unreasonable. For example, if we found no difference in the number of new positions to be created between responding small and large hospitals over the next 2 years, it would make sense to assume that nonresponding small and large hospitals are also similar on this variable. The downside, if we expect no response bias, is that we will be assigning the very same value to each of the nonresponding cases. This will reduce the variation in your variable because many cases will be clustered directly at the mean, making the statistical properties of the variable less desirable.

If you do find evidence of response bias, as we did between small and large hospitals on this variable, imputing the mean for the full sample can seriously bias your results. We found that small hospitals were much less likely to respond to our survey, and the small hospitals that responded were adding fewer new positions than large hospitals. If we assigned the mean for the full sample (10.5 new RN FTEs over 2 years), we would probably overestimate the true number of new FTEs we could expect in North Carolina hospitals over the next 2 years. We have not yet used enough information to make a reasonable guess for each case.

We can use more information with conditional mean imputation. In this strategy, the value we impute for a given case will vary depending on the characteristics of the case. In the simplest form of conditional mean imputation, we would use a single variable to provide direction on the value to impute for each case. If we know, for example, that large hospitals expect to add a larger number of new positions, we might impute the mean of responding large hospitals for nonresponding large hospitals. Similarly, we would impute the means for responding medium and small hospitals to medium and small nonresponding hospitals, respectively. This is a definite improvement over simple mean imputation, but even still, we are imputing only three different values across all cases missing data on this variable—our variance is reduced.

An extension of using a single variable, of course, is to use more than one variable. This multivariate imputation strategy may take a number of forms, but one commonly used technique for imputing continuous variables—those measured at the interval/ratio level and containing many discrete values across all cases—is the ordinary least squares regression model. These models are fairly easy to implement with most statistical packages, and their results are easily transformed into predictions to make imputations for missing data. Using our example of growth in staff size, we might choose to use information on hospital size, metropolitan status, region of the state, and HPSA status to predict growth. The equation would be as follows: RNgrowth = intercept + B_1size + B_2metro + B_3region + B_4HPSA + e, where B_1, B_2, B_3, and B_4 indicate slope coefficients for each variable, and e indicates residual error unexplained by the model. When this equation is estimated by your statistical software, you will have values for the intercept and slope coefficients that can be used to predict growth for your nonrespondents.

The second step in this process is to ask your statistical software to do the predictions. If you are using a package that is code-based or can be used in code-based form (such as SAS, SPSS, or STATA), the commands will be some variant of the following:

1   If RNgrowth is missing, then assign the value using the equation below:
2   RNgrowth = –6.16 + 0.11*size + 0.03*metro + 0.24*region + 0.10*HPSA

The values used in equation 2 would be drawn directly from your estimates using complete cases. The equation would assign new values to your incomplete cases using the existing data you have for those cases on the other variables.

Using more information is usually better, and the regression-based conditional imputation described here gives the analyst a great deal of control over the imputation. The analyst can select as many variables as are necessary to adequately describe the things that influence, or create, RN demand in hospitals. The variable combinations used also mean that a larger number of values are imputed across the missing cases. The value changes with each possible combination of the independent variable values in your equation. One caveat is that regression equations may be specified incorrectly such that your efficiency in predicting the dependent variable actually declines as you add independent variables. You can use model fit statistics, such as the R-squared statistic and statistical significance of parameter estimates, to judge the adequacy of your model. The biggest weakness of this method is that it takes more time to implement than the other methods, and it requires proficiency in multivariate analysis.

RECENT DEVELOPMENTS IN MISSING DATA TECHNIQUES

Although it is beyond the scope of this chapter to describe more complex methods in great detail, nurse workforce researchers should be aware of some of the latest developments for dealing with missing data and resources they can use to learn more about them.

Maximum likelihood estimation has been used for some time to estimate regression models with nonlinear dependent variables. It is the preferred method for estimating logistic regression models, where the dependent variable is binary. The general idea of maximum likelihood (ML) is fairly intuitive: the goal of the process is to reproduce with as much precision as possible the actual value of a dependent variable given information on each of the independent variables. A researcher has data, for example, on each dependent and independent variable for each complete case, and he or she can estimate a series of coefficients that predict some dependent variable using the independent variables of choice. The question is, if those coefficients are used to predict the value of a dependent variable for each case, how close do the predictions come to the actual value of the dependent variable for each case?

ML essentially maximizes the fit of the coefficients so that the dependent variable can be predicted with the most accuracy. To accomplish this, ML uses an iterative procedure—essentially trial and error—until the coefficients it is trying are the best possible coefficients. When additional iterations yield no further improvements in the coefficients, the process stops, and the researcher has the best possible coefficients. The computational power needed to implement maximum likelihood would have been prohibitive decades ago, but modern computing power and updated statistical software packages make this a plausible solution for model estimation. Statisticians have also discovered that ML is excellent at handling missing data in many cases. For a review of ML approaches to missing data, see Vach (1994), McLachlan and Krishnan (1997), and Little and Rubin (2002).

A second development in approaches to missingness is *multiple imputation*. Compared with the single imputation approaches reviewed in the previous section, multiple imputation (MI) recognizes the uncertainty associated with a single imputed value for each case. Instead of imputing a single value, the process creates multiple complete case data sets with different imputed values. In analysis, the multiply imputed data sets are combined so that a single estimate can be generated. Researchers using SAS can easily accomplish MI using two procedures: PROC MI (to create the data sets) and PROC MIANALYZE (to combine and analyze the data sets). See the SAS online documentation at http://support.sas.com/onlinedoc/913/docMainpage.jsp for more details.

Imputation Results From the NC Nurse Employer Survey Using Multiple Methods

Figure 5.1 compares the projected growth in RN FTEs over a 2-year period in North Carolina hospitals using no imputation and four different imputation methods. Note that in this case, the worst possible projection is one in which missing data are ignored. Responding hospitals planned to grow their RN staffs by 1,013.4 FTEs, but this estimate ignores the growth that is likely to occur in nonresponding hospitals and those that did not answer the items on projected growth.

If simple mean imputation is used—assigning the average amount of growth to all cases missing data on that variable—the projected growth increases to 1,664.4 FTEs. As noted earlier, this may overestimate growth given that small hospitals were less likely to respond to the survey and tended to project a smaller number of new RN positions. When hospital size is taken into account, the growth drops to 1,508.6 FTEs, as expected. However, when our projections take into account other information we had about nonresponding hospitals, such as their metropolitan status, region of the state, and HPSA (using multiple regression), the estimate is back up to 1,668.6 FTEs. And finally, when multiple imputation is accomplished, the number of FTEs stands in the middle at 1,625.1 FTEs.

Which of these imputation results is most accurate? This is an impossible question to answer because we do not know how much

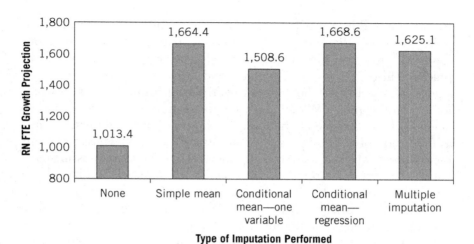

Figure 5.1 Projected RN FTE growth in NC hospitals, 2004–2006

nonresponding hospitals will grow. It is reasonable to assume, however, that they *will* grow. Each of the imputation procedures is within 160 FTEs of all others, which is a reasonable range of estimates for workforce planning purposes. In our judgment, given the uncertainty associated with imputation, the most reasonable reporting approach was to provide the range of estimates and average them for a point estimate: 1,600.8 new RN FTEs over a 2-year period.

CONCLUSIONS

The techniques discussed in this chapter will vary in their appropriateness for a given analytic problem. There is no "magic bullet" for missing data problems. Fortunately, there are many bullets, and the modern researcher typically has access to all of them. The point of this chapter has not been to advocate for a specific technique but rather to arm the nurse workforce researcher with an array of techniques appropriate for different situations. What should be emphasized, however, is that the problem of missing data must be considered. It should be a routine part of the researcher's analytic work.

Most social science and medical research has real-world implications, whether for public policy or for the practice of health professions. Because of this, missing data and their effects on the conclusions researchers draw from their studies are not simply statistical problems—they can create policy problems. Biased research results may yield inappropriate solutions for social problems, incomplete knowledge of drug side effects or poor practices in the provision of medical and nursing care. In the research study discussed here, the concern over biased results relates to workforce planning policy. Without an accurate projection of nurse workforce needs, policies designed to increase the supply of licensed nurses—such as expansion of nursing program capacity or loan forgiveness programs for nursing students—may come up short. Had we ignored missing data, our assessment of future workforce needs in hospitals would have been several hundred RN FTEs fewer than what will likely be needed.

Researchers should begin the process of correcting for missing data by thinking through the potential policy implications of bias for the research question under consideration. A second step is to consider what types of bias are most likely, given the research question and knowledge of the sample members' motivations to respond or refuse participation in the study. Once these conceptual considerations have been made, the appropriate course of action will be much clearer. Although approaches to missing data are statistical in nature, the real-world causes and implications of missing data are what drive the choice of an approach.

NOTES

1. It is important to note that tests of statistical significance do not account for survey or item nonresponse. They merely describe the probability that a randomly selected sample accurately describes a population.
2. Throughout this chapter, statistical significance is ignored because the study being described is a census (a study of the entire population) rather than a random sample survey.

REFERENCES

Allison, P. D. (2002). *Missing data.* Thousand Oaks, CA: Sage.

Dillman, D. A. (2007). *Mail and Internet surveys: The tailored design method* (2nd ed.). Hoboken, NJ: Wiley.

Horton, N. J., & Kleinman, K. P. (2007). Much ado about nothing: A comparison of missing data methods and software to fit incomplete data regression models. *The American Statistician, 61*(1), 79–90.

Little, R. J., & Rubin. D. B. (2002). *Statistical analysis with missing data* (2nd ed.). Hoboken, NJ: Wiley.

McLachlan, G. J., & Krishnan, T. (1997). *The EM algorithm and extensions.* New York: Wiley.

North Carolina Center for Nursing (NCCN). (2005a). *Nurse employer survey 2004: Study design and methods.* Raleigh, NC: Author. Retrieved September 18, 2007, from http://www.ga.unc.edu/NCCN//research/empsurv2004/study%20methods.pdf

North Carolina Center for Nursing (NCCN). (2005b). *Evidence of increasing demand for nursing personnel in North Carolina.* Raleigh, NC: Author. Retrieved September 18, 2007, from http://www.ga.unc.edu/NCCN/research/empsurv2004/demand% 20expect%20statewide.pdf

Penn, D. A. (2007). Estimating missing values from the General Social Survey: An application of multiple imputation. *Social Science Quarterly, 88*(2), 573–584.

Pigott, T. D. (2001). A review of methods for missing data. *Educational Research and Evaluation, 7*(4), 353–383.

Vach, W. (1994). *Logistic regression with missing values in the covariates.* New York: Springer-Verlag.

SECTION II. TOWARD EVIDENCE-BASED POLICY: LESSONS LEARNED

Linda Flynn

Researchers rely on data as the bases for analyses and interpretation that provide the foundation for their findings. In our context of the research to policy-connection, their findings are the evidence needed to construct policy recommendations and create a policy agenda that demands attention by policymakers.

Methods used to supply the data are multiple and encompass both quantitative and qualitative methods. In this section, seasoned nurse researchers have shared their experiences, tips, skills, and humor regarding the design and implementation of rigorous, policy-influencing research. They covered the use of focus groups, primary data collected by surveys, secondary data analysis, and how to address a problem that plagues most researchers—missing data. Each section in this book closes with the lessons learned, so follow along to see what we think are some lessons learned from these experienced researchers.

LESSON 1. CAREFULLY DEVELOP YOUR RESEARCH QUESTIONS

In chapter 3, we learned from Patricia Moulton that the first step in this important process is to clarify what is it that you want to know. Has this question already been explored? If so, what measures and methods were used, and have study results been published? Are findings from previous studies applicable to the current context, target population, and time period? In short, a thorough review of the literature either may prevent you from reinventing the wheel or may guide you in the design of a relevant and timely study.

LESSON 2. FOCUS GROUPS ARE HELPFUL RESOURCES

Moulton suggests that focus groups, conducted with representatives of your target sample, may also be helpful in framing and refining your research question. Second, and most important, focus groups can also be useful in constructing survey items or measures for key study variables.

121

We also learned that focus groups could be a useful technique for clarifying the results of a survey, when evidence seems to be contradictory. These are important lessons learned about the use of qualitative methods.

LESSON 3. HOW TO DEVELOP SURVEY QUESTIONS

We also learned that surveys are a particularly useful approach to collecting data that have the potential to influence organizational, professional, or public policy. Regarding the development of survey questions, Linda M. Lacey shared her valuable tips for the proper construction of nonambiguous survey items, cautioning against the use of jargon and double-barreled questions—questions that combine two choices or two questions into one. She guided us through the process of designing response categories that make sense to the respondent and that are both comprehensive and exclusive, making every possible response available to the respondent without the possibility of overlap. We learned that we might inadvertently introduce bias into participants' responses by using words such as "agree" or "disagree" in the construction of scale items, and we learned about the need to ground respondents in time and place by developing items in ways that create a shared reference point.

LESSON 4. HOW TO FIELD A SURVEY

Once the survey instrument has been designed, the researcher needs to ensure that the survey packet reaches its intended recipients and that they complete and return the survey instrument. A comprehensive process developed by Donald Dillman (2000, 2006) provides a step-by-step guide to fielding your survey and obtaining a high response rate. Consequently, I described in chapter 3 how I used Dillman methodology in a survey of more than 44,000 registered nurses to obtain a 50% response rate. I highlighted strategies that are essential to success, as well as pitfalls to avoid.

LESSON 5. THE DEVIL IS IN THE DETAILS

Likewise, two expert survey researchers, Christine Tassone Kovner and Carol S. Brewer, shared their recent experiences in fielding a large, multistate survey. They discussed the lessons learned as they encountered issues with state files, incorrect addresses, missing zip codes, and the use of incentives, to name a few. Importantly, their experience teaches us to expect that, despite careful planning, things will go wrong; the key to success, however, is to problem solve and persevere—remembering that details are important.

LESSON 6. SECONDARY DATABASES CAN BE CHALLENGING AND REWARDING

In addition to the collection of primary data, secondary analyses of existing data files can be another important approach to providing policy-influencing evidence. Because legislators respond to numbers, the forecasts of nurse demand and supply have been very effective in focusing policy makers' attention on the escalating nurse shortage. In chapter 4, Lynn Unruh and Valerie Danesh provided an excellent and comprehensive tutorial on how to use national models to forecast state-level nurse supply and demand.

We learned that although promising, this process is challenging because state-level data required in forecasting models are not always readily available. The nonexistence of state-level data is a challenge, and there are areas where one might need to use the national default data. However, all states have some data, and that data can be more accurate than the national forecasts using the default data as a template. Although completing the analyses was somewhat time-consuming and challenging, the authors concluded that it was worth the effort and encouraged others to try it. Using examples from the models' handbooks, their carefully delineated process will make the task doable—a helpful lesson.

LESSON 7. METHODS FOR DEALING WITH MISSING DATA

Regardless of whether you are analyzing primary data that you have collected or are conducting secondary analyses of existing data files, every researcher must deal with the problem of missing data. In chapter 5, Jennifer Nooney provided a crash course on techniques for handling missing data, using real-life examples from a study of nurse employers in North Carolina. She explained how some missing data, if ignored, could potentially bias findings and result in the inadvertent presentation of misleading information to policy makers. The use of simple mean imputation, conditional mean imputation (both univariate and multivariate), and multiple imputation are reviewed and compared.

In summary, the proper collection and management of data is essential to producing trustworthy findings with the potential to inform policy decisions. Yet whether you are conducting focus groups, developing questions, fielding surveys, mining records from state and federal agencies, or imputing missing data, collecting and managing data will always be a challenge. In the research enterprise, as in most areas of life, anything that can go wrong probably will go wrong. Learning from the experiences of a variety of researchers, we can conclude that the successful researcher (a) commits to the ongoing refinement of his or her skills and knowledge, (b) develops contingency plans, (c) seeks expert advice when needed, and last, but certainly not least, (d) perseveres in the face of obstacles.

Research and Workplace Policy

INTRODUCTION

Geri L. Dickson

Many studies have identified the workplace of nurses as an area in great need of change through evidence-based policies. These chapters continue the theme of the book, *Nursing Policy Research: Turning Evidence-Based Research Into Health Policy,* by investigating the impact of the workplace on the nurse shortage. This is the beginning of exploring nurse work-related studies and of the dialogue about how nurses and research may begin to shape evidence-based policies.

Cyclic nurse shortages have been the norm since nursing education changed from a model in which care was given by student nurses around the clock in hospitals to one in which learning and reflective practice became the focus of education. At the same time, the nation's hospital infrastructure grew, and allopathic medicine became the standard of medical care, thereby increasing the demand for nurses.

The current shortage, although of major concern in hospitals where 56% of RNs are employed, is also problematic in nonhospital settings. As the current prospective system of payment for health care emerged, for economic reasons the length of stay was decreased for patients. As the length of hospital stay decreased, the increased acuity of patients required more intensive nurse care, whether in the hospital or in the community.

The increased demand for nurses' care continues to grow, just as the nurse workforce is on the cusp of massive retirements in the baby boom generation. Complicating an already complex problem is the much smaller potential pool of health care workers available to fill the void between the supply and demand of workers as the baby boomers leave the workforce. Further, policies focused on retaining experienced nurses in the health care workforce are an essential strategy toward reducing the projected shortage and providing mentors for the novice nurses.

The severity of the current and projected nurse shortages requires serious thought to develop research-based strategies for retaining experienced nurses in the workforce, while at the same time looking at the efficiencies of the work of nurses. The development of research-based retention policies, designed to create a productive and healthy workplace for nurses and their patients, are crucial to the overall health of the health care system.

In the first chapter of this section, Brewer and Kovner present the results of their research relating factors in the work environment to the work satisfaction of acute care nurses. In the following chapter, Flynn outlines the variables, such as quality of care, that play a major role in the job satisfaction of home care nurses. The research by Erickson in chapter 8 then addresses the emotional toll experienced by practicing nurses in today's health care environment. Presenting her findings using both words and numbers, Erickson supplements the numbers with stories of nurses, a good method to catch the attention of policy makers.

A moving example of policy change in the hospital environment, this time by newly empowered direct-care nurses, can be found in a project funded by the Robert Wood Johnson Foundation. For information about the program, Transforming Care at the Bedside, please see chapter 14. The research in these chapters and their exemplars of policy recommendations can serve as a stimulus for more research to delineate a process of using research to foster workplace policy change at the organizational, professional, and public policy levels.

6

Work Satisfaction Among Staff Nurses in Acute Care Hospitals

CAROL S. BREWER AND CHRISTINE TASSONE KOVNER

With reports of registered nurse (RN) shortages continuing, information about RNs' work satisfaction is crucial to an understanding of its impact on RN turnover. The federal government's 2004 National Sample Survey of Registered Nurses (NSSRN) (Steiger, Bausch, Johnson, & Peterson, 2006) is the most recent study commonly used to describe working RNs. Unfortunately, that survey is conducted only every 4 years and does not include detailed questions, particularly about work attitudes and RNs' work life. Other studies that include such detailed questions are limited to individual hospitals or groups of hospitals.

Getting a grasp on what staff RNs find satisfying about their jobs could provide information about how to change the work environment in ways that would improve staff RNs' work life and reduce turnover. Job satisfaction is an important issue to RNs and managers, in part because of their relationship with organizational commitment and RN turnover

This manuscript was supported in part by the Agency for Healthcare Research and Quality, Grant R01HS01132002, and the Robert Wood Johnson Foundation. The authors of this manuscript are responsible for its contents. No statement in this manuscript should be construed as an official position of the Agency for Healthcare Research and Quality or the Robert Wood Johnson Foundation.

We would like to acknowledge the assistance of Kellie Hoerter, MA, for her skills in data analysis and editorial support throughout this project, and Ying Cheng, MA, for her coordination of the analysis with that of the larger national RN R01 study.

(Francis-Felsen et al., 1996; Gurney, Mueller, & Price, 1997; Ingersoll, Olsan, Drew-Cates, DeVinney, & Davies, 2002; Lake, 1998; Larrabee et al., 2003; Prevosto, 2001; Shader, Broome, Broome, West, & Nash, 2001). Although the relationships among RN satisfaction, organizational commitment, and intent to leave have been the subjects of study (Lum, Kervin, Clark, Reid, & Sirola, 1998; Tett & Meyer, 1993), it is clear that satisfaction is a major precursor to turnover and also holds promise for employers as a way to affect the outcomes of RNs' work decisions.

This study of the predictors of RN staff nurse satisfaction is based on the theoretical model proposed by Price (2001) that suggests precursors of satisfaction include the following: (a) work attitudes, such as kinship responsibility, job involvement, positive/negative affectivity, autonomy, distributive justice, job stress, pay, promotional chances, variety, and social support; and (b) perceived job opportunities for employment elsewhere. Additionally, we included (c) personal demographic characteristics, such as education and gender; (d) relevant work characteristics, such as setting, shift, and injuries; and (e) variables suggested to be important by other research, such as family and work conflict (Frone, 2003).

Last, we concluded that it was important to control for job market indicators across Metropolitan Statistical Areas (MSAs) in order to isolate the influence on job satisfaction of work attitudes, perceived job opportunities, demographic variables, and work characteristics. These job market indicators, such as RN-to-population ratio, unemployment rate, and size of the MSA, have been found in previous research (Brewer et al., 2006) to create movement constraints on RNs not considered by Price in his original model. Consequently, they may have an indirect impact on RN job satisfaction through their effects on nurse supply or demand.

The purpose of this study is to test the Price model, which proposes that a variety of attitudes as well as perceived job opportunities are related to work satisfaction. The Price model is well tested; thus, we are particularly interested in the additional contribution of local job market conditions to RN satisfaction.

SAMPLE

The sample included 553 staff RNs who work in inpatient settings in hospitals in a random sample of MSAs in the United States. More than 1.36 million RNs worked in hospitals (including clinics and other parts of hospitals) in the United States in 2004. Of these hospital-based nurses, about 1,211,632 were staff RNs. A total of 80% of all RNs were working in MSAs (Brewer et al., 2006; Steiger et al., 2006). This analysis is part of a larger study examining the work participation of a national sample of RNs who work in MSAs. The sample design was a cross-sectional, two-stage sample with RNs nested in MSAs. The sample for this analysis was a random subsample of the one recruited by the Center for Studying Health System Change (2000) for their Community Tracking Study (CTS). The final sample in the current analysis included RNs from 29 states (AL, AR, AZ, CA, CO, CT, FL, GA, IL, IN, KY, LA, MA, MD, MI, MO, NC, NJ, NV, NY, OH, OK, PA, SC, TN, TX, VA, WA, and WV) and the District of Columbia.

We delimited the list of licensed RNs in each state to those RNs who lived in the subsample of MSAs that were randomly chosen for inclusion from the 51 MSAs stratified by size and randomly chosen for the Health System Change Study. From this sampling frame we then randomly selected RNs from each MSA to receive a mailed survey. The number of RNs randomly selected from each MSA was in proportion to the MSA's total population. In all, a total of 4,000 RNs were selected to receive a survey. A total of 1,907 survey recipients returned a completed survey, for a response rate of 48%. From those 1,907 respondents we chose for inclusion in this current study all RNs who noted that they worked in inpatient hospital settings and indicated that their position was staff nurse or nurse clinician. Nurses employed in these positions were included based on the assumption that they provided direct patient care. Thus, the final analytic sample consisted of the 553 RNs who indicated they were employed in a hospital as a staff nurse or nurse clinician. Response rates from the different MSAs varied from a low of 30% from Phoenix, Arizona, to a high of 51% from Greensboro/Winston-Salem, North Carolina.

METHODS

Data were collected using a 12-page mailed survey with up to six subsequent follow-up mailings. In addition, a follow-up phone call was made to nonresponders for whom telephone numbers were available, urging them to complete the mailed survey.

We obtained information about four groups of variables as follows: (a) work attitudes and settings (e.g., staffing levels, shift work, autonomy); (b) demographic (e.g., age, race); (c) movement constraints, including the RNs' perceptions of job opportunities in both the local geographic area and other geographic areas; and (d) county-level variables that indicate characteristics of the job market (e.g., unemployment rate, hospital beds per 1,000 population).

The nurse variables were measured with reliable scales that were used in previous research. For example, work attitudes and job opportunity were measured with scales used in previous research (Carlson & Frone, 2003; Gurney, 1990; Price, 2001, Quinn & Staines, 1979; Spector & Jex, 1998). Satisfaction was measured using the five-item Quinn and Staines satisfaction scale, but with modified response items. Assessing validity of the instrument, Quinn and Staines reported that scores on the Facet-Free Job Satisfaction instrument significantly and negatively correlated, as expected, with role ambiguity ($r = -.22$) and positively correlated, as expected, with facet-specific job satisfaction ($r = .55$), thus supporting the validity of the instrument. On the other hand, Quinn and Staines reported that there was also a positive correlation with depressed mood at work ($r = .43$), which is opposite of what we would expect from a valid satisfaction scale. Job opportunity was measured using two scales from previous research (Price). Family and work conflict were measured using scales developed by Carlson and Frone. Work characteristics were measured using items developed by the researchers, most of which were modeled on items from the National Sample Survey (Steiger et al., 2006). All scales were Likert-type scales and varied in the number of items from 3 for work–family conflict to 10 for organizational constraint.

Reliabilities for the scales ranged from a low of .70 for variety to .95 for supervisory support. Usually, it is desirable to have an internal consistency of .80 or above. In practice, researchers may compromise and have internal consistency as low as .70. Confirmatory factor analysis was conducted on all scales by the research team as part of the larger research project. The factor structure was supported in all cases except organizational constraint. After removing one item from the scale, a one-factor solution was supported.

Statistical analysis included chi-squares, t-tests, and ordinary least squares regression. The findings are presented in the next section, including the predictors from the regression analysis.

FINDINGS

About 44% of the respondents worked part-time (PT), and 56% worked full-time (FT). We used the RNs' self-definition of PT or FT to create a dichotomous variable, and if the data were missing, we substituted a value based on the hours worked reported by the respondents. PT was defined as those who worked fewer than 35 hours per week, and FT was defined as 35 hours or more, which is the Bureau of Labor Statistics (BLS) definition (Ehrenberg & Smith, 2006).

Personal Demographic Characteristics

Most respondents were white (93.1%), non-Hispanic (84%), and married (67.5%). More of the FT than PT RNs were male. Only 6.9% of the hospital RNs providing direct care were male, and 16% were non-white. Less than 3% of hospital RNs were Hispanic, and more Hispanic hospital RNs worked PT than FT (4.6% versus 1.3%, although these numbers are small). Although 67.5% were married, an additional 17.8% had been married in the past; a higher percentage of PT RNs were married. Only 18.2% of the hospital RNs had children under age 6, and 19.7% had children ages 6 to 11 years living with them. FT RNs were more likely (87%) to have children under 6, but otherwise FT and PT RNs did not differ. The mean age was 42.6 (SD = 10.2) years and did not differ by work status.

Most of the RNs were educated in the United States (92.8%) and were quite well educated, with 41.8% having at least a baccalaureate degree as their highest degree. This proportion of baccalaureate-educated RNs is somewhat higher than the 34.2% reported in the 2004 National Sample Survey of RNs. A higher percentage of PT RNs had a baccalaureate degree as both their basic and their highest degree. Almost 8% of the RNs were enrolled in a formal education program or were nationally certified in a specialty practice area. Of those with a degree in a discipline other than nursing (37.8%), about one-third reported having a non-nursing degree related to health. They reported that religious beliefs were moderately to extremely important (83.5%).

On average, the RN respondents were experienced, although they had worked for only a limited number of employers (1.9, SD = 1.1). Having graduated on average almost 15 years (SD = 10.7) earlier, they had over 14 years of experience (.5 SD). Not surprisingly, because of the way the sample was chosen, these staff RNs had experienced approximately only one promotion in their career (SD = 1.2) and had worked for slightly less than two employers (SD = 1.1) on average.

Work Characteristics

Most RNs (96.1%) had been employed on the same date 1 year prior to responding to the survey. However, about 15% had changed their work status from the previous year, more RNs shifting from working FT to working PT than from working PT to FT. About 18.4% of the RNs held more than one position, with most (88%), but not all, of those second positions in nursing. With an average income from the primary position of a PT RN of $43,000 per year, the annual income of PT RNs was, as expected, significantly lower, yet their hourly wages were significantly higher than those of FT RNs. Not surprisingly, the partners of those RNs who worked PT also had higher yearly income than the partners of FT RNs.

In addition to salary, the RNs had a variety of non-compensation benefits, with 87.2% having medical insurance, although only 21.1% used it; 87.3% reported retirement benefits, but only 8.6% used them. Benefits varied by PT and FT work status, with PT RNs generally having and using fewer benefits. Almost 84% of the RNs reported that benefits were somewhat or very important. The mean number of benefits was also significantly higher for FT RNs (7.1 versus 5.8).

The average scheduled work hours per year for respondents employed in FT principal nursing positions, including paid vacations, holidays, and sick leave, were estimated to be 2,047 hours; for PT workers it was 1,254 hours. A comparison of the number of scheduled hours and actual hours showed that 65.1% of FT RNs actually worked the hours scheduled to work, but about 32.6% of them worked more hours than they were scheduled. Only 13.2% of RNs worked a regular 8-hour day shift. Ten- to 12-hour shifts were reported to be the norm by 50.2% of PT RNs and 68.8% of FT RNs; 27.3% of RNs worked the night shift. More PT (15.6%) than FT (9.6%) RNs worked flexible or rotating shifts. Clearly, many of the RNs were unhappy with the number of hours they worked: 30.3% reported that they preferred to work fewer hours next year.

The RN respondents worked in a variety of units providing direct patient care. Almost a quarter of all RNs worked in intensive care units, and almost a third worked in general or specialty care units. In addition to working in a variety of units, 11.8% had transferred to another work unit within the organization in the previous 12 months, and 35.2% of all RNs had experienced a change in supervisors. Of those who had not moved, 29.9% had still experienced a change in supervisors.

Injuries were commonplace for hospital RNs, but no differences were found according to FT or PT status. Just over 30% reported at least one needlestick injury in the last year, and over 57% reported at least one strain or sprain. In addition, 32.3% reported one or more cuts or lacerations, and 63.4% reported bruises or contusions. Only a few reported injuries such as broken bones or head injuries. In contrasting those with injuries and their overall health, we found that 57.2% of those who had never had a strain or sprain reported excellent health, whereas only 18.1% of those with multiple strains or sprains felt they had excellent health. Interestingly, neither FT/PT work status nor work schedule was significantly related to injuries.

Work Attitudes

More than 34% of RNs viewed their jobs as a career, whereas only 29% of the RNs said their spouses viewed the spouses' jobs as a career. Although the majority of RNs intended to continue working, stay in the same type of position, and remain at their current organization in the next year, 23.1% planned to leave their organization, 22% planned to leave their position, and 30% preferred to work fewer hours in the near future. About 13% of RNs expected it unlikely to be working for the same organization in 12 months.

Surprisingly, there were few differences between FT and PT RNs in their perceptions of their working conditions, and there were few differences in work attitudes between FT and PT RNs. The only exception was that FT RNs thought there were higher levels of organizational constraint and quantitative workloads than PT RNs. The hospital staff RNs in this sample were slightly less satisfied than the sample of RNs who worked in all types of settings (Brewer et al., 2006). Hospital staff RNs viewed themselves as quite autonomous, with the mean at almost 4 (SD = .65) on a scale ranging from 0 to 5, and reported a high degree of work group cohesion, as indicated by a mean of 3.78 (SD = .84), also measured on a scale ranging from 0 to 5. On the other hand, they viewed themselves as having a high quantitative workload, as indicated by a mean of 4.23 (SD = 1.01) on a scale of 1 to 6.

We conceptualized work/family conflict as two variables; work interferes with family (work–family), and family interferes with work (family–work) (Frone, 2003). Family–work and work–family conflict did not vary by FT and PT status. RNs reported low family–work conflict and moderate work–family conflict.

Perceived Job Opportunities

FT and PT RNs perceived the same local and nonlocal job opportunities (how easy it was to find a job locally or nonlocally). Job opportunities

were influenced by the market factors discussed in the following para-
graphs.

Objective Job Market Indicators

In addition to their immediate employment settings, the RNs worked
in communities that had different influences on the supply and demand
for nurses. Although the mean unemployment rate of the MSA populations was 5.6% (SD = 1.0), more than 68% worked in MSAs where
the unemployment rate was 1% above or below that rate. The RN-to-
population rate, size of MSA, index of competition, and percentage of
HMO Medicare patients also varied between PT and FT RNs, as did
the RNs' perception of the job opportunities, both within the immediate
geographic area and outside the area.

Analyses of Relationships Among Variables

Understanding the relationship of these various demographics, working
attitudes, job opportunities, and market indicators to satisfaction is key
to improving RN retention rates in hospitals. To identify which variables
were associated with work satisfaction, we conducted an ordinary least
squares regression in which we entered the variables in groups, based
on a model of work participation and satisfaction developed by Brewer
et al. (2006), which was derived from Price's (2001) earlier work. In this
model, satisfaction is standardized. We entered the variables from those
that were least changeable (e.g., age) to those that were most changeable
(e.g., autonomy at work). We entered them in the following order: personal demographics, job market indicators, job opportunity, and workplace characteristics and attitudes.

Results in Table 6.1 show the relationships between the predictor variables and job satisfaction. The model explained 51% of the variance in job
satisfaction. Most of the variance in the model was explained by working
conditions, although the RNs' health, race, and whether he or she attended
a nursing program in the United States were also related to satisfaction.
Black RNs were less satisfied in comparison with white RNs. Those RNs
with good health, in comparison with those with very good health, were
less satisfied. RNs educated outside of the United States were also less
satisfied than those educated within the United States. Those RNs who
considered themselves more career-oriented than other nurses were more
satisfied than those who considered themselves about average in their

Table 6.1

PREDICTORS OF JOB SATISFACTION

PREDICTORS' LABEL (REFERENCE)	UNSTANDARDIZED COEFFICIENTS B	P VALUE
Health (very good)		
Poor or fair	−.193	.050
Good	−.137	
Excellent	−.008	
Race (White)		
Black	−.296	.037
Asian	−.183	
Other	−.016	
Basic nursing program in United States (Yes)		
No	−.346	.012
Compared to other people, extent view job as a career (Same as others)		
Less than others	−.172	.008
More than others	−.170	
Distributive justice	.148	.000
Word group cohesion	.101	.022
Work–family conflict	−.059	.024
Organizational constraint scale	−.198	.000
Quantitative workload inventory	−.086	.019
Supervisory support	.090	.011

Note: R^2 = .51, Adjusted R^2 = .431. Nonsignificant variables not shown in table: highest degree related to nursing, enrolled in a formal education program, national certification, religious beliefs, gender, number of children who live with you, years experience in nursing, partner's yearly income, age, primary care practitioners per 1,000 population, paid through fee schedule, inpatient days ratio/pop, index of competition, RNs/per 1,000 population, more than one position for pay, work schedule, transferred to another unit within the organization, change in the past 12 months of supervisor, ethnicity, compared to other people's views of job as a career, needlestick injury, strains benefits, paid time off, medical insurance, retirement, tuition reimbursement, income from principal position, number of benefits, autonomy, family–work conflict, mentor support, promotional opportunities, variety, work motivation.

career orientation. In all, demographic variables explained 9% of the variance in satisfaction. None of the income, benefits, or market-level characteristics were significantly related to satisfaction, nor were the movement constraints.

More than 37.8% of the variance in satisfaction was explained by the various work attitude scales. Distributive justice, group cohesion, and supervisor support were positively related to satisfaction, and work/family conflict, organizational constraint, and quantitative workload were negatively associated with satisfaction.

In terms of compensation, contrary to findings from some other studies (Gurney et al., 1997; Ingersoll et al., 2002), wages and benefits were not associated with satisfaction. However, distributive justice, which asks about the fairness of pay, was negatively related to satisfaction. The day shift and shift length were not related to satisfaction. The quantitative workload of RNs was negatively related to satisfaction. Thus, RNs who said that they had high workloads were less satisfied than those who said that they had low workloads. RNs can get support at work through three groups: peers, mentors, and supervisors. In this study, work group cohesion and supervisory support were significant predictors of job satisfaction.

Conflicts between work and family have been reported as related to work satisfaction. When work interfered with family, RN work satisfaction was lower. When family interfered with work, however, there was no relationship to work satisfaction.

DISCUSSION

In this study, we examined a nationally representative sample of hospital staff RNs in MSAs. Our sample was demographically comparable to the sample of working hospital RNs from the 2004 NSSRN survey (Steiger et al., 2006): respectively, male (7.0% vs. 5.8%), white (84.0% vs. 86.7%), and married RNs (67.5% vs. 70.5%). The mean age in our sample (M = 42.6) was somewhat less than the mean age of RNs in the National Sample Survey who were working in the hospital (M = 46.8) (Steiger et al., 2006). The educational preparation of our sample was 14.2% diploma, 42.1% associate's degree, and 43.6% baccalaureate or higher, whereas Steiger et al. (2004) reported educational preparation to be 25.2% diploma, 42.4% associate's degree, and 31.0% baccalaureate or higher degree.

As predicted by Price (2001) in relation to turnover models, demographic variables have little explanatory power (about 9%) when work attitude variables are included. In addition, the MSA level variables were not significant, suggesting that indeed they do not directly impact satisfaction but rather may impact the likelihood of working in comparison with not working. Consequently, they may be shown to be important in predicting intent to work and turnover (Brewer et al., 2006). It is also possible, although we have not as yet tested this hypothesis, that MSA level variables directly affect *perceived* job opportunity, which contributed 2.4% of the variance of satisfaction in this study. Because this is the first major national study to include such variables, the exact relationships are still under consideration in our large sample.

There are some disturbing trends in terms of RNs' work intentions, in that RNs were more likely to decrease their work participation (FT to PT) from the previous year than to increase it from PT to FT. Moreover, if working FT, many wanted to work fewer hours. Given the number of RNs working overtime, and the indicated work–family conflict, this is not surprising. Univariate analysis showed that benefits were much more important to FT than PT RNs, and PT RNs clearly did not have as many benefits. Benefits, however, did not affect satisfaction in the multivariate analysis, so RNs may be choosing their level of work participation knowledgeably. An interesting finding is that 32.6% of RNs work more than they were scheduled. This may be because of mandatory or voluntary overtime or on-call hours.

A quite striking descriptive finding is that of the reported change or discontinuity among nurses' supervisors. Although there has been much written about the need for RNs to have support from mentors (Prevosto, 2001), this was not related to satisfaction. Kirpal (2004) discusses the increasingly important role for entrepreneurial employees of work groups and professional allegiance rather than organizational allegiance (commitment) in retention. If RNs with good work group cohesion and support are more satisfied, it follows that they may be more committed and less likely to leave. Given the importance of various kinds of support in retention, the frequent change of supervisor could be destructive to the organizational bonds that employers would like to develop with their staff. There is no indication from these data whether the changes experienced by the RNs are voluntary or involuntary, or whether the change is perceived as positive or negative. A longitudinal study would be needed to explore these questions.

Injuries were very common yet had no impact on satisfaction. It may be that injuries directly impact intentions to leave or other factors rather than satisfaction. It may be that RNs accept injuries as "part of the job." Alternatively, it may be that RNs perceive that it is not the injuries themselves that are dissatisfying, but in contradistinction, the way in which they are handled by management. These perceptions, however, were not explored in the current study and remain the topic of future research.

POLICY IMPLICATIONS

The following policy recommendations are grounded in the findings of this study that provided the evidence for policies in hospitals (see Exhibit 6.1). Suggestions to employers as to ways that may have an impact on nurse satisfaction include instituting policies that relate directly to keeping nurses safe from injuries, providing competent and stable managers, and implementing fairness in salaries for nurses.

Exhibit 6.1 Key Findings

---

1. Hospital staff RNs' work satisfaction is related to their working conditions. More than 37.8% of the variance in satisfaction was explained by working conditions. Distributive justice (whether the employer rewards fairly), group cohesion, and supervisor support were positively related to satisfaction, and work/family conflict, organizational constraint, and quantitative workload were negatively associated with satisfaction. All of these factors are under the control of employers.

2. Hospital staff RNs who were educated outside of the United States are less satisfied than those educated in the United States. Slightly over 7% of the staff RNs were educated outside of the United States, and those RNs were less satisfied than RNs educated in the United States.

3. Income and benefits were not related to hospital staff RNs' work satisfaction, but the RNs reported that the benefits are important to their staying in their job. With an average income of more than $53,000 per year for full-time RNs and $43,000 for part-time RNs from their principal positions, 75% of the part-time RNs and 90% of the full-time RNs reported that having benefits is somewhat to very important to their staying in their jobs.

4. Staff nursing in hospitals is dangerous work The hospital staff RNs (31%) reported that they had had at least one needlestick injury, and 57% said they had had at least one work-related strain or sprain in the last 12 months. For the same time period, 63% reported at least one bruise or contusion, and 33% reported at least one cut or laceration. A much smaller percentage had other injuries such as fractured bones, dislocated joints, and head injuries.

5. Change in supervisors is a common experience for hospital staff RNs. Although almost 12% of hospital staff RNs transferred to another work unit within the organization in the 12 months prior to the survey, more than 35% of all staff RNs experienced a change in their immediate supervisor during that time period.

6. Hospital staff RNs work more hours than they are scheduled to work. Full-time staff RNs who on average were paid to work 2,040 hours per year (which includes sick time and vacation) worked an average of 100 hours (at least 2½ weeks) more per year than they were scheduled to work. Part-time RNs worked an average of 70 hours (almost 2 weeks) more per year than scheduled to work.

7. Hospital staff RNs plan to make changes in their choice of work. Almost all staff RNs (96.7%) planned to continue to work 12 months from when they answered the survey, but 23% planned to leave the organization in which they worked, and 28% planned to change their position. Of those who planned to leave their organization, almost 25% planned to no longer work in nursing.

Safety in the workplace has been an important policy concern since the release of the Institute of Medicine's report *Keeping Patients Safe: Transforming the Work Environment of Nurses* (2003). Our data suggest that although injuries are very common, they do not seem to be related to satisfaction. The level of injuries, however, is important for other reasons. For example, in addition to the potential impact on patient safety, nurses with injuries may be absent from work. This in turn could create a cascade of staffing issues such as the need for additional or agency staff or, alternatively, short staffing if additional staff are not available. RNs may accept injuries as part of the job, but how injuries are handled by the administration may create problems for RNs. There could be inadequate access to lifting devices or other equipment that help prevent injuries, an issue related to adequate time off for recovery, or pressure to work while injured because of the difficulty of replacing an injured staff member. The poor handling of injuries may thus be reflected in less satisfaction with management rather than issues directly related to the injuries.

The RNs reported a tremendous amount of change and discontinuity with respect to the supervisors to whom they report. Some of this change was related to the nurses moving and thus working under new managers. Yet some was clearly related to turnover among the managers themselves. This degree of change is disruptive to the RNs as well as to the management of units and may result in perceived lack of supervisor support. Overtime, workgroup cohesion, organizational constraints, and quantitative workload are also very much under the purview of management. Thus, it is not surprising that many RNs planned to make changes in their employment, with far too many planning to leave nursing altogether. Giving nurses more control over their schedules and creating systems of support that allow them to do their jobs more easily and with fewer injuries would likely result in better RN satisfaction.

Last, it should be noted that money alone is not enough to solve the nurse shortage problem. Hospital RNs in general are not dissatisfied with their pay. Money is unlikely to help satisfaction—but fairness matters, and benefits are important too. Whether any RNs can feel that they are rewarded fairly, regardless of the objective data, is an interesting conundrum in workforce research. There has been so much publicity about the nursing shortage and how underpaid RNs are that even if RN wages compared favorably to other occupations, it is possible that RNs in general would answer negatively to the fairness-in-pay issue. For example, examining salaries on www.salary.com reveals that staff RNs in

Buffalo, New York, in late 2007 earned a median income of $59,515, and with benefits these earnings ranged up to $84,554. High school teachers earn, respectively, $50,467 and $72,974, whereas engineers earn $54,932 and $79,197. If this example is at all representative, then objectively nurses are doing quite well in comparison with at least these two professions. The implication for employers is that the RNs must feel that what they earn is fair. Determining how to accomplish that could be a major challenge for health care leaders.

CONCLUSION

Understanding factors that influence RNs' satisfaction provides important evidence that points to improvements that employers can make to increase RN satisfaction. The connection between satisfaction and turnover is well established and provides opportunities to build relationships between the employer and nurse. For example, tying work rewards to work efforts in ways that are perceived as fair is more important to satisfaction than the actual pay. Likewise, a stable leadership and adequate work group cohesion and supervisory support are well within the purview of employer influence.

REFERENCES

Brewer, C. S., Kovner, C. T., Wu, Y., Greene, W., Liu, Y., & Reimers, C. W. (2006). Factors influencing female registered nurses' work behavior. *Health Services Research, 41*(3), Part 1, 860–866.

Carlson, D. S., & Frone, M. R. (2003). Relation of behavioral and psychological involvement to a new four-factor conceptualization of work-family interference. *Journal of Business and Psychology, 17*(4), 515–535.

Ehrenberg, R. G., & Smith, R. S. (2006). *Modern labor economics: Theory and public policy* (9th ed.). Boston: Pearson/Addison Wesley.

Francis-Felsen, L. C., Coward, R. T., Hogan, T. L., Duncan, R. P., Hilker, M. A., & Horne, C. (1996). Factors influencing intentions of nursing personnel to leave employment in long-term care settings. *Journal of Applied Gerontology, 15*(4), 450–470.

Frone, M. R. (2003). Work–family balance. In J. C. Quick & L. E. Tetrick (Eds.), *Handbook of occupational health psychology* (pp. 143–162). Washington, DC: American Psychological Association.

Gurney, C. A. (1990). *Determinants of intent to leave among nurses with doctoral degrees.* Urbana: University of Illinois Press.

Gurney, C. A., Mueller, C. W., & Price, J. L. (1997). Job satisfaction and organizational attachment of nurses holding doctoral degrees. *Nursing Research, 46*(3), 163–171.

Ingersoll, G. L., Olsan, T., Drew-Cates, J., DeVinney, B. C., & Davies, J. (2002). Nurses' job satisfaction, organizational commitment, and career intent. *Journal of Nursing Administration, 32*(5), 250–263.

Institute of Medicine. (2003). *Keeping patients safe: Transforming the work environment of nurses.* Washington, DC: The National Academies Press.

Kirpal, S. (2004). Work identities of nurses: Between caring and efficiency demands. *Career Development International, 9*(3), 274–304.

Lake, E. T. (1998). Advances in understanding and predicting nurse turnover. *Research in the Sociology of Health Care, 15FF,* 147–171.

Larrabee, J. H., Janney, M. A., Ostrow, C. L., Withrow, M. L., Hobbs, G. R., Jr., & Burant, C. (2003). Predicting registered nurse job satisfaction and intent to leave. *Journal of Nursing Administration, 33*(5), 271–283.

Lum, L., Kervin, J., Clark, K., Reid, F., & Sirola, W. (1998). Explaining nursing turnover intent: Job satisfaction, pay satisfaction, or organizational commitment? *Journal of Organizational Behavior, 19*(3), 305–320.

Prevosto, P. (2001). The effect of "mentored" relationships on satisfaction and intent to stay for company-grade U.S. army reserved nurses. *Military Medicine, 166*(1), 21–26.

Price, J. L. (2001). Reflections on the determinants of voluntary turnover. *International Journal of Manpower, 22*(7), 600–624.

Quinn, R. P., & Staines, G. L. (1979). *The 1977 quality of employment survey: Descriptive statistics, with comparison data from the 1969–70 and the 1972–73 surveys.* Ann Arbor: Survey Research Center, Institute for Social Research, University of Michigan.

Shader, K., Broome, M. E., Broome, C. D., West, M. E., & Nash, M. (2001). Factors influencing satisfaction and anticipated turnover for nurses in an academic medical center. *Journal of Nursing Administration, 31*(4), 210–216.

Spector, P. E., & Jex, S. M. (1998). Development of four self-report measures of job stressors and strain: Interpersonal conflict at work scale, organizational constraints scale, quantitative workload inventory, and physical symptoms inventory. *Journal of Occupational Health Psychology, 3*(4), 356–367.

Steiger, D. M., Bausch, S., Johnson, B., & Peterson, A. (2006). *The registered nurse population: Findings from the March 2004 National Sample Survey of Registered Nurses.* Research Triangle Park, NC: U.S. Department of Health and Human Services, Health Resources and Services Administration, Bureau of Health Professions.

Tett, R. P., & Meyer, J. P. (1993). Job satisfaction, organizational commitment, turnover intention, and turnover: Path analyses based on meta-analytic findings. *Personnel Psychology, 46*(2), 259–293.

7

Workload, Quality of Care, and Job Satisfaction in Home Health Nurses

LINDA FLYNN

The United States is facing a registered nurse (RN) shortage of unprecedented proportions. The U.S. Department of Health and Human Services (DHHS) estimates that by 2020 the deficit between RN demand and RN supply will be close to 1 million RN full-time equivalents (2002). Although much attention has been focused in recent years on the impact of such RN staffing deficits in acute care settings, national estimates indicate that a severe shortage of home health nurses is, likewise, on the horizon. An aging population is sparking an escalated demand for chronic or non-acute health care services. Consequently, between 2000 and 2020 the demand for home health nurses is expected to double (DHHS). Unfortunately, a national shortage of nurses makes it unlikely that the home health nurse workforce will be sufficient to meet this increased demand. Consequently, shortages of home health nurses may very well jeopardize older patients' access to those community-based nursing services that would allow them to be maintained in their homes. Therefore, it is essential to recruit and retain an adequate supply of RNs in the increasingly important home health practice sector. Toward that end, in this chapter we examine the relationships among workload, quality of care, and job satisfaction among RNs practicing in home health.

BACKGROUND AND SIGNIFICANCE

In the midst of a growing nurse shortage, reported trends indicate that home health care settings are already experiencing difficulties in recruiting and retaining home health nurses. Nationwide, the attrition rate among home health RNs is estimated at 21% with a vacancy rate of approximately 18% (United States General Accounting Office, 2001). These national estimates are consistent with reports from a variety of state nursing workforce centers, which indicate turnover rates among home health RNs currently range from 14.4% to 25.7% (Burton, Morris, & Campbell, 2005; Lacey & McNoldy, 2007; Palumbo, 2003; Smith-Stoner & Markey, 2007). Similarly, in a recent survey of Medicare-certified home health agencies in New Jersey, 62% of agencies reported that recruitment of home health RNs was more difficult than in the previous year (Flynn & Mazzella-Ebstein, 2007).

Although multiple factors may be contributing to these recruitment and retention difficulties, lack of job satisfaction among home health RNs is a problem that warrants further attention. According to the 2004 National Sample of Registered Nurses, only 79% of home health RNs indicated they were satisfied with their jobs. Conversely, 21% of home health RNs surveyed were either dissatisfied with their jobs or unsure about their job contentment. In comparison with other practice settings in the national survey, the proportion of home health RNs satisfied with their jobs was just slightly higher than RNs working in nursing homes, who were the least satisfied nurses with only 73.8% reporting satisfaction (Steiger, Bausch, Johnson, & Peterson, 2006).

Clearly, in order to enhance the recruitment and retention of home health nurses, it is important to understand those factors that significantly influence job satisfaction and turnover in this crucial practice setting. Existing theoretical models identify a plethora of variables proposed to contribute to satisfaction and retention, including salary, autonomy, staff interaction, professional status, task requirements, and organizational policies (Stamps & Piedmonte, 1986); workload, coworker relationships, educational opportunities, and professional support (Chou, Boldy, & Lee, 2002); individual factors, organizational structure factors, and economic factors (Irvine & Evans, 1995); and family/work conflict, mentor support, work variety, promotional opportunities, organizational constraint, other job opportunities, and distributive justice (Gurney, Mueller, & Price, 1997; Kovner, Brewer, Wu, Cheng, & Suzuki, 2006). Specific to home health nurses, factors proposed to influence job satisfaction directly include autonomy, group cohesion, stress, workload, salary and benefits, and other employment opportunities (Ellenbecker, 2004).

Among the variety of proposed predictors, however, nurse workload emerges as a factor that is frequently included across theoretical models as an important determinant of job satisfaction and retention (Chou et al., 2002; Ellenbecker, 2004; Kovner et al., 2006). Recent studies have quantified the impact of workload on job satisfaction in that high patient-to-nurse ratios have been associated with increased odds on job dissatisfaction in samples of hospital-based nurses (Aiken, Clarke, & Sloane, 2002; Aiken, Clarke, Sloane, Sochalski, & Silber, 2002).

Yet in proposing the essentials of organizational magnetism, McClure and Hinshaw (2002) explain that the organization's ability to support and deliver high-quality patient care is paramount to nurses' job satisfaction and the ability of the organization to recruit and retain nurses. Organizational traits such as manager support, autonomy, collaborative working relationships, and even nurse staffing levels—or workload—influence nurses' job satisfaction in large measure *because* they influence the delivery of quality patient care. Based on decades of research, the nursing organization and outcomes model (Aiken et al., 2002) likewise proposes that these supportive organizational traits enhance nursing processes of care, including care quality, and it is through the high-quality care processes that superior nurse and patient outcomes are achieved.

Therefore, it appears that the level of nurse-assessed quality of care provided within the nurse's organization is, ultimately, an important determinant of nurse job satisfaction and retention. Consequently, it seems that nurse-assessed quality of care should be explicitly included in job satisfaction and retention models. Few studies, however, have investigated the relationship between quality-care processes and job satisfaction among home health nurses. Of those that have been conducted, findings from qualitative studies indicate that agencies' dedication to the delivery of quality patient care is a highly important contributor to nurses' job satisfaction (Flynn, 2003; Flynn & Deatrick, 2003). A recent quantitative study, however, yielded contradictory results (Stone, Pastor, & Harrison, 2006). Therefore, the purpose of this study was to quantify the relationships among nurses' workload, quality-care processes, and job satisfaction in a sample of home health staff nurses. The impact of selected variables on nurses' intentions to leave their jobs was also explored.

METHOD

The sampling frame consisted of subscribers to a popular, professional journal for home health nurses. A total of 645 subscribers were selected randomly to receive a survey packet, which was mailed to their home. Of the surveys mailed, 25 were returned by the post office as undeliverable, resulting in a total of 620 delivered surveys. Of these, 325 surveys were completed and returned for a response rate of 52.4%. Among the 325 nurse respondents, 137 respondents from 38 states indicated they were employed as home health staff RNs, and they made up the sample for this analysis. Sample characteristics are presented in Table 7.1.

The study utilized a descriptive, correlational design, and the protocol was approved by the university's institutional review board prior to data collection to ensure the protection of human subjects. In accordance with a modified Dillman (2000) survey method, a reminder postcard was

Table 7.1

SAMPLE CHARACTERISTICS ($n = 137$)

VARIABLE	M	SD
Age	50.35	9.29
Years at employing agency	9.92	7.67

	N	%
Gender		
Female	134	97.80
Male	3	2.20
Race		
Caucasian	121	88.30
African American	6	4.40
Hispanic	2	1.50
Asian/Pacific Islander	4	2.90
Native American	2	1.50
Not reported	2	1.50
Nursing Education		
Diploma	17	12.40
Associate's degree	44	32.10
BSN	53	38.70
MSN or higher	22	16.10
Not reported	1	0.70

mailed 1 week after the initial survey packet was sent, a repeat survey packet was mailed to nonrespondents 2 weeks after the initial survey mailing, and a final reminder postcard was mailed to remaining nonrespondents 4 weeks after the initial survey mailing.

The survey consisted of a variety of measures related to workplace characteristics and nurse-reported patient events (Flynn, 2007b). Job satisfaction was measured by an item asking nurses to rate their job satisfaction on a 4-point scale ranging from 1 (very dissatisfied) to 4 (very satisfied). Nurses were asked to rate the overall quality of care provided by their agency using a four-4 scale ranging from 1 (poor) to 4 (excellent). As another indicator of quality care, nurses were asked to report the degree to which the "nurse dose," or frequency of nursing visits, provided to their patients was appropriate to patients' skilled nursing needs (visit adequacy). The three response categories included (1) fewer visits than necessary, (2) more visits than necessary, and (3) visits appropriate to need. As a third indicator of quality, an item asked the nurse to rate, on a scale of 1 (never) to 4 (frequently) the frequency with which patients or their families lack the preparation to manage their care at the time of discharge from home health. For measures of workload, home health nurses reported (a) the total number of patients they had scheduled to visit on their most recent full day of work, (b) the total number of patient visits they actually made during their most recent full day of work, and (c) the total number of patients in their current caseload.

FINDINGS

A total of 30% of home health nurses in the sample indicated they were dissatisfied with their job, and 26% reported they were planning to leave their job within the next 12 months. Although only 8% of nurses rated the quality of care provided by their agency as fair/poor, fewer than one-half (46.7%) rated the quality of care at their agency as excellent. A total of 11.9% of nurse respondents indicated the quality of care provided by their agency had deteriorated over the last year. Surprisingly, although 21.2% of home health staff nurses reported that their patients received fewer nursing visits than the nurse felt was necessary, no respondents indicated that patients received more visits than were necessary. A total of 14.1% reported that their patients were frequently unprepared for discharge. The mean number of patient visits that nurses reported scheduled on their most recent full day of work ranged from 1 to 15, with a mean of 5.23 (SD = 1.99). The number of patient visits actually made ranged from 1 to 10 with a mean of 5.06 (SD = 1.68). These reports of visit productivity from nurses in this sample are consistent with the mean of 5.13 patient visits per day by home health RNs nationwide, as reported by the National Association for Home Care and Hospice (2007). The average caseload reported by home health nurses in this sample consisted of 20.69 patients (SD = 11.80), with a range from 1 to 62 patients.

Because demographic characteristics are theoretically associated with job satisfaction, correlation coefficients and analysis of variance were used to determine relationships between demographic variables such as age, years of nursing experience, years of experience in current job, race/ethnicity, gender, highest level of nursing education, and nurses' ratings of their job satisfaction. There were no significant relationships between any demographic variables and job satisfaction in this sample.

Correlation coefficients were then determined among workload measures, two of the three quality care indicators, and job satisfaction. The size of the current caseload, as an indicator of workload, was not significantly associated with either job satisfaction or quality of care, and no measures of workload were significantly associated with job satisfaction in this sample of home health nurses. In contrast, however, higher ratings of nurse-assessed quality of care were associated with higher job satisfaction ($r = .355$, $p = .000$), and conversely, patients' lack of preparation for discharge was associated with lower job satisfaction ($r = -.253$, $p = .003$). Logistic regression was then used to estimate the effect of visit adequacy on the odds on nurses' job satisfaction. Home health staff nurses who reported that their patients' visit frequencies were appropriate to their skilled nursing needs were almost three times as likely to be satisfied with their jobs than nurses who felt their patients were receiving fewer visits than needed: $O.R. = 2.94$ (1.25, 6.94), $p = .013$.

Although workload measures were not correlated with job satisfaction, Table 7.2 indicates that two indicators of workload, number of visits and the number of scheduled patients, were inversely associated with nurse-rated quality of care. All three measures of workload, including (a) the number of patients in nurses' caseloads, (b) the number of patients scheduled, and (c) the number of visits actually conducted, were associated with a higher frequency of patients' lack of preparedness for discharge. These findings indicate that, in accordance with models of organizational magnetism, workload may have an indirect effect on job satisfaction by negatively influencing quality-care processes.

Table 7.2

CORRELATIONAL COEFFICIENTS OF WORKLOAD VARIABLES AND QUALITY INDICATORS ($n = 137$)

	UNPREPARED AT DISCHARGE	# SCHEDULED PATIENTS	# VISITS CONDUCTED	# PATIENTS IN CASELOAD
Quality of care	−.372**	−.352**	−.268**	NS
Unprepared at discharge		.224*	.204*	.214*

NS = not significant; *$p < .05$; **$p < .01$ (2-tailed).

Last, logistic regression models estimated the unadjusted or individual effects of workload and quality indicators on nurses' intentions to leave their jobs. As presented in Table 7.3, two of the three quality-care indicators and two of the three workload indicators were significantly associated with intent to leave the job. Results indicate that the higher the ratings of quality of care within their agencies, the lower the odds on

Table 7.3

ODDS RATIOS ASSOCIATED WITH UNADJUSTED EFFECTS OF WORKLOAD AND QUALITY INDICATORS ON HOME HEALTH NURSES' INTENTIONS TO LEAVE THEIR JOBS

PREDICTOR	GROSS EFFECT OR (95% CI)	P VALUE
Quality indicators		
Quality of care	.33 (.17, .64)	.001
Unprepared at discharge	2.29 (1.03, 5.08)	.041
Visit adequacy	_____	NS
Workload indicators		
# of scheduled patients	1.30 (1.03, 1.63)	.024
# of visits conducted	1.32 (1.00, 1.73)	.044
# patients in caseload	_____	NS

NS = not significant.

nurses' intent to leave. In contrast, nurses who indicated their patients were occasionally/frequently unprepared for discharge were more than two times as likely to be planning to leave their jobs. Regarding workload indicators, higher numbers of scheduled and visited patients were associated with higher odds on intent to leave.

A final logistic regression model was estimated to determine the effects of visits conducted, as a workload indicator, controlling for overall ratings of quality of care. When quality of care was added to the model, the effect of workload on intent to leave was not significant, $p = .382$. Quality of care, however, remained significantly associated with intent to leave, $O.R. = .367\ (.17, .75)$, $p = .007$, indicating that quality of care may mediate the effect of workload on intent to leave.

POLICY IMPLICATIONS

It is troubling that 30% of the home health staff RNs in this geographically diverse sample representing 38 states reported that they were dissatisfied with their jobs. It is equally disturbing that 26% of the home health staff RNs were planning to leave their job within the next year. This finding, however, is consistent with trends reported over the last several years that estimate job dissatisfaction and attrition rates to be 20% or more among RNs working in home health care. Clearly, RN job dissatisfaction and attrition are serious problems that must be addressed by the home health sector if an adequate home health nursing workforce is to be maintained. Findings from this study indicate that home health nurses' assessment of the overall quality of care provided by their agency is positively associated with their job satisfaction.

Findings from this study are consistent with the tenets of the nursing organization and outcomes model (Aiken, Clarke, & Sloane, 2002) and the essentials of organizational magnetism, as described by McClure and Hinshaw (2002). Findings reveal that indicators of patient care quality were paramount in influencing nurses' job satisfaction and intentions to leave their job in this sample of home health staff nurses. Specifically, lower ratings of quality care and poor care practices, such as providing patients with fewer visits than needed and lack of preparation for discharge, were associated with nurses' job dissatisfaction, intent to leave, or both. Considered individually, higher workloads were also associated with nurses' intentions to leave. However, when quality-of-care ratings were controlled, workload effects were not significant.

This finding does not negate the potentially harmful impact of workload on nurses. Indeed, the literature is replete with empirical findings that link oppressively high nurse workloads to job dissatisfaction, role strain, and burnout. Rather, this finding highlights one operant mechanism through which higher nurse workloads are proposed to predict job dissatisfaction and attrition—simply stated, higher nurse workloads negatively impact the quality of patient care; poor quality of care leads to nurse job dissatisfaction and turnover.

Building on this evidence, it behooves agency managers and administrators to develop policies to enhance the adequacy of their staffing and the quality of their care processes. Implementing these policies is crucial to retain and to promote job satisfaction among home health staff nurses. A growing number of reports indicate that home health nurses feel pressured to curtail visit frequencies and shorten patients' episodes of care (Dombi, 2006). Although the current Medicare prospective payment system may provide agencies with financial incentives to reduce the number of home visits per patient, shorten home health lengths of stay, and cut staffing levels, the short-term financial gains may well be offset by costs incurred through nurse turnover and escalating vacancy rates. Recent studies support a rising concern among home health nurses regarding inadequate service provision and the premature discharge of patients from their agencies (Eaton, 2005; Flynn, 2007a). Findings from this study indicate that nurses associated these impaired care processes with poor care quality, which in turn was associated with job dissatisfaction and plans to leave.

For recruitment and retention of home health care nurses, policies are needed that focus efforts on enhancing and maintaining care quality and a culture of excellence. For example, home health managers and administrators might examine some of the strategies adopted by acute care facilities in their attempts to create magnetic organizations. Although home health is a practice setting uniquely different from acute care, a growing body of research indicates that nurses from home health and acute care share a core set of nursing values that includes the preeminence of quality patient care as a professional priority and an affinity for those organizational traits that support the delivery of quality patient care (Flynn, 2003; Flynn, Carryer, & Budge, 2005). Therefore, it is not surprising that in a recent study, acute care RNs and home health RNs agreed on seven of the eight essential attributes of organizational magnetism as being important in their ability to provide quality care (Mensik, 2007). Home health leaders and administrators should no longer allow reported differences between acute care and home care settings to prevent them from pursuing cultures of excellence as described by the magnetism movement (McClure & Hinshaw, 2002) and accreditation programs, such as the American Nurses Credentialing Center's Magnet Recognition Program. Hospitals have long recognized that magnetic organizations, characterized by those traits that support nursing practice and care quality, have a distinct advantage in recruiting and maintaining a nursing workforce. In the face of an escalating nurse shortage, home health leaders can ill afford to ignore the lessons learned by their counterparts in acute care.

CONCLUSION

The demand for home health nurses is rising at a time when the nation is facing an escalating shortage of nurses in all practice settings. For an adequate home care workforce to be maintained, it is imperative that agencies address the troubling prevalence of job dissatisfaction and attrition among home health staff nurses. The evidence from the findings of this study, consistent with the tenets of organizational magnetism, indicate that nurses' assessments of the overall quality of care provided by their organizations are an important determinant of the nurses' job satisfaction and decision to stay or leave their employer. These findings imply that policies related to organizational processes and structures that support nursing practice and, thereby, enhance the quality of patient care are essential in improving the job satisfaction and retention of staff nurses in home health.

REFERENCES

Aiken, L. H., Clarke, S. P., & Sloane, D. M. (2002). Hospital staffing, organization, and quality of care: Cross-national findings. *International Journal for Quality in Health Care, 14*(1), 5–13.

Aiken, L. H., Clarke, S. P., Sloane, D. M., Sochalski, J., & Silber, J. H. (2002). Hospital nurse staffing and patient mortality, nurse burnout, and job dissatisfaction. *Journal of the American Medical Association, 288*(16), 1987–1993.

Burton, D. A., Morris, B. A., & Campbell, K. K. (2005). *A report on Oregon's registered nurse workforce.* Portland: Oregon Center for Nursing. Retrieved January 2, 2008, from http://www.oregoncenterfornursing.org/documents/OCNReportWEB.pdf

Chou, S. C., Boldy, D. P., & Lee, A. H. (2002). Measuring job satisfaction in residential aged care. *International Journal of Quality Health Care, 14*(1), 49–54.

Dillman, D. A. (2000). *Mail and Internet surveys: The tailored design method.* New York: Wiley.

Dombi, W. A. (2006). Revisiting patient admission and discharge processes in today's homecare environment. *Caring, 25*(2), 30–33.

Eaton, M. K. (2005). The influence of a change in Medicare reimbursement on the effectiveness of stage III or great decubitus ulcer home health nursing care. *Policy, Politics, & Nursing Practice, 6*(1), 39–50.

Ellenbecker, C. H. (2004). A theoretical model of job retention for home health nurses. *Journal of Advanced Nursing, 47*(3), 303–310.

Flynn, L. (2003). Agency characteristics most valued by home care nurses: Findings from a nationwide study. *Home Healthcare Nurse, 21*(12), 812–817.

Flynn, L. (2007a). Discharged from home health: A quiet threat to patient safety? *Home Healthcare Nurse, 25*(3), 184–190.

Flynn, L. (2007b). Extending work environment research into home health settings. *Western Journal of Nursing Research, 29*(2), 200–212.

Flynn, L., Carryer, J., & Budge, C. (2005). Organizational attributes valued by hospital, home care, and district nurses in the United States and New Zealand. *Journal of Nursing Scholarship, 37*(1), 1–6.

Flynn, L., & Deatrick, J. A. (2003). Home care nurses' descriptions of important agency attributes. *Journal of Nursing Scholarship, 35*(4), 385–390.

Flynn, L., & Mazzella-Ebstein, M. A. (2007). *Survey of Medicare-certified home health agencies in New Jersey.* Unpublished data.

Gurney, C. A., Mueller, C. W., & Price, J. L. (1997). Job satisfaction and organizational attachment of nurses holding doctoral degrees. *Nursing Research, 46*(3), 163–171.

Irvine, D., & Evans, M. G. (1995). Job satisfaction and turnover among nurses: Integrating research findings across studies. *Nursing Research, 44,* 246–253.

Kovner, C., Brewer, C., Wu, Y. W., Cheng, Y., & Suzuki, M. (2006). Factors associated with work satisfaction of registered nurses. *Journal of Nursing Scholarship, 38*(1), 71–79.

Lacey, L. M., & McNoldy, T. P. (2007). *Turnover rates in NC home health and hospice agencies.* Raleigh: North Carolina Center for Nursing. Retrieved December 31, 2007, from http://www.ga.unc.edu/NCCN/research/EmpSurvey2006/Turnover%20-%20Home%20Health.pdf

McClure, M. L., & Hinshaw, A. S. (2002). *Magnet hospitals revisited: Attraction and retention of professional nurses.* Washington, DC: American Nurses Publishing.

Mensik, J. (2007). Impact of organizational attributes on nurse satisfaction in home health. *Home Health Care Management & Practice, 19*(6), 456–459.

National Association for Home Care and Hospice. (2007). *Basic statistics about home care.* Washington, DC: Author. Retrieved on January 1, 2008, from http://www.nahc.org/facts/07HC_Stats.pdf

Palumbo, M. (2003). *Home health nursing pilot study.* Burlington: Office of Nursing Workforce Research, Planning, and Development, College of Nursing and Health Sciences, University of Vermont. Retrieved December 31, 2007, from http://www.choosenursingvermont.org/reports/Summaries/hhnrs.html

Smith-Stoner, M., & Markey, J. (2007). Home healthcare nurse recruitment and retention: Tips for retaining nurses: one state's experience. *Home Healthcare Nurse, 25*(3), 198–205.

Stamps, P., & Piedmonte, E. (1986). *Nurses and work satisfaction.* Ann Arbor, MI: Health Administration Press Perspectives.

Steiger, D. M., Bausch, S., Johnson, B., & Peterson, A. (2006). *The registered nurse population: Findings from the March 2004 national sample survey of registered nurses.* Table 33. Retrieved December 31, 2007, from http://bhpr.hrsa.gov/healthworkforce/rnsurvey04/appendixa.htm#33

Stone, P., Pastor, D. K., & Harrison, M. I. (2006). Organizational climate: Implications for the home healthcare workforce. *Journal for Healthcare Quality, 28*(1), 4–11.

U.S. Department of Health and Human Services. (2002). *Projected supply, demand, and shortages of registered nurses: 2000–2020.* Table 7. Rockville, MD: National Center for Health Workforce Analysis, Health Resources and Services Administration.

United States General Accounting Office. (2001). *Nursing workforce: Emerging shortages due to multiple factors* (No. GAO-01-944). Washington, DC: Author.

8

The Emotional Demands of Nursing

REBECCA J. ERICKSON

Today I am no longer in bedside care. I work in an office, writing nursing research reports. I still feel about nursing as I always have, that it is an honorable and noble profession, affecting countless lives by providing a caring, honest, human touch in times of great distress. I love nursing. I just can't do it anymore.

(Bingham, 2001, p. 217)

These sentiments expressed by Ray Bingham reflect the emotional toll being paid by many registered nurses (RNs) working in today's demanding care environment. Such experiences are by no means limited to one person, one state, or even one nation. Despite the frequency with which nurses may recognize and share the emotional demands they face, the extent to which such demands are influencing nurse well-being and their decisions to leave jobs in acute care settings remains unexplored. The purpose of this chapter is to examine the emotional dimensions of the nursing work environment in an effort to illustrate its significance for the development of effective policies targeting job burnout and, ultimately, the retention of nurses in bedside care. The broader relevance of this study must be understood, however, in light of the current nursing shortage.

A CRISIS IN NURSE STAFFING

In 2003 the World Health Report stated, "The most critical issue facing healthcare systems is a shortage of people who make them work" (2003, p. 110). Among the most critical facets of this shortage is the lack of sufficient nursing staff. Given that nurses remain the largest group of health care providers and are on the front lines of health care delivery, a continuing shortage of nurses has the potential to severely compromise health care systems across the globe (Stone et al., 2003). Within the United States, the nurse shortage that began toward the end of the last century continues today, and the Health Resources and Services Administration (HRSA, 2004b) projects that by the year 2020, the shortage of nurses will grow to more than one million in the United States. The effects of the shortage are substantial, ranging from increased costs to hospitals for recruitment and training of new nurses to deteriorating working conditions and lower overall staffing levels that have the potential to compromise the provision of safe and effective patient care (Aiken, Clarke, Sloane, Sochalski, & Silber, 2002; Hassmiller & Cozine, 2006).

Although there has been some indication that the reentry of older nurses into the workforce and the successful efforts to recruit foreign-born nurses have helped ease the shortage, scholars continue to project that the combination of forces influencing this trend are unlikely to abate the projected shortage (Auerbach, Buerhaus, & Staiger, 2004; Buerhaus, Donelan, Ulrich, Norman, & Dittus, 2006; Larkin, 2007). One of the unique facets of the current shortage is that it is both a supply and a demand problem.

As the population ages and levels of acuity increase, the demand for quality nursing care is expected to remain high in both hospitals and nursing homes (Atkinson, 2005; Buerhaus, Staiger, & Auerbach, 2000; Hatcher, 2006; Hecker, 2001). Unfortunately, although there is an increased interest in nursing, the schools of nursing now lack the capacity to enroll more nursing students because of a shortage of nurse faculty. At the same time, fewer individuals are choosing nursing as a career, the most experienced nurses are quickly approaching retirement age, and others have been leaving the profession before they reach retirement age, citing poor workplace conditions (Buerhaus et al., 2007; Gordon, 2005).

Given the complexity of the current shortage, the need for systematic empirical understanding of the factors contributing to its continuation has never been greater. To be sure, steps have been taken in a number of areas. Congress invested in the Nurse Reinvestment Act and increased the budget of the National Institute of Nursing Research, Johnson & Johnson continues their recruitment efforts through their Campaign for Nursing's Future, and the Robert Wood Johnson Foundation has sought to develop strategies to retain the most experienced nurses in the workforce (Hatcher, 2006).

Although much of the research and media attention has been directed toward the need to recruit new nurses—thus emphasizing the need to expand enrollment capabilities and to increase the number of nurse faculty (Berlin & Sechrist, 2002; Yordy, 2006)—similar emphasis needs to be placed on retaining qualified nurses in direct patient care. As one nurse has commented, "you can recruit 'til the cows come home...but until you can stop the bleeding, they're coming in the front door and leaving out the back" (McPeck, 2004). The importance of developing effective retention policies has been echoed by Buerhaus et al. (2006), who indicate that despite some positive signs in shortage statistics, employers should work to develop policies that entice nurses to remain employed in direct patient care.

Larkin (2007) notes, however, that achieving such goals is complicated by the fact that a lack of research exists on how to retain experienced bedside nurses. One study indicates that in 2002 and 2004, 89% of direct care nurses and 86% of direct care nurses, respectively, identified an "improved working environment" as the strategy they believed would have the greatest influence on the nursing shortage (Buerhaus, Donelan, Ulrich, Norman, & Dittus, 2005). Consequently, it appears that research that promotes improved working conditions or that evaluates the effect of initiatives on nurse retention is particularly needed. In sum, solving the nation's crisis in nurses' working conditions requires that we develop a more complete understanding about the factors underlying nurses' decisions to leave direct patient care.

WHY NURSES LEAVE DIRECT PATIENT CARE

As Mary Foley (2000) indicated during her terms as president of the American Nurses Association (ANA), money is not the primary force driving nurses away; the work environment is—an environment characterized by increased patient loads, increased floating between departments, decreased support services, and frequent demands for mandatory overtime. Given these conditions, it is not surprising that Aiken and her colleagues reported that more than 40% of American nurses were dissatisfied with their jobs as compared to 15% of workers in the general population (Aiken et al., 2001). Further, in a report on the nursing shortage issued by the United States General Accounting Office (2001), job dissatisfaction was cited as a major factor causing nurses to leave patient care for reasons other than retirement.

In a study conducted by the Federation of Nurses and Health Professionals (FNHP, 2001), those who had left nursing in the previous 4 years identified the demands and stresses of the job as being the central reasons for their departure. These factors were also named by 50% of those who had recently considered leaving the profession (FNHP). Fully three in four of these potential leavers indicated they would consider continuing in patient care if conditions at their job improved. A NurseWeek/American Organization of Nurse Executives (AONE) (2002) study further reported that "a less stressful work environment" was cited as the most likely condition to cause those who are not currently working as a nurse to consider returning to the workforce. In addition, an "improved working environment" was cited by 83% of all nurses surveyed as helping "a great deal" to solve the nursing shortage (p. 5).

Stressful working conditions not only lead to dissatisfaction but also increase burnout. The Nurse Week/AONE study reports that 59% of nurses say that their job is often so stressful that they feel burned out, and more than half of those surveyed by the ANA (2001) reported experiencing stress-related illnesses in the past 2 years. Most frequently cited in this regard is the study conducted by Aiken et al. (2001), which found that 43% of American nurses reported experiencing significantly higher rates of burnout than would be expected for medical workers. Because job burnout is named by the ANA as the condition that most often leads the average American nurse to leave hospital employment after 4 years, it is a particularly critical process to understand and disrupt (Foley, 2001; O'Sullivan, 2001). Developing a more complete understanding of the burnout process is thus critical to the development and implementation of organizational policies and educational initiatives that seek to improve both retention and patient care quality over the long term.

THE EMOTIONAL FOUNDATIONS OF BURNOUT

Resulting from chronic interpersonal and emotional stressors associated with one's job, the experience of burnout is a unique type of stress syndrome that is fundamentally characterized by "emotional exhaustion" (Cordes & Dougherty, 1993; Maslach, Schaufeli, & Leiter, 2001). Because of the nature of their work, health care professionals are at especially high risk for experiencing burnout. Research by Aiken and her colleagues has demonstrated that not only are nurses experiencing burnout at a significantly higher rate than is expected for medical workers, but 43% of nurses reporting high burnout said that they intended to leave their jobs within the next 12 months, compared to just 11% of those who were not burned out (Aiken et al., 2001; Aiken et al., 2002).

What leads to the experience of burnout? Many suggest that workload is the primary correlate of feeling burned out. For example, nurses working in hospitals with the highest patient-to-nurse ratios are more than twice as likely to experience job-related burnout as nurses with the lowest ratios (Aiken et al., 2002). Generally, studies suggest that nurses' negative feelings about their jobs, including their feelings of burnout, tend to be influenced more by the organizational practices governing the workplace than by the challenges inherent in caring for others (Aiken et al., 2001; Aiken et al., 2002; Hinshaw & Atwood, 1984). Supporting this view, the National Sample Survey of Registered Nurses (HRSA, 2001, p. 31) found that it was the "structure of the job, rather than the composition of the work" that influenced nurses' job satisfaction (Aiken & Sloane, 1997).

Although most agree that consideration of the structural organization of work must be included in any comprehensive strategy to address the emerging national crisis in nurse staffing, little is known about the mechanisms through which the hospital work environment comes to affect nurses' well-being (Aiken et al., 2002). Understanding *how* structural conditions lead to heightened feelings of burnout requires a program of research aimed at understanding how nurses themselves experience the burnout process. Given that burnout's most fundamental attribute is "emotional exhaustion," *developing an understanding of how nurses become burned out requires knowledge of the emotional components of their daily work experiences.*

The ANA staffing survey (2001) asked nurses how they felt when they left their jobs each day. The following were the four most frequent responses: exhausted and discouraged (50%); discouraged and saddened by what I could not provide for my patients (44%); powerless to effect change necessary for safe, quality patient care (40%); and frightened for patients (26%). Exhausted, discouraged, saddened, powerless, frightened—these are the emotions experienced by nurses on a daily basis. Recognizing that burnout is rooted in such intense emotional experiences is integral to preventing its occurrence. This is especially true in the case of nursing, a profession whose "ethic of care" is central to its claim for professional distinctiveness (Leininger, 1980; McCance, McKenna, & Boore, 1999) and in which the ability to manage effectively one's own and others' emotions is integral to the provision of excellent patient care. Although the experience and management of emotion is critical to nursing practice (Bolton, 2000; deCastro, Agnew, & Fitzgerald, 2004; James, 1992; Smith, 1992), the human cost to the provider of care has generally been overlooked (Smith). The disproportionate rates of burnout experienced by nurses may be one continuing consequence of this oversight.

Clearly, there have been recent strides in identifying those factors that contribute to the burnout phenomenon. Examinations of the effects of emotional experiences and management among a broad range of workers have demonstrated that the experience and management of anger and irritation are significantly related to increased feelings of burnout (Erickson & Ritter, 2001), inauthenticity and depression (Erickson & Wharton, 1997), job satisfaction, turnover intentions (Côté & Morgan, 2002; Zerbe, 2000), and other indicators of physical and psychological well-being (Bulan, Erickson, & Wharton, 1997; Grandey, 2000; Pugliesi, 1999). Despite these advances in general understanding, more research is needed to specify the structural, cultural, and interpersonal conditions under which these negative emotions arise and translate into negative mental health outcomes among registered nurses.

The findings of previous research suggest the need for identifying the facets of nurses' everyday work environment that lead to the frequent experience and management (i.e., suppression, evocation, modification) of intense emotion (Erickson & Ritter, 2001; Morris & Feldman, 1996). In so doing, researchers would be specifying the conditions that influence the performance of emotional labor and its effects on well-being. In the context of nursing, *emotional labor* has been defined by Smith (1992) as the work of inducing or suppressing feeling in order to make others feel cared for and safe, irrespective of one's actual feelings (Bono & Vey, 2005; Hochschild, 1983). The facets of the care environment that require nurses to manage feelings of exhaustion, sadness, frustration, powerlessness, and fear ultimately result, along with the management process itself, in increased job burnout. Interestingly, these are the same "workplace issues" that others have suggested cause nurses to leave direct patient care and that tend to discourage long-term commitment to nursing as a career (American Association of Colleges of Nursing, 2001).

In sum, acquiring greater knowledge about the emotional demands experienced by nurses is an essential step in the development of policies and practices that can lead to higher rates of retention in acute care settings. As Henderson (2001) observed, "It may be particularly crucial, in these days of increasing patient acuity, nurse shortages...and an aging nurse population, to recognize the impact of emotional work on nurses" (p. 137). Nurses themselves are vitally aware of the emotional engagement that is necessary to be an excellent nurse. Efforts seeking to improve nurse retention need to recognize explicitly the emotional labor being performed by nurses and must be targeted toward the development of systems of care delivery that support nurses' ability to experience and manage emotion in ways that improve the quality of patient care at the same time that they reduce the incidence of burnout.

Evidence From the Field

The whole environment...causes a lot of emotion and stress....I feel that I'm always in the middle of this whirlwind of emotion.
                                                    —CAARE Project nurse

The data presented in this chapter are from the baseline phase of a longitudinal, multimethod project (i.e., The CAARE Project, Changing Attitudes About Retention and Emotion; see http://careproject.org) that examined how the emotional demands of nursing were related to the experience of burnout among RNs working within two acute care hospitals in the Midwest. The results presented here suggest that future examinations of the nursing work environment should explicitly account for the emotional demands nurses face and that policies developed with the intention of lowering burnout should include specific consideration of such demands. To provide support for these suggestions, I urge nursing researchers and administrators to become familiar with the dimensions and effects of the emotional context of care.

The emotional context of care has three conceptual components: emotional experience, emotional labor, and emotional labor requirements or feeling rules. In attending to the first dimension, emotional experiences, one seeks to understand the range of feelings experienced by nurses on the job (e.g., happiness, pride, anger, frustration, sadness, guilt, etc.). The second dimension, emotional labor, refers to the *work* of managing one's feelings and emotional expressions in order to convey the emotion that is expected during a particular interaction. Here it is important to recognize that emotional labor refers to the effort involved in managing the emotion rather than the extent to which this management is successful (Hochschild, 1983). The final dimension, feeling rules, does not refer to what nurses actually do during their workplace interactions but to the rules or guidelines they are expected to follow in order to emit the appropriate emotional display. For example, professional and organizational norms or rules are likely to prescribe that nurses try to hide their anger or disgust from patients and that they appear sympathetic to the pain of others. As one nurse in Smith's (1992) study describes it,

> I've found that at work well you've almost got to be, well people expect you to be happy and not cross. And you can't be cross even though you feel like wringing someone's neck! You've got to be reasonably under control and of course everybody suffers when you go home... I think you learn to stop that, you learn to switch off and be different, forget about work when you go home, I mean you've got to. (p. 14)

Although this nurse was still in the training stage of her nursing career, she vividly illustrates her growing understanding of the feeling rules she must follow in order to provide for both her patients and her own well-being. In doing so, she aptly demonstrates the emotional demands that nurses face on a daily basis but that often go unacknowledged or undiscussed.

To understand each of these dimensions further, and to determine their relevance to the emotional facets of the care environment, I now turn to a more detailed discussion of the current study. In doing so, I address three research questions:

1   What influences burnout among registered nurses?
2   Which, if any, facets of the emotional context of care contribute to our understanding of burnout over and above the effect of individual and occupational characteristics?
3   What are the implications of the findings on policy and practice?

METHODS

I think a lot of our frustration comes from just having to be calm in chaos.

—CAARE Project Nurse

Data and Sample

As noted, the data for this study were collected from RNs employed at two urban hospitals located in a Midwestern city. The hospitals were owned and operated by a single health care system. This chapter presents results from the baseline phase of the projects and focuses on findings from the nurse survey, though a few illustrative quotes from the baseline focus groups also are used (for more information on focus group methodology and results, please see http://caareproject.org). Questions elicited nurses' responses on a variety of topics regarding the hospital work environment, work and family relationships, mental and physical well-being, and demographics, as well as burnout and measures of the emotional context of care.

In the spring of 2004, a complete listing of nursing personnel was obtained from the health system's human resources department, and a written questionnaire was distributed to all registered nurses employed by each of the two hospitals (N = 1,443). Eighty-one percent of the nurses returned a completed questionnaire without substantial missing data (n = 1,169). Nine individuals were dropped from the analyses as a result of large amounts of missing data; for those missing one or two scale items, mean substitution was used.

Of the remaining 1,158 RNs for whom complete data were available, 96% were female, and 95% were white. In regard to education, 33% had earned a diploma of nursing, 11% had earned an associate's degree in nursing, 49% held a bachelor's degree in nursing, and 7% had earned a graduate degree in nursing. Seventy-five percent of the respondents were married, and 65% had children living at home. The mean age of respondents was 43 years old, with an average of 17 years of experience as a registered nurse. Twelve percent of the sample were under age 30, and 43% were over age 45. These demographics are generally consistent with national averages for gender and age. However, the current sample underrepresents minority nurses and overrepresents those who are married with children (HRSA, 2004a). Although these demographics are representative of nurses employed by the health system studied, nurses holding bachelor's degrees (56%) are also overrepresented in this sample compared with hospitals nationally (HRSA, 2001, 2004a). The average nurse in this sample worked 34 hours per week, with 21% working a night shift. Among clinical areas of employment, 21% of the nurses in this longitudinal sample were employed in medical-surgical units, 29% in critical care, 16% in operating or recovery units, 17% in maternity, and 17% in psychiatric, home health, or other units.

Measures

The standardized emotional exhaustion dimension of the Maslach Burnout Inventory (MBI) was used to assess job burnout (Maslach, Jackson, & Leiter, 1996) and served as the dependent variable for the study. The key independent variables were the dimensions of the emotional context of care, each of which were measured separately. The operationalization of emotional experiences builds on prior measurement strategies (Erickson & Ritter, 2001), as well as information obtained in preliminary focus groups with RNs from both hospitals (n = 96). The resulting list included the following 15 emotions: afraid, angry, anxious, ashamed, calm, excited, frustrated, guilty, happy, helpless, irritated, proud, relaxed, sad, and surprised. In answering the survey, nurses were asked to think about the last week at the hospital and to indicate how strongly or intensely they felt each of the identified emotions on an 8-point scale (0 = Not at all; 1 = Very Slightly; 4 = Moderately; 7 = Very Intensely). Using factor analysis, three groups of emotions emerged. *Agitated emotions* included feelings of anger, frustration, and irritation (Cronbach's alpha reliability = .89). *Negative emotions* included afraid, ashamed, and guilty (Cronbach's alpha = .60). And *positive emotions* included calm, happy, excited, proud, and relaxed (Cronbach's alpha = .78). The following quotations from nurses in the CAARE Project focus groups provide further insight into the types of situations that trigger particular emotions and the implications that these experiences have for the well-being of nurses over time. For example, the following nurses express agitated emotion.

> I feel overwhelmed, frustrated. There are any number of good days, but there are an equal number of days that are not good. You know, you start out on a good foot and then, a few hours later, you're just frustrated.

> You're getting this admission and this admission and then you have to discharge this patient and you're being called non-stop. And it's like you're just having a huge meltdown right there in the middle of the hallway. It's frustrating.

Examples of negative emotions can be found in the following words spoken by nurses in the focus groups.

> Sometimes you're doing other things, those little things that you just want to do, but you can't do. You go home feeling guilty because you can't do enough.

I feel like I let my patients down.

It's terrible. They [patients] look so disappointed looking at you. You just feel disgust that you can't do anything for them. Like you're just trying to ignore them and leave the room. It makes me feel bad because I want to be there for all of them.

On the other hand, the following quotations emphasize the positive emotions that nurses may experience.

We're very fortunate because it's usually almost always a daily experience where you make somebody feel significantly better and there's nothing cooler. They come in and they're blue or they're in agony or they're not even talking to you at all, and within an hour, they roll back up and actually smile at you and tell you "Thank you." There's nothing like it…and that's why I think I stay in [it] because there's nothing like it.

There are very rare moments where I get to go out there and be with the patient. It's wonderful, but it doesn't happen very often.
Like today, I took care of a patient and they were so nervous beforehand and afterwards they said, "Oh, you were great." He goes, "You put me right at ease," and, I mean, I just felt so good. I mean, I felt good that I could make him, you know, more comfortable. It was just a happy feeling.

The second dimension of the emotional context of care, emotional labor, was measured using three items; two capture the performance of what Hochschild (1983) refers to as "surface acting," and one relates to the performance of "deep acting." Surface acting takes place when a person changes his or her outward emotional display in an effort to conform to relevant feeling rules. This can be done in two ways. The first way is for a person to disguise or suppress what he or she feels and is traditionally measured by questions related to masking or covering up emotions that are at odds with feeling rules (Erickson & Ritter, 2001; Erickson & Wharton, 1997; Hochschild, 1983; Lively, 2000). The second form is a more active process in which the individual attempts to generate visible signs of expected feeling. Based on these conceptual differences, the first indicator of surface acting asked nurses to indicate on a 5-point scale the frequency with which they covered up their true feelings at work with each set of role-related interactional partners: patients, patients' families, physicians/residents, unit managers/directors, nursing coworkers, and non-RN staff (1 = never, 5 = every day; adapted from Brotheridge & Lee, 2003).

For the second indicator of surface acting, respondents were asked to report the frequency with which they pretended to have feelings that were expected but that they did not really feel when interacting with members of each of the previously identified groups (1 = never; 5 = every day; adapted from Brotheridge & Lee, 2003). In both cases, the items were summed to form an index where higher scores indicate more attempts to cover up feelings or pretend to feel the expected emotions.

Whereas surface acting refers to the effort of trying to *appear* to be experiencing the required emotion, deep acting requires that individuals work on their emotions in a direct attempt to actually experience the expected emotion (Hochschild, 1983). To measure deep acting, nurses were asked to indicate the frequency with which they made an effort to actually feel the emotions they are expected to display with each group (1 = never, 5 = every day; adapted from Brotheridge & Lee, 2003). Again responses were summed, with higher scores indicating more frequent deep acting efforts. Quotations from nurses in the focus groups illustrate the time, energy, and skill that underlie the performance of emotional labor.

> Wear that smile. That's what I tell myself. That comes right into my head just like a character. Put on that pseudo smile and just go. Nobody can know that anything bothered you. They don't need to know that you have three other call lights and the family is waiting to talk to you because you're the person that is in front and the nurse at that time... it's hard by the end of the day to keep that focus like you have all the time in the world for them and that smile on your face.

> You know how, some days, when you smile, then all of a sudden you're happier. If you don't smile, then you're like HMMMMMMM. I feel that, for me, a good strategy is to sort of force myself to do that and then you start feeling better and forget about the bad.

> You can't show all of your emotions, you have to work, you have to deal with it. Function. And a bad part is, I mean, you know, with...what all we go through here and the frustrations and things that go on, I guess, whatever happens to be happening, you still have all the stressors at home that you might be dealing with...you have to also shut them away while you are here doing your job.

Positive and negative feeling rules constitute the final measures of the emotional context of care. To provide quality care, nurses are

often expected to work actively toward the creation of positive interactional contexts and to neutralize negative ones (Boykin & Schoenhofer, 2001; Mitchell & Grippando, 1993). The operationalization of
feeling rules used in this study attempted to capture both aspects of
these professional expectations. Positive feeling rules were measured
by summing the responses to the following question: To be effective
in your job, to what extent are you required to (a) reassure patients
who are distressed or upset; (b) express feelings of sympathy; and
(c) express friendly emotions? (Cronbach's alpha = .73; adapted from
Best, Downey, & Jones, 1997). Negative feeling rules included requirements
that nurses (a) hide anger or disapproval about something someone has
done; (b) remain calm even when they are astonished; (c) hide disgust
over something someone has done; and (d) hide fear of someone who
is threatening (alpha = .85; adapted from Best et al., 1997). For both
of these scales, higher scores indicate that nurses perceived that they
must follow more of these requirements to do their job effectively. The
following quotations from the nurses in the focus groups demonstrate
the extent to which they are keenly aware of the professional norms that
require them to manage their emotional experiences and displays in
particular ways.

> You have to watch every facial expression, the tone of your voice, at least
> the nurses do. I can't say that the physicians do that, but I have to say that,
> as nurses, we have to do that. And maybe that's how you feel at the mo-
> ment, but it's part of your professionalism that you have to maintain that
> perception of everything's okay and you have everything under control.

> It's the environment... I don't care whether it's the patient to the nurse, the
> family to the nurse, the physician to the nurse, [or] the administration to
> the nurse; it comes from every direction. As soon as somebody's unhappy,
> it's the nurse that's here the most directly with the patient and she's the
> one in the line of fire. And while that is all going on, the underlying stream
> is "you should not be concerned about these things because you need to
> be altruistic. You are out there doing a nurturing thing. You are caring for
> people, so you should not be concerned about... all these other things that
> are on the outside."

> Oh sure. If someone comes in, you're supposed to be Florence Nightingale.
> She would never get upset at a family member for being totally irrational
> and throwing things at you from across the room. She would very calmly
> deal with that. So why would you have any emotion other than "everything
> you do and say is fine because I realize you're upset." You know, though,

somewhere inside you realize that you're still human too and sometimes you are just off the wall nuts.

Control Variables

Although the focus of this study is on the relationship between the emotional context of care and burnout, individual and occupational characteristics known to be related to these variables of interest must be included in the equation for full understanding of the effect of emotional context of care on the burnout phenomenon. In the discussion of final results, ordinary least squares (OLS) regression was used to determine not only what had the greatest impact on burnout but also the extent to which the emotional context of care was associated with burnout over and above the influence of more traditional individual and occupational characteristics.

To determine the control variables used in the regression analysis, a series of correlation analyses were conducted. The resulting controls included all variables that were significantly correlated with burnout or any of the measures of the emotional context of care. The individual characteristics controlled were gender, race, marital status, income, education, and years of experience as an RN.[1] The other facets of the nursing work environment included were as follows: managerial status, division (e.g., medical/surgical, critical care), hours worked per week, shift worked, patient load, number of patients perceived to have high acuity, workload and job autonomy (Karasek, 1979), the environment as measured by the Practice Environment Scale (Lake, 2002), perceived value congruence between nurse and organization, equitable distribution of resources, and nurses' sense of community or teamwork (Leiter & Maslach, 2004).

RESULTS

I think some days I am asked to do the impossible. Most days.
—CAARE Project Nurse

The primary goal of these analyses was to identify what influences burnout among registered nurses and to what extent the emotional context of care is part of this equation. To this end, a few descriptive relationships are worth noting before moving on to the results of the multivariate analysis. To get a sense of the scope of burnout in this sample and the extent to which the emotional context of care might be related to it, each measure was recoded into high and low groups. Following Aiken et al. (2001; Sean Clarke, personal communication, 2007), nurses with high levels of burnout scored over 27 on the MBI on a scale from 0 to 42. This is the level of burnout that is associated with negative occupational and health outcomes (Ashforth & Humphrey, 1993; Bono & Vey, 2005; Morris & Feldman, 1996). Because there are no standard metrics for the emotion measures, each was divided at the median to create the groups.

Overall, 37% of RNs in this sample reported experiencing high burnout. Although this is less than the 43% reported by Aiken et al. (2001), it still constitutes a significant problem. Perhaps most problematic from a long-term retention perspective is that 42% of nurses under age 30 reported these high levels of burnout, in comparison with just 32% of nurses within all other age groups. Moreover, initial analyses indicate that nurses reported experiencing each facet of the emotional context of care quite frequently. As shown in Figure 8.1, more than 95% of nurses report experiencing agitated and positive emotions and attempts to cover up their true feelings. Eighty-nine percent also report engaging in the other two forms of emotional labor—pretending to have feelings that were expected but not actually felt and making an effort actually to feel the emotions they were expected to display. Similarly, 99.8% and 98.9% of nurses also report needing to follow positive and negative feelings rules in order to be effective in their job.

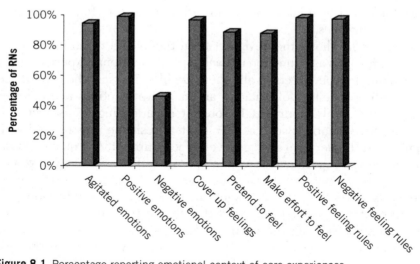

Figure 8.1 Percentage reporting emotional context-of-care experiences

The one measure whose frequency differed significantly from the others was the experience of negative emotions (i.e., fear, guilt, and shame). Even here, however, 47% of nurses in this sample reported experiencing these emotions during the past week at work. Clearly, the emotional context of care is a pervasive feature of the nursing work environment. Although merely preliminary, the results suggest that in considering the nursing work environment, policies that fail to take the emotional context of care into account are missing a critical facet of nurses' daily work experience.

WHAT INFLUENCES BURNOUT AMONG REGISTERED NURSES?

Turning to the results of the regression analysis, when all variables are included in the model, workload clearly has the strongest influence on the experience of job burnout ($b = 1.515, \beta = .394, p < .001$). These results are consistent with those of other researchers who have consistently showed workload to be the primary predictor of burnout (Maslach et al., 2001). The effect of burnout is nearly three times stronger than the next most influential variable, the experience of agitated emotions ($b = 2.871$, $\beta = .138, p < .001$). Although workload remains the strongest predictor of burnout, the next six most significant variables (all at the $p < .001$ level except for pretending to feel at $p = .003$) are those for emotional experience and emotional labor. No significant effects were found for either set of feeling rules.

Figure 8.2 shows the deviation from the overall mean level of job burnout for RNs as a function of each type of emotional experience and controlling for the effects of all other variables. Nurses who experience fewer intense feelings of agitation and negative emotions report lower than average levels of burnout. In contrast, experiencing intense agitation and negative emotions such as fear, guilt, and shame is associated with significantly higher than average levels of job burnout. As expected, positive emotional experiences have the opposite effect. Nurses who report few intense feelings of positive emotions (e.g., happiness, pride, excitement) also report significantly higher than average levels of burnout.

In contrast, nurses who report that they experienced intense positive emotional feelings during the previous week at work experienced significantly lower levels of job burnout—not only in comparison with those experiencing few positive feelings but also in comparison with the level of burnout reported by the average nurse.

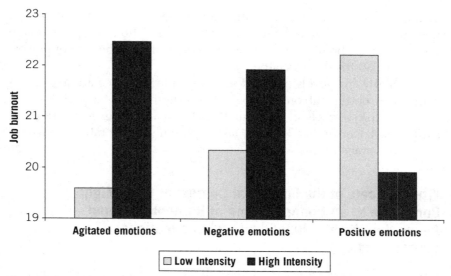

Figure 8.2 Job burnout regressed on emotional experience

Figure 8.3 presents the results for the performance of emotional labor. Consistent with the findings originally reported by Hochschild (1983), each type of emotional labor performance is positively associated with higher levels of job burnout. These results suggest that both surface

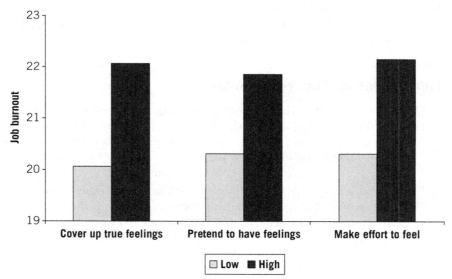

Figure 8.3 Job burnout regressed on emotional labor

acting (i.e., covering up and pretending to feel) and deep acting (i.e., making an effort to actually feel the expected emotion) are problematic for nurses' well-being. In each case, high rates of emotional labor performance are positively associated with burnout.

Similarly, low levels of emotional labor performance are associated with much better outcomes. Not only do these nurses experience significantly lower levels of burnout than those who engage in frequent surface and deep acting, but they also experience lower rates of burnout than the average nurse.

Which Facets of the Emotional Context of Care Might Contribute to an Understanding of Burnout Over and Above the Effect of Individual and Occupational Characteristics?

Based on the preceding results, the full range of emotional experiences and emotional labor performance were associated significantly with burnout, over and above the effect of workload and all of the other individual and occupational characteristics. When the dimensions associated with the emotional context of care were entered into the regression model, the amount of variance explained also increased significantly from .47 to .55, an increase of 15%. In sum, these results provide support for the claim that the emotional context of care constitutes a significant facet of the nursing work environment and, as such, should be carefully considered in the development of research and policy aimed at reducing the incidence of burnout among nurses.

Implications for Policy and Practice

> Well, how many of you have ever felt, "You know, if my manager could just shadow me for one day and see what I have to do," you know? I know I feel that way all the time because they make decisions that impact how I do my job and yet they've never done my job.

> I think, to me . . . [what's] always bothered me about higher administration— generally those who aren't nursing, particularly, I guess—is that they tend to take the opinion of consultants for how they should fix problems rather than looking at their own managers and staff and say, "What would you do to fix this problem?" or "How do you think we could fix this problem?"
> —CAARE Project Nurses

Data from the CAARE Project focus groups and written question-naires demonstrate the broad range of emotional demands nurses face on a daily basis. They further demonstrate that emotional experiences and emotional labor have a significant impact on the experience of job burnout over and above the influence of other individual and occupational characteristics. Although these results may not be news to those in sociology and organizational psychology (Erickson & Ritter, 2001; Grandey, 2003; Gross & Levenson, 1997), the emotional demands of nursing have not as yet been widely acknowledged or examined for the impact on job burnout, particularly within nursing research and policy in the United States.

As others have reported (FNHP, 2001; Lafer, 2005; NurseWeek/AONE, 2002), the association between workload and burnout was found to be particularly strong. Nonetheless, all of the emotional experience and emotional labor variables demonstrated stronger association with burnout than any of the other controls. This further indicates the relative importance of accounting for the emotional dimensions of care in developing further studies of burnout among nurses and developing effective and efficient policies to combat burnout within acute care settings. Although this study did not examine the relationship between the emotional context of care and retention, the connection between these two outcomes implies the potential significance of the emotional context of care for helping to address the retention side of the nursing shortage in the years to come. Given that burnout levels were higher among younger nurses, attending to their emotional experience may be particularly consequential. For example, Erickson and Grove (2007) demonstrated that these relationships can be quite complex. They reported that although nurses under age 30 report experiencing significantly higher levels of agitation and burnout than their older counterparts do, they do not engage in as much emotional labor. Although there has been a tendency, particularly among sociologists, to examine the effects of emotional labor on worker health outcomes, Erickson and Grove's findings suggest that what younger nurses are *feeling* may play a greater role than their management of these feelings in understanding their higher burnout rates.

Considering that Buerhaus et al. (2005, 2006) indicate that approximately 40% of the RN workforce will be over age 50 by the year 2010, employers should take advantage of the experience and effective coping strategies used by many older nurses to develop *emotional* mentors for younger nurses. Such mentorship would place particular emphasis on helping novice nurses recognize and understand the emotional demands they are likely to face as they transition into the clinical workforce. Given that over 95% of all nurses in the current sample report experiencing agitation and performing all forms of emotional labor, such mentorship activities should not be relegated only to oncology or critical care (Smith, 1992). Instead, acknowledging the pervasive presence of the emotional context of care, in all its forms, should become a central feature of nursing education and mentorship (Staden, 1998; Woodward, 1997).

This raises the more general policy implication of the current study, recognizing the emotional demands of nursing. Based on my experience with the CAARE Project, nurses have an intuitive understanding of these demands. However, few researchers, educators, administrators, or policy makers have systematically considered the influence and effects of the emotional context of care. As this pervasive feature of the nursing work environment continues to be ignored, changes to hospital policies or the development of new initiatives aimed at retaining novice and experienced nurses are not as effective or efficient as they might be. As the quotations at the beginning of this section imply, the most beginning step is to develop a more complete understanding of the emotional facets of nursing by truly listening to what nurses have to say and by carefully observing what they do on a daily basis.

In today's acute care settings, this is much easier said than done. The development and implementation of policies that successfully account for the emotional context of care require a series of ongoing changes at the unit, division, and organizational levels. Unit-level conversations must take place in which nurses identify and discuss the specific emotional rewards and demands they experience. The structure and culture of medical-surgical units are vastly different from those of critical care units—it should not be assumed that "one size fits all" in the development of emotionally sensitive policies. In addition, unit managers and nursing and hospital administrators must seek to understand fully the emotional dimensions of nursing practice. For managers this requires a *consistent* physical presence on the unit—something that can be hampered by meetings and paperwork. For administrators this requires that visits to the unit include attempts to increase understanding of the emotional demands of the job. To the extent that managers and administrators can walk in the shoes of nurses both physically and emotionally, these efforts toward increased understanding are likely to be more effective.

Because the emotional demands faced by nurses are not the same for each patient and their family, policies related to patient assignments should recognize the need to share the emotional burden, as well as issues of continuity, expertise, and patient acuity. Because the single most important trigger for positive emotional experiences is time spent with patients, organizations should seek creative, and potentially unit-specific, means of increasing the amount of time that nurses are able to spend with patients. Finally, managers, administrators, and nursing colleagues should work toward the development of policies that facilitate the formal and informal recognition of nurses who handle the emotional demands of their jobs well. Patients and their families will be thankful for it—and so will the nurses.

NOTE

1. Both age and years of experience were significantly related to the variables of interest. However, these two variables were also highly correlated with one another ($r = .81$). To avoid problems of multicollinearity, only years of experience was retained in the final models (Belsley, Kuh, & Welsch, 1980).

REFERENCES

Aiken, L. H., Clarke, S. P., Sloane, D. M., Sochalski, J. A., Busse, R., Clarke, H., Giovannetti, P., Hunt, J., Rafferty, A. M., & Shamian, J. (2001). Nurses' reports on hospital care in five countries. *Health Affairs, 20,* 43–53.

Aiken, L. H., Clarke, S. P., Sloane, D. M., Sochalski, J., & Silber, J. H. (2002). Hospital nurse staffing and patient mortality, nurse burnout, and job dissatisfaction. *Journal of the American Medical Association, 288,* 1987–1993.

Aiken, L. H., & Sloane, D. M. (1997). Effects of organizational interventions in AIDS care on burnout among urban hospital nurses. *Work & Occupations, 24,* 453–477.

American Association of Colleges of Nursing. (2001). *Strategies to reverse the new nursing shortage.* Retrieved April 8, 2003, from http://www.aacn.nche.edu/Publications/positions/tricshortage.htm

American Nurses Association. (2001). *Analysis of American Nurses Association staffing survey.* Retrieved April 28, 2008, from http://www.nursingworld.org/MainMenuCategories/ThePracticeofProfessionalNursing/workplace/Workforce/ShortageStaffing/Staffing/SatffingSurvey.aspx

Ashforth, B. E., & Humphrey, R. H. (1993). Emotional labor in service roles: The influence of identity. *Academy of Management Review, 18,* 88–115.

Atkinson, M. (2005). RNs: Understaffing hurts care. 6–7.

Auerbach, D. I., Buerhaus, P. I., & Staiger, D. O. (2004). Better late than never: Workforce supply implications of later entry into nursing. *Health Affairs, 26,* 178–185.

Belsley, D. A., Kuh, E., & Welsch, R. E. (1980). *Regression diagnostics: Identifying influential data and sources of collinearity.* New York: Wiley.

Berlin, L. E., & Sechrist, K. R. (2002). The shortage of doctorally prepared nursing faculty: A dire situation. *Nursing Outlook, 50,* 50–56.

Best, R. G., Downey, R. G., & Jones R. G. (1997, April). *Incumbent perceptions of emotional work requirements.* Paper presented at the 12th annual conference of the Society for Industrial and Organizational Psychology, St. Louis, Missouri.

Bingham, R. (2001). Leaving nursing. *Health Affairs, 21,* 211–217.

Bolton, S. C. (2000). Who cares? Offering emotion work as a "gift" in the nursing labour process. *Journal of Advanced Nursing, 32,* 580–586.

Bono, J. E., & Vey, M. A. (2005). Toward understanding emotional management at work: A quantitative review of emotional labor research. In C. E. J. Härtel, W. J. Zerbe, & N. M. Ashkanasy (Eds.), *Emotions in organizational behavior* (pp. 213–233). Mahwah, NJ: Erlbaum.

Boykin, A., & Schoenhofer, S. O. (2001). *Nursing as caring: A model for transforming practice.* Boston: Jones & Bartlett.

Brotheridge, C. M., & Lee, R. T. (2003). Development and validation of the emotional labour scale. *Journal of Organizational and Occupational Psychology, 76,* 365–379.

Buerhaus, P. I., Donelan, K., Ulrich, B. T., Norman, L., DesRoches, C., & Dittus, R. (2007). Impact of the nurse shortage on hospital patient care: Comparative perspectives. *Health Affairs, 26,* 853–862.

Buerhaus, P. I., Donelan, K., Ulrich, B. T., Norman, L., & Dittus, R. (2005). Is the shortage of hospital registered nurses getting better or worse? Findings from two recent national surveys of RNs. *Nursing Economic$, 23,* 61–71, 96.

Buerhaus, P. I., Donelan, K., Ulrich, B. T., Norman, L., & Dittus, R. (2006). State of the registered nurse workforce in the United States. *Nursing Economic$, 24,* 6–12.

Buerhaus, P. I., Staiger, D. O., & Auerbach, D. I. (2000). Policy responses to an aging registered nurse workforce. *Nursing Economic$, 18,* 278–303.

Bulan, H. F., Erickson, R. J., & Wharton, A. S. (1997). Doing for others on the job: The affective requirements of service work, gender, and emotional well-being. *Social Problems, 44,* 235–256.

Cordes, C. L., & Dougherty, T. W. (1993). A review and an integration of research on job burnout. *Academy of Management Review, 18,* 621–656.

Côté, S., & Morgan, L. M. (2002). A longitudinal analysis of the association between emotion regulation, job satisfaction, and intentions to quit. *Journal of Organizational Behavior, 23,* 947–962.

de Castro, A. B., Agnew, J., & Fitzgerald, S. T. (2004). Emotional labor: Relevant theory for occupational health practice in post-industrial America. *American Association of Occupational Health Nursing Journal, 52,* 109–115.

Erickson, R. J., & Grove, W. J. C. (2007). Why emotion matters: Age, agitation, and burnout among registered nurses. *Online Journal of Issues in Nursing.* Retrieved April 28, 2008, from http://nursingworld.org/MainMenuCategories/ANAMarketplace/ANAPeriodicals/OJIN/TableofContents/Volume62001/Number1January2001/Why EmotionsMatterAgeAgitationandBurnoutAmongRegisteredNurses.aspx

Erickson, R. J., & Ritter, C. (2001). Emotional labor, burnout, and inauthenticity: Does gender matter? *Social Psychology Quarterly, 64,* 146–163.

Erickson. R. J., & Wharton, A. S. (1997). Inauthenticity and depression: Assessing the consequences of interactive service work. *Work and Occupations, 24,* 188–213.

Federation of Nurses and Health Professionals. (2001). *The nurse shortage: Perspectives from current direct care nurses and former direct care nurses.* Retrieved April 4, 2003, from http://www.aft.org/pubs-reports/healthcare/Hart_Report.pdf

Foley, M. E. (2000). *ANA calls hospital staffing practices unsafe: Nurses being forced to regularly work excessive over time.* Retrieved April 4, 2008, from http://www.needle stick.org/pressrel/2000/pr0420b.htm

Foley, M. E. (2001). Statement of the American Nurses Association before the Committee on Education and Workforce on the nursing shortage: Causes, impact and innovative Remedies. Retrieved March 13, 2003, from http://www.kaisernetwork.org/health_cast/uploaded_files/09.25.01__transcript.pdf

Gordon, S. (2005). *Nursing against the odds: How health care cost cutting, media stereotypes, and medical hubris undermine nurses and patient care.* Ithaca, NY: Cornell University Press.

Grandey, A. A. (2000). Emotional regulation in the workplace: A new way to conceptualize emotional labor. *Journal of Occupational Health Psychology, 5,* 95–110.

Grandey, A. A. (2003). "When the show must go on": Surface acting and deep acting as determinants of emotional exhaustion and peer-rated service delivery. *Academy of Management Journal, 46,* 86–96.

Gross, J. J., & Levenson, R. W. (1997). Hiding feelings: The acute effects of inhibiting negative and positive emotion. *Journal of Abnormal Psychology, 106,* 95–103.

Hassmiller, S. B., & Cozine, B. (2006). Addressing the nurse shortage to improve the quality of patient care. *Health Affairs, 25,* 268–274.

Hatcher, B. J. (Ed.). (2006). *Wisdom at work: The importance of the older and experienced nurse in the workplace.* Princeton, NJ: Robert Wood Johnson Foundation.

Health Resources and Services Administration. (2001). *The registered nurse population: Findings from the national sample survey of registered nurses.* Retrieved March 18, 2007, from http://bhpr.hrsa.gov/healthworkforce/reports/nursing/samplesurvey00/default.htm

Health Resources and Services Administration. (2004a). *The registered nurse population: Findings from the 2004 national sample survey of registered nurses.* Retrieved March 18, 2007, from http://bhpr.hrsa.gov/healthworkforce/rnsurvey04

Health Resources and Services Administration. (2004b). *What is behind HRSA's projected supply, demand, and shortage of registered nurses?* Retrieved May 24, 2007, from ftp://ftp.hrsa.gov/bhpr/workforce/behindshortage.pdf

Hecker, D. E. (2001). Occupational employment projections to 2010. *Monthly Labor Review, 124,* 51–84.

Henderson, A. (2001). Emotional labor and nursing: An under-appreciated aspect of caring work. *Nursing Inquiry, 8,* 130–138.

Hinshaw, A. S., & Atwood, J. R. (1984). Nursing staff turnover, stress, and satisfaction: models, measures, and management. *Annual Review of Nursing Research, 1,* 133–153.

Hochschild, A. R. (1983). *The managed heart: Commercialization of human feeling.* Berkeley: University of California Press.

James, N. (1992). Care = Organization + physical labour + emotional labour. *Sociology of Health and Illness, 14,* 488–509.

Karasek, R. A. (1979). Job demands, job decision latitude, and mental strain: Implications for job redesign. *Administrative Science Quarterly, 24,* 285–306.

Lafer, G. (2005). Hospital speedups and the fiction of a nursing shortage. *Labor Studies Journal, 30,* 27–46.

Lake, E. T. (2002). Development of the practice environment scale of the Nursing Work Index. *Research in Nursing & Health, 25,* 176–188.

Larkin, Michelle. (2007). Shortage strategies: Retaining the experienced nurse. *Journal of Nursing Administration, 137,* 162–163.

Leininger, M. M. (1980). *Caring: A central focus of nursing and health care services.* Westport, CT: Technomic.

Leiter, M. P., & Maslach, C. (2004). Areas of worklife: A structured approach to organizational predictors of job burnout. In P. L. Perrewe & D. C. Ganster (Eds.), *Research in occupational stress and well being: Vol. 3. Emotional and physiological processes and positive intervention strategies* (pp. 91–134). Oxford, UK: JAI Press/Elsevier.

Lively, K. (2000). Reciprocal emotion management: Working together to maintain stratification in private law firms. *Work and Occupations, 21,* 32–63.

Maslach, C., Jackson, S. E., & Leiter, M. P. (1996). *The Maslach Burnout Inventory* (3rd ed.). Palo Alto, CA: Consulting Psychologists Press.

Maslach, C., Schaufeli, W. B., & Leiter, M. P. (2001). Job burnout. *Annual Review of Psychology, 52,* 397–422.

McCance, T. V., McKenna, H. P., & Boore, J. R. P. (1999). Caring: theoretical perspectives of relevance to nursing. *Journal of Advanced Nursing, 30,* 1388–1395.

McPeck, P. (2004, February 23). Can we fix it? Accessed April 22, 2008, from http://www.nurseweek.com/news/features/04-02/shortages.asp

Mitchell, P. R., & Grippando, G. M. (1993). *Nursing perspectives and issues* (5th ed.). Albany, NY: Delmar.

Morris, J. A., & Feldman, D. C. (1996). The dimensions, antecedents, and consequences of emotional labor. *Academy of Management Review, 21,* 986–1010.

NurseWeek/American Organization of Nurse Executives. (2002). *NurseWeek/American Organization of Nurse Executives national survey of registered nurses.* Retrieved on April 4, 2003, from http://www.nurseweek.com/survey/

O'Sullivan, A. (2001). *Statement for the Committee on Governmental Affairs Subcommittee on Oversight of Government Management, Restructuring, and the District of Columbia on addressing direct care staffing shortages.* Retrieved March 13, 2003, from http://www.needlestick.org/gova/federal/legis/teon/2001/govaref.htm

Pugliese, K. (1999). The consequences of emotional labor: Effects on work stress, job satisfaction, and well-being. *Motivation and Emotion, 23,* 135–154.

Smith, P. (1992). *The emotional labour of nursing.* London: Macmillan.

Staden, H. (1998). Alertness to the needs of others: A study of the emotional labor of caring. *Journal of Advanced Nursing, 27,* 147–156.

Stone, P. W., Tourangeau, A. E., Duffield, C. M., Hughes, F., Jones, C. B., O'Brien-Pallas, L., & Shamian, J. (2003). Evidence of nurse working conditions: A global perspective. *Policy, Politics, & Nursing Practice, 4,* 120–130.

United States General Accounting Office. (2001). *Nursing workforce: Recruitment and retention of nurses and nurse aides is a growing concern.* Washington, DC: U.S. Government Printing Office.

Woodward, V. M. (1997). Professional caring: a contradiction in terms? *Journal of Advanced Nursing, 26,* 999–1004.

World Health Organization. (2003). *World health report.* Retrieved May 24, 2007, from http://www.who.int/whr/2003/en/whr03_en.pdf

Yordy, K. D. (2006). *The nursing faculty shortage: A crisis for health care.* Princeton, NJ: Robert Wood Johnson Foundation.

Zerbe, W. J. (2000). Emotional dissonance and employee well-being. In N. M. Ashkanasy, C. E. Hartel, & W. J. Zerbe (Eds.), *Emotions in the workplace: Research, theory and practice* (pp. 189–214). Westport, CT: Quorum Books.

Geri L. Dickson

A nurse quoted in Erickson's study summed up what many nurses feel about the workplace in which they work, be it a hospital or a home health agency. She said, "I think somedays I am asked to do the impossible. Most days." Yet this area of research that provides evidence for us (and policy makers) about the work life of nurses—and its impact on nurses and their patients' lives—is a relatively new phenomenon.

Today, however, we have not only nurse researchers who have active programs of research focused on the relationship of the work environment and nurses' satisfactions with their work, but also researchers who directly link the nurse practice environment, plus the nurses' characteristics and care within that environment, to patient outcomes. Sean Clarke, one of those researchers, provides the foundation in chapter 2 for this collection of scholarly works.

LESSON 1. FAIRNESS IN COMPENSATION

So what have we learned from these chapters in Section III? If you look closely at the studies, you will see some similarities as well as some differences among their findings. For example, Brewer, Kovner, and Flynn all agree that money alone will not keep nurses in their current jobs or even in the profession. However, as Brewer and Kovner's research suggests, fairness matters in terms of salaries. Does the new nurse start at a higher salary than the experienced nurse? Am I, the experienced nurse, rewarded with a retention bonus just the same as the new nurse who receives a sign-on bonus? There is research evidence in this section to support institutional policies that outline just and fair guidelines for salary compensation for all nurses. One way to implement this strategy is for employers to have a clinical ladder in place that fairly rewards nurses for gaining education or certification to enhance their practice of patient care. But above all, nurses want just and fair policies in place that will determine their remuneration.

LESSON 2. AGE MATTERS IN NURSE BURNOUT

Another area explored in these studies was the relationship of demographic variables to job or work satisfaction and, subsequently, the intent to leave.

179

Although there was no significant relationship found between demographic information and satisfaction, Erickson reported that age mattered. In her study of burnout (emotional exhaustion) among hospital nurses, Erickson found that a higher percentage of younger nurses reported burnout than did older nurses: 42% of RNs under the age of 30 reported high levels of burnout, in comparison with 32% of nurses in all other age groups. Although all nurses, to a degree, experience stress in their work environments, the nurse under 30 reported the highest levels of burnout. To address this troubling and significant finding, policies can be developed that provide programs for new nurses to help ease the transition from the culture of school to the culture of the workplace. Developing new mentor roles for experienced nurses, as some employers have done, may ease the transition for recent graduates. Policies that directly affect the stressful work environment and the work that confronts nurses today need to be developed, implemented, and evaluated—a lesson whose time has come.

LESSON 3. PROMOTING A CULTURE OF NURSE EXCELLENCE

Policies that address these issues may be in place in some practice settings. One suggested policy arising from these studies could be creation of a culture of magnetism, as Flynn suggests. Implementing the principles inherent in the American Nurses Credentialing Center (ANCC) Magnet status may be one way to develop cohesion among staff nurses and administrators, to reduce the environmental stress that Brewer and Kovner identified. Flynn advocates for this policy change, heretofore found only in acute care facilities, for home health agencies. Her research has suggested that the elements of magnetism are just as relevant to home care agencies and the nurses' workplace as they are to hospital nurses. The essential principles of magnetism, however, can be implemented without the accreditation of Magnet status by the ANCC. Magnetism acknowledges and promotes excellence in the nursing profession, as well as inclusion of nurses in all aspects of leadership in magnet institutions—a lesson embedded in these findings.

LESSON 4. NURSE MANAGERS MAKE A DIFFERENCE

In these three chapters, the roles and relationships of nurses and their managers were important to nurses' work satisfaction. The nurses in

Brewer and Kovner's study reported a great deal of change and discontinuity of managers, which they described as destructive to the organizational culture. To address this issue, Erickson suggests that to understand the work life of nurses, managers and administrators "walk in the shoes" of nurses both physically and emotionally. Extant research literature is replete with studies regarding the importance of a competent and well-educated nurse manager. It is time to address this lesson learned by establishing organizational policies about the qualifications and experiences of a nurse manager and to take seriously the role of the manager in retaining nurses.

LESSON 5. QUALITY OF CARE AND NURSE SATISFACTION

Flynn's findings suggest that there is a significant relationship between the quality of care perceived by home health nurses and the nurses' satisfaction with their jobs. Flynn points out that savings realized from reduced turnover and vacancies among the nurse staff could reduce the cost to agencies of the amount of nursing services provided to patients by nurses, thereby increasing the quality of care. In a similar vein, nurses in Erickson's study reported that the single most important trigger for positive emotional experiences was time spent with patients. Policies rethinking the RNs' role and carefully determining the economic savings of providing quality care, along with satisfied nurses, are long overdue—a lesson learned.

LESSON 6. STRESSFUL WORK ENVIRONMENT

A survey, cited by Erickson, of nurses who were no longer working in nursing identified a "less stressful work environment" as the number one condition that would bring them back to work. By the same token, another survey of nurses revealed that over 80% of RNs suggested "improved working environment" as the strategy they believed would have the greatest influence on the nurse shortage. There is consensus among these studies that RNs' work/job satisfaction is related to workplace conditions, such as quantitative workload, quality of patient care, and organizational culture. This is not a new lesson, but it is crucial that we determine what we can do to create organizational, professional, or public policies to improve the workplace for nurses. The lesson learned here is that to stem the tide of dissatisfied nurses leaving the workplace, safety and quality strategies to improve the work environment must be developed. Careful study of the most efficient care provided by RNs is a necessary precursor to developing a new and important care delivery system. Professional organizations or accrediting bodies may play a role in carefully crafting and implementing care delivery guidelines based on input from direct care RNs.

LESSON 7. NURSE SAFETY

Brewer and Kovner describe staff nursing in hospitals as dangerous work. Though this was not a predictor of satisfaction, in their study, between one-third and two-thirds of nurses reported that they had suffered a workplace injury in the past year, such as bruises/contusions, cuts/lacerations, needlestick injuries, and strain/sprains. A small percent had more serious injuries such as fractured bones, dislocated joints, and head injuries. In addition to causing pain to the individual, these injuries, which result in nurses' absence from the workplace, can cause a cascade of staffing issues, including short staffing or the added expense of supplemental nurses. These incidents of workplace injuries are documented in the literature, and it is time to develop a body of evidence through multiple studies that address appropriate policy changes. For example, other research evidence points to the benefits of using easily operated and readily available lifting devices to help save nurses' backs. This, as well as other safety issues, has been identified for a long time but often is not addressed by appropriate policy changes. On the other hand, another safety strategy has entered the practice arena because of a public policy that mandated "needleless" syringes be used in practice. Can we advocate for a safer environment for nurses?

In sum, each of the studies in this section has quite impressive references for you to mine. Perhaps you may want to continue your research or use the existing literature to advocate for your patients. Most importantly, these studies may provide an opportunity to identify changes that make a difference in nurses' work. Continuing on to Sections V and VI, you will find examples of how nurses may obtain funding for their research and how nurses can—and should—advocate for policy changes.

In closing, I leave you with these words from a nurse in Erickson's study: "There are very rare moments where I get to go out there and be with the patients. It's wonderful, but it doesn't happen very often." Can you help make that happen?

INTRODUCTION

Geri L. Dickson

Weaving the theme of the research to policy connection throughout the chapters, we now turn our attention to the preparation of nursing students to enter the workforce. For the public, the nursing educational system is not easy to understand. Historically, nurses were educated in hospitals in which they performed most of the work of caring for patients. Based on the Nightingale model of nurse education, student nurses lived in hospital quarters under the watchful eyes of housemothers and were governed by strict rules appropriate for young single women at that time.

As time went on, many leaders of U.S. nursing worked diligently to move nursing education from the hospital to institutions of higher learning. The first professor of nursing, M. Adelaide Nutting, was installed at Teachers College, Columbia University, in 1907. Slowly teachers of nursing began to become college educated.

After World War II, the first severe nurse shortage arose, and thought was given to a new kind of nurse who could fill the void when many nurses left their work behind to raise families. Mildred Montag, at Teachers College, conducted research and in 1952 developed a curriculum for a new nurse—the technical nurse. Hence, the associate degree (AD) nurse was born. At that time then, there were nurses educated in hospitals who received a diploma on graduation and nurses who were educated in 2-year community or junior colleges who received an associate's degree. Little by little, baccalaureate education for nurses also expanded, and a degree was awarded to students graduating from a 4-year college or university. All three of these educational programs prepared students to sit for the same state board examination to become registered nurses. This system still exists today, although many states no longer have hospital diploma schools.

Currently, reports from the National League for Nursing and the American Association of Colleges of Nursing, which separately accredit nursing schools, indicate that nationwide, numerous qualified students are being denied admission to all types of schools of nursing because the schools lack the educational capacity to increase enrollments. Further, one of the major obstacles is lack of qualified faculty, but to a lesser degree, clinical placements, adequate learning resources laboratories and classroom space also contribute to the lack of educational capacity.

Recruitment efforts, such as the mass media campaigns of Johnson & Johnson, have had a degree of success, with greater numbers of students interested in nursing today, in comparison with a decade ago. Nationwide, the number of graduates from associate degree, hospital diploma, or baccalaureate schools who were eligible to enter the workforce reached a peak in 1994 and then decreased dramatically until a plateau was reached about 2002. Since that time, the graduates have gradually increased, and the numbers of graduates now approximate those of 1994. Overall, the rise in graduates has slowed somewhat since a massive growth between 2002 and 2004. Further, the schools have expanded greatly their capacity to educate students, without a comparative increase in numbers of faculty positions, thereby exacerbating the faculty shortage by increasing workloads.

In this section, you will find three studies exploring some of the current issues in nursing education: (a) recruiting high school students into nursing, (b) addressing issues of a faculty shortage, and (c) incorporating the use of high-fidelity simulation models into nursing education. In chapter 9, Rudel and Moulton describe the unique historical background of North Dakota regulation. North Dakota was the only state to change its regulation of nurses to require an associate's degree to sit for the licensed practical nurse examination and a baccalaureate degree with a nursing major to sit for the registered nurse examination.

In reaction to fears of a nurse shortage, the legislation establishing these regulations was repealed in 2003. At the same time, the North

Dakota Nursing Needs Study was mandated in their new 2003 Nurse Practice Act. To fulfill this mandate, the Board of Nursing contracted with the University of North Dakota, Center for Rural Health, to conduct a state nursing needs study. In addition to eliciting data regarding a shortage of nurses in North Dakota, the study mandate also included a stipulation with regard to informing stakeholders about the recruitment of future nurses.

In chapter 9, then, you will find a description of the resulting North Dakota High School Survey, as well as a literature review of how students come to make career choices. The online survey and analyses yielded interesting results about high school students' perspective on nursing as a career choice. The authors provide food for thought, as well as policy recommendations based on their findings.

Moving on to issues related to a faculty shortage, Cleary and her team from the North Carolina Center for Nursing, the first such center in the nation, relate shortage issues to faculty retirements and a shortage of baccalaureate-prepared nurses and develop interesting faculty-shortage projection scenarios. Based on the retirements and these three faculty projections providing differing student–to–clinical faculty ratios, they present policy recommendations to increase the efficiencies of nurse faculty.

Last, in chapter 11, Lashley and Nehring, experts in the use of simulation models in nursing education, present the background and future of their use in better preparing nursing students. They identify the pros and cons of the use of simulation models, plus describe how they are, or may be, used as a means to ameliorate the nurse faculty shortage. They identify potential policy issues related to recognizing simulation practice and evaluation as clinical experience.

Together these three chapters outline the important factors relating to recruitment of students and nurse education, plus the underlying reasons for the nurse faculty shortage. Some states are moving forward in collaborative ways to address the nurse and nurse faculty shortage, such as a major project in Oregon: the Oregon Consortium for Nursing Education. They are working toward a standardized curriculum, dual admission of students into both associate and baccalaureate nursing schools, plus a major change in clinical education (for more information, see chapter 15 or http://www.OCNE.org). Now is the time for *change!*

You must be the change you want in the world.

Mahatma Gandhi

9

Nursing's Long-Term Pipeline: A Study of High School Students Using a Unique Data Collection Approach

REBECCA RUDEL AND PATRICIA MOULTON

The future of health care in the United States increasingly pivots on a sufficient supply of appropriately educated and skilled professional registered nurses (RNs). Shortage statistics do vary widely, but as we fully appreciate, all shortage projections are alarming. According to the latest projections from the U.S. Bureau of Labor Statistics' *Occupational Outlook Handbook,* more than one million new and replacement nurses will be needed by 2020 (2006–2007). For the first time ever, the U.S. Department of Labor has identified registered nursing as the profession that is expected to experience the most job growth through the year 2012. This chapter is a segmented accounting of our state's dance with the nurse shortage.

The purposes of the study of high school students reported here were (a) to increase understanding of how the potential North Dakota labor pool views the nursing profession and (b) to identify themes to encourage young people to consider a career in nursing. To begin, we contextualize this work by offering a brief accounting of how this unique study was mandated. The historical context of North Dakota and its journey in changing the educational entry into practice provided the background for this study.

NORTH DAKOTA'S UNIQUE NURSING EDUCATION HISTORY

For nearly a century, the educational preparation for RNs has been a contentious issue. As far back as 1922, Josephine Goldmark in the Goldmark Report examined issues facing the nursing profession and established recommendations for minimum educational standards at the level of a "dignified college education" (Goldmark, 1922). In 1965, using the Goldmark report as the foundation, the American Nurses Association (ANA) published its first position paper on nursing education, titled *Educational Preparation for Nurse Practitioners and Assistants to Nurses: A Position Paper.* The position paper described two levels of nursing: (a) baccalaureate education for professional nursing practice and (b) associate degree education for entry to technical nursing practice (ANA, 1965). In 1978 the ANA set forth the mandate that by 1985, all RNs would have a minimum of a baccalaureate degree (Lewis, 1985). By 1985, not one state had yet adopted the ANA recommendation.

Against this background, the North Dakota Board of Nursing (NDBON) established new rules for entry into North Dakota nursing practice in 1987. North Dakota then became the first state to standardize two educational requirements for entry levels of nursing practice—the associate degree for licensed practical nurses (LPNs) and the baccalaureate degree for RNs. In these rules, North Dakota nurses who had graduated from nursing programs prior to 1987 were "grandfathered," and nurses moving in from out of state were be given provisional licensure with 4 years to achieve their respective educational degree.

In 1987, North Dakota colleges and universities readily responded to the entry-into-practice mandate. However, there were those few who believed that this "entry" deterred nurses from neighboring states from considering employment in North Dakota. Responsively, by 1992 the NDBON had begun long-range planning to review the North Dakota Nurse Practices Act for potential revision. In time, a draft was completed, public forums were held, and consensus building happened. In 1995 the NDBON introduced the legislative bill to revise the Nurse Practices Act. In that session, the board presented testimony to continue support of the 1987 educational standards, but with changes to the 1987 rules to remove the 4-year educational time frame for out-of-state nurses (Haagenson, 1995; Rose, 2006). Including these educational levels in the Nurse Practices Act, rather than in the administration rules, was a major successful revision to the act in 1995.

In the following decades, legislative changes were proposed and some implemented—for example, removing the educational requirement for out-of-state nurses and replacing it with 30 continuing education hours. In the 2003 state legislative session, the long-term care and hospital associations ramped up their opposition to the educational requirements in the Nurse Practices Act. Although other states (Oregon, Maine, and Montana) had been strongly considering baccalaureate entry, North Dakota was still the only state with higher educational requirements for nursing practice.

However, the increased warnings of a national shortage of nurses created a focusing factor. Although there were no true shortage statistics available for North Dakota, the associations made their stand to policy makers: North Dakota's entry into practice was a factor in creating a nursing shortage in North Dakota. Meanwhile, the North Dakota Nurses Association (NDNA) developed its solution to the issue by creating legislative language believed to remove the debate about nursing education requirements from the legislative arena. In addition, in that 2003 session, the NDNA introduced a bill that would remove the power of the NDBON to approve nursing programs and transfer that power to approve nursing programs to the North Dakota State Board of Higher Education, perceiving that the Board of Education did not endure the scrutiny of the legislature (Rose, 2006).

In short, throughout the North Dakota 2003 legislative year, even further confusion and fragmentation within the state nursing leadership and the nursing community ensued (Rose, 2006). Kingdon (1995), in his policy work, concluded that the fragmentation of a policy system affects the stability of the agenda within that system. Fragmentation within the nursing community carried heavy consequences and opened a policy window of opportunity for advocates to strengthen the push for removal of the 1987 nursing education requirements for the state. By then, many of North Dakota's community colleges had joined the long-term care and hospital associations, resulting in the North Dakota legislators repealing the 1997 Nurse Practices Act in 2003 (Rose).

The North Dakota Nursing Needs Study

Amid this saga and the 2003 repeal, the North Dakota Nursing Needs Study was mandated in the new 2003 NDCC Nurse Practices Act (2003). The North Dakota Board of Nursing was directed to address issues of supply and demand for nurses including concerns of recruitment, retention, and utilization of nurses. The Board of Nursing contracted with the Center for Rural Health (University of North Dakota) to conduct the state Nursing Needs Study, a study that was funded for 10 years. The overall Nursing Needs Study was designed and implemented with three primary goals: (a) to provide a more accurate picture of the APN, RN, and LPN workforce in both rural and urban areas of North Dakota, (b) to compare these data with existing national data, and (c) to inform policy for needed change.

The first biennial North Dakota needs study, which was conducted in 2003, reported four counties in the state to have RN shortages at 6%–9%, six counties with shortages at 10%–14%, and two counties at 14% or greater. In subsequent biennial reports, these figures have remained relatively constant. North Dakota has a population of approximately 635,000 people, of whom 632 are advanced practice nurses, 8,468 are RNs, and 3,365 are LPNs (Moulton, 2006). Although the results are not nearly as dramatic as those seen in some counterpart state reports, North Dakota definitely has concern for nursing care delivery, particularly for the aged, the rural, and the more remote citizens of this lightly populated state. In 2003 the state nurse shortage approximated 500 RNs, which was projected to increase to a shortage of about 2,000 RNs by 2013. By 2005, the statewide vacancy rate for RNs had risen 9% in one year. In that year, the state RN turnover rate was 20% (increase from 15% in 2003). Considering demographics (an aged state) and out-migration trends, it is predicted from the study data that nearly one in four nursing positions will remain open in North Dakota by year 2020.

Indirectly, the High School Student Study resulted from this entry-into-practice history; the study was one of the Nursing Needs Study strategies to inform stakeholders about concerns of recruitment for future nurses. The purposes of the study of high school students were to (a) increase understanding of how the potential North Dakota labor pool views the nursing profession and (b) identify themes to encourage young people to consider a career in nursing.

The study was conducted in 2006. Students (grades 9–12) were surveyed through a unique voluntary online process, with the largest sample recorded in related literature ($N = 571$ students), representing 25 high schools. We continue this chapter with a literature review on career decision making of our developing youth, followed by an accounting of the North Dakota High School Student Survey and subsequent recommendations for action. The intent is to offer enlightenment related to the recruitment and retention of young people as an issue for nursing in North Dakota, in the United States, and around the world. The long-term future of the nursing profession depends on the recruitment and retention of young people in nursing.

TOMORROW'S NURSING PIPELINE: A LITERATURE REVIEW

Early Age-Related Perceptions of Nursing

For most people, career development is a lifelong process of engaging with the work world through choosing among many available employment opportunities. Each individual in the process is influenced by many factors, including the person's personal aptitude, the context in which he or she lives, and his or her educational attainment (Bandura, Barbaranelli, Caprara, & Pastorelli, 2001). Career choices involve physical, emotional, intellectual, and value development processes that begin early in life (Leonard & Iannone, 2000). By primary school age, a child's perceptions relating to career choices have actually begun to develop. Nurse visionaries have advocated for programs to encourage young children to consider nursing as a career for over a decade (Alexander & Fraser, 2001; Beck, 2000; Blasdell & Hudgins-Brewer, 1999; Mignor, Cadenhead, & McKee, 2002; Pellman & Meyer, 2000; Reiskin & Haussler, 1994; Tomey, Schwier, Marticke, & May, 1996).

As children age, negative attitudes about nursing reportedly increase. Costello's report (2002) confirmed that even second grade children perceived no reason to become a nurse, and when they were interested in health care, it was only to become a doctor. Older grade-school children reported the sense that nursing was associated with unfavorable hours, tasks, schedules, and stresses (Costello). These findings are similar to those from earlier work by Tomey et al. (1996), who reported that as young children mature, a gap of perceptions emerges between ideal careers and nursing career choices.

Middle School Students and Career Considerations

In middle school, students begin to explore various career options, with most fashioning their attitudes related to learning, work, and related adult values (Toepfer, 1994). Job shadowing, exposure to new interests, the chance to try on new roles, community service, and mentoring relationships are strategies that help middle school adolescents make the decisions that will affect career options (Benz, 1996; Lozada, 2001;

Wright, 2001). Middle school students' exposure to nurses and positive nursing images are an essential step to increasing recruitment into the profession. Related findings of significance for middle school students led to several recommendations by Cohen, Palumbo, Rambur, and Mongeon (2004):

1   Target boys in recruitment during early adolescence.
2   Emphasize what is accurate about nursing and what early adolescents reportedly want: opportunities for autonomous decision making and varying (practice) environments within nursing.
3   Power, leadership, and being influential are important to the career vision of middle school youth.
4   Youth in middle school want to feel as though they will make a difference.

Decision Making in High School

In educational research in the recent past, student decision making about college education choices has attracted a great deal of attention. Peters and Marshall (1996) termed students as "autonomous choosers" in this decision-making process. Subsequent reports strongly challenged this idea, pointing out that some students have no choice at all—opportunity is not the same for all groups and types of people, and in most cases, the institution selects students; they do not select the institution. There are also studies showing that decision making is not the rational, linear process it is perceived to be (Tyler, 1998). Perna's work (2000) certainly challenges econometrics models in her measurement of social and cultural capital as requisites for expectations, preferences, tastes, and uncertainty in career and collegiate aspirations. Student decision making is "a complex nexus in which habitus, personal identity, life history, social and cultural contexts, action and learning are inter-related" (Bloomer & Hodkinson, 1997, p. 46).

Leach and Zepke (2005) orchestrated an extensive review of the educational literature that offers condensed insight as to how prospective high school students make career decisions. Their findings are presented around four themes, briefed and further supported here:

Theme 1: Decisions. Decision making is a complex process and can be captured in one of many model examples; the most used is a three-stage model with predisposition, search, and choice phases.

Decision making starts very early, much earlier than grades 11 and 12 (Cabrera & La Nasa, 2000; Harker, Slade, & Harker, 2001).

Theme 2: Factors influencing choice. Socioeconomic status is arguably the strongest predictor of whether students enter the college environment. Other important factors influencing students' decisions are the parents' influence on decisions, a student's academic aptitude and achievement, subject area interest, school experiences, and the total cost of attending college.

Theme 3: Information. Family experiences inform decisions; if a family has prior experience of higher education; children are more likely to navigate postsecondary education. Interestingly, the most effective information delivery mode is interpersonal; the effect of mass marketing is overrated. Information is most effective when constantly exchanged between families, schools, and college representatives. Peers of decision makers are also recognized as strong members of this complex web of interpersonal information networks (Christie, Munro, & Fisher, 2004).

Theme 4: Diversity. A diverse range of people have traditionally been underrepresented as minorities or nontraditional students in higher education. Relatively little data are available on the decision making of these nontraditional students, and all factors are complex. Socioeconomic class and membership of "at risk" groups were major influences on decision making. Ethnicity and age have some influence, and data on gender actually suggested that this variable has little effect. For nontraditional students, a key decision-making factor centers on the needs of the family and the community (Leach & Zepke, 2005).

NURSING AS A SPECIFIC CAREER VISION IN HIGH SCHOOL

By high school, a very small percentage of our youth reportedly view nursing as a viable career. High school students have indicated they want more appreciation, money, safety, and power than they perceive as attainable in nursing. In 1989 Grossman, Arnold, Sullivan, Cameron, and Munro warned that less than 15% of high school juniors surveyed believed that nursing would provide what those youth wanted: opportunity for leadership, for teaching in higher education, to be an executive, or to be involved in research. Others followed with the message of discrepancy between what high school students consider an ideal career and their perceptions of nursing, such as independence, respect, appreciation, and safe working environments (Hemsley-Brown & Foskett, 1999; May, Champion, & Austin, 1991; Stevens & Walker, 1993; Tomey et al., 1996). By high school age, more and more students want less caring for people, less hard work, less working with their hands, less being busy, and more ability to work with high technology than what they perceive is available to them in the nursing profession.

Many studies have been undertaken with nursing students to understand further the factors that influence the decision to choose nursing over the innumerable other career options. Overall, it appears that students who did elect nursing as their career goal desired human contact, wanted to help others, and wanted job security (Larsen, McGill, & Palmer, 2003; Rognstad, Aasland, & Granu, 2004; Williams, Wertenberger, & Gushuliak, 1997). Past experiences with illness, health care work, or family members as nurses also have been found to be important motives for those who do choose nursing as a career goal (Beck, 2000; Ditommasso, Rheaume, Woodside, & Gautreau, 2003). Power and empowerment were resounding themes in a grounded theory study exploring why women chose a career in nursing (Boughn & Lentini, 1999).

Summary of Factors Influencing Students' Career Choice

Occupational choice is influenced by many factors, such as a predisposition toward higher education, the search process, and choices available. The decision-making process is complex, and meeting this developmental milestone is critical. Though the literature is relatively sparse, researchers have clearly warned that few young people seem to view nursing as an ideal career option. Contemporary nursing calls for the very roles and responsibilities that achieving youth desire, yet students in that pipeline are not fully appreciative of the real nursing roles. There is a lack of essential congruence between the high school students' preferred career and nursing as a career.

THE HIGH SCHOOL STUDENT SURVEY

Consequently, the high school student survey was designed to examine education and career plans of North Dakota's high school students (grades 9–12). The study's key aim was to determine what affected students' decision making regarding the selection of nursing or another health profession as an occupational choice.

Method

Procedure and Participants

The survey was developed using questions based on multiple journal articles (Buerhaus, Donelan, Norman, & Dittus, 2005; Grossman & Northrop, 1993; Stevens & Walker, 1993), the North Dakota Healthcare Association (2002) study of health care career perceptions, and the North Dakota Nursing Needs Study survey (Moulton & Speaker, 2004). Questions included inquiries about demographic information, future career plans including career choice, and perception of the nursing field and specific written questions regarding barriers to choosing nursing that led to a qualitative analysis of the responses.

Sample

A stratified sample of 25 schools representing North Dakota's urban and rural counties was selected to represent the eastern and western halves of the state. Participant recruitment began with a phone call to the administrator of each potentially participating school. Once interest was affirmed, these administrators received an e-mail describing the study process. In response, the administrators provided the total number of their high school student body and a written confirmation of their permission for the researchers to solicit student participation. Without exception, administrators returned these letters of permission, and the process continued.

Unique Data Collection

We wanted a large cross section of student participants representing a rather diverse state and knew that a traditional mailed-survey approach would be challenging because of several issues, including Institutional Review Board approval for research with minors, concerns about a poor survey-in-envelope response rate, and cost. Our study population was the "Net Generation." Grunwald (2003) writes that teenagers want "new information" from the Internet, and they report they want to "learn more or to learn better." We also know that the use of the Internet to learn is not limited to schoolwork—today's students are often informal learners, seeking information on a variety of topics, such as personal health. Other common activities involve participating in online communities, showing others what they can do, or voicing their opinions. Thus, we opted to take advantage of that Net Generation mindset and put forth a request for an online survey to students. Through this indirect sampling method proposal, we readily obtained approval from the University of North Dakota Institutional Research Review Board, including a waiver of consent required from both parents and children.

Each participating school received a mailing of student participant recruitment flyers, which were distributed to the grades 9–12 students while they were in class. These flyers invited the students to go online for this survey, assured the students that study participation was anonymous (and thus, confidential), and explained that participants would be rewarded with a chance to be in a drawing to win an iPod nano. With this, consent was implied when the student went online, read the consent information, and completed the survey. Again, a waiver for signed consent was granted, and 571 students from selected schools across North Dakota participated in the study.

Results

Descriptions. Participating students represented a strong cross section of North Dakota's youth in urban, rural, and frontier sections across the state. The average age of respondents was 16.16 years, and the average reported grade point average (GPA) was 3.29 on a 4-point scale. Typical of our rather homogeneous state, almost all of the respondents were Caucasian (92%), and slightly more respondents were female (53%) than male (48%).

Ninety-three percent of student respondents indicated that they had begun to think about a possible career. The majority (70%) planned to pursue a 4-year college education. Of students with a GPA of at least 3.00, 78% planned to pursue a college education. Students were asked who had had the most influence on their decisions about future career plans. Over half of students (55%) indicated that their parents were the most influential; friends ranked second in influence, and teachers and counselors were rated as least influential at 3%.

Similar to the findings of the North Dakota Healthcare Association study (2002), 38% of students indicated an interest in health care (n = 216 students). However, nearly half (46%) of those students indicated an interest in more than one profession (e.g., health care and sciences). Business, technology, and engineering were strong interest vocations for a large percentage of these respondents.

Of those respondents potentially interested in health care, about one-third ($n = 120$) reported that they were interested in nursing along with other health care professions (e.g., interested in being a nurse or a physician). For other areas of health care interest, interest in medicine and in physical therapy followed nursing. Eighty-two of the students clearly intended to study nursing. Of those, 33% planned to obtain a baccalaureate degree as their highest degree. Interestingly, 25% of those interested in nursing indicated that they would like to obtain a PhD in nursing. Students most frequently indicated that the reasons they did not want to go into nursing were that they disliked nursing settings, found the work to be unpleasant, or hated blood or because of poor salary (see Figure 9.1).

Students were asked whether they agreed or disagreed with a variety of statements designed to evaluate their perceptions of nursing as a career option. The majority of respondents indicated that nursing is an important profession (84%), and nurses care for people in their time of need (82%). Fewer students felt that nursing is a good career for men (54%) and that nurses make a lot of money (56%) (see Figure 9.2).

Students who planned on pursuing a nursing career were asked to rate the importance of several factors in their decision. On average, the opportunity to make a difference in people's lives was rated as the most important factor in their nursing career interest, and the opinion or experience of a teacher or counselor was rated as the least important factor. Of those planning to go into nursing, most (91%) chose hospital as the employment setting in which they would most like to work; 19%

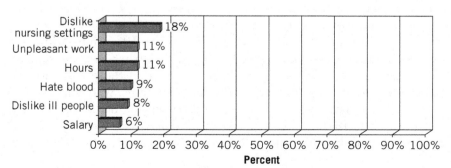

Figure 9.1 Reasons for not planning for a nursing career

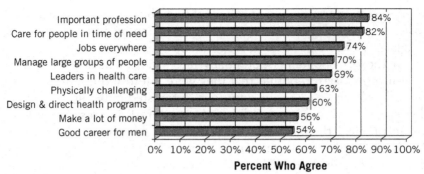

Figure 9.2 Students' agreement with perception statements

desired to be in nursing education, and long-term care settings were least desirable (11%).

Buerhaus et al. (2005) conducted a national survey of nursing students, asking similar questions. Unlike North Dakota high school students, 90% of those nursing students surveyed agreed that nursing is a good career for men and that nursing is physically challenging. Grossman and Northrop (1993) surveyed high school students in Florida and found that 72% believed that nurses managed large groups of people, 66% believed that nurses were leaders in directing and influencing national health policy and legislation, and 80% believed that a nursing career could be financially successful. Substantially fewer North Dakota students agreed that nurses earn a strong salary. Although the time difference between the two studies could be a consideration, there is an obvious disconnect between perception and truth related to nurses' salaries.

Findings from the current study indicate that among the North Dakota students who planned to go into nursing, 87% personally knew someone who works in the field. Presumably, those students have derived some information about nursing from this relationship. Additionally, 88% of students who wanted to go into nursing as a career had taken care of an ill person. In contrast, however, of those who did not plan to go into nursing, 86% personally knew someone who works in the field—the assumption being that this relationship could have influenced negatively a decision to pursue nursing as a career. Additionally, 73% of students who did not want to go into nursing as a career had taken care of an ill person.

Stevens and Walker (1993), in their study of high school students' opinions of nursing, found that knowing a nurse or the experience of caring for an ill individual was correlated significantly with interest in nursing as a career. These results did not correspond with the information gathered from North Dakota high school students. The two groups (interested in nursing and not interested in nursing) reported nearly equal rates of personally knowing a nurse. It is likely that students who are interested in nursing-type careers are more willing to care for someone; it cannot be inferred that experience caring for an ill individual leads to interest in a nursing career.

North Dakato students in the current study were asked to provide their own original responses to the following question: "When you think of nursing as a possible career choice, what is the ONE thing that would discourage you from obtaining a career in that field?" Responses were thematically coded, and major themes emerged: (a) the nature of the work, (b) competing interests, (c) educational demands, (d) schedules and shifts, and (e) other.

1 *Nature of the work.* Various job activities were listed as discouraging factors by 29% of respondents. Blood was mentioned very frequently, and responses involving needles, surgery, germs, and caring for sick or elderly patients were included in this category.

2 *Competing interests.* Sixteen percent of respondents indicated a lack of interest in nursing or that they were more interested in other occupations. These included responses such as "If I was a nurse, I wouldn't be able to be a teacher" and "I wouldn't want to be a nurse."

3 *Educational demands.* Some respondents (12%) indicated no desire for the necessary education or knowledge nursing requires. Many of these responses mentioned a requirement to go to school for a long time or no desire to acquire scientific knowledge or "learn big words."

4 *Schedules and shifts.* Beliefs about the schedule nurses work discouraged 11% of respondents. Many mentioned nights and weekends, as well as desiring flexibility for family life.

5 *Other.* Fewer respondents (4% each) indicated they would not like to pursue nursing because of the inevitable experience with death, the social interactions involved, the stress and responsibility, and the belief that nursing was a female job.

DISCUSSION

The nursing shortage is real; the long-term pipeline numbers are alarming. Across the nation, and in North Dakota, the future adequacy of the nursing workforce is disconcerting. Although the need for nurses is soaring, many applicants to nursing schools are not qualified for admission, and there is a nationwide lack of further educational capacity (National League for Nursing, 2005). This study suggested that, at best, 15% of high school students in North Dakota (82 of 571) might consider nursing as a career path in their future.

Considering our expected and traditional out-migration of youth, the prospective nurse workforce projections are shocking to North Dakota leaders. Most of the research suggests that those students who do choose nursing as a career do so mainly because of their desire for human contact and caring. These motives have not changed significantly over the past decade and were reflected in this study. Concern remains as to how to encourage more young people to consider the right path to nursing education and to launch their career trajectory by choosing nursing.

Hospitals continue to struggle with shortages of RNs (American Hospital Association, 2006). In independent national random sample surveys conducted recently, the vast majority of RNs, physicians, hospital executives, and chief nursing officers reported a nursing shortage in the hospitals where they admitted patients or were employed (Buerhaus et al., 2007). Moreover, aging is among the more powerful and omnipresent structural trends occurring in North Dakota and throughout the United States. To maintain the current ratio of paid long-term care personnel to the oldest of the elderly (those over 85), the long-term care workforce would need to grow by 2% per year from now until 2050, adding more than four million new long-term care personnel (Friedland, 2004). Government estimates for eldercare nursing shortages are even higher (Levy et al., 2005). The Institute for the Future of Aging Services (2007) is a policy research institute whose mission is to create a bridge between the practice, policy, and research communities to advance the development of services for America's aging population. Their 2007 report provides strong challenges as we consider how the United States will choose to meet growing demand for long-term care nursing in the near future. Moreover, the list of arenas for nurses in practice goes on and on.

The findings from this study indicate that more and more, nursing is not perceived as a positive career option. Could it be that young people who do not choose nursing view the career as being more negative than it actually is? Hemsley-Brown and Foskett (1999) suggest that young people tend to exaggerate the negative attributes of options they have not chosen. Alternatively, is it that nursing is just not seen as "cool"? There are many negative impressions of nurses' work. There are certainly misconceptions about the work of a nurse. In many ways, the nursing profession can offer the exact work that young people report they aspire to: work that enables them to be leaders, change agents, problem solvers, autonomous workers, caregivers, teachers, policy makers, career climbers, and those who earn a rewarding income stream. Students need to know the roles of nurses in a way that makes sense for them.

Policy Impact of the High School Student Survey

The survey information provided the evidence base for North Dakota leaders to plan action steps designed to influence the career choices of high school students. The process of developing action steps to increase the number of students interested in health care careers began when the survey results were presented to the North Dakota State Legislative Council Interim Healthcare Budget Committee during a presentation on the status of the health care workforce. Although the original intent of the survey was to look at nursing recruitment, it has provided a wealth of information about a wide range of health- and non-health-related occupations. This information also was used to inform a statewide North Dakota Health Workforce Summit in December 2006, which involved 200 individuals representing state government, statewide health care organizations, economic development commissions, health care employers, and education programs.

The Health Workforce Summit resulted in several action steps related to introduction of health care careers for elementary and high school students (Amundson, Moulton, Wakefield, Beattie, & Gibbens, 2007). One of the action steps was to develop a curriculum plan and design a workshop to engage parents, given that they are influential in the choice of future careers. Educators (including K–12 and higher education programs) will work with health care providers in order to include exposure to clinical experiences (e.g., job shadowing) for students in concert with workshops for parents to provide more information about health careers. Another action step is program development that uses existing community resources (health care employers, etc.) to market career opportunities, increase student experiences, and create resources for use by career counselors and teachers. This may include encouraging health care providers or education programs to adopt a K–12 class as a community service project. They could provide tours, presentations, and experiences related to introducing students to the health professions. These ideas could also be used in other states that are interested in increasing the recruitment of students into health careers, and North Dakota will certainly gain by considering additional recruitment efforts reported by state nursing centers in states across the nation.

Further Policy Recommendations

The Pew Health Professions Commission (Coffey-Love, 2001) stressed that there must be an increase in enrollment of students in nursing colleges to prevent a future worsening of the nursing shortage crisis. They suggested the initiation of a collaborative approach between nursing, the community, academia, professional organizations, and governments in order to develop early educational outreach programs for stimulating young people's interest in nursing (Nevidjon & Erickson, 2001). The following recommendations are offered:

- *Translate the existing research.* The literature reported within this chapter stands for the continuous challenge: translate the research into action! For over a decade, visionaries have forecast this nursing shortage crisis and have offered recommendations for long-term action for the long haul. Within this chapter, there is much to consider from former admonitions regarding youth and for influencing career choices. Essentially, parents, teachers, and counselors must hear the strong message of satisfaction from choosing a nursing career because parents, teachers, and counselors, in that order, have influence on the career choices of our youth.
- *RNs: Be positive messengers.* We know that students who choose nursing are largely influenced by a nurse in practice; we also know that students who do not choose nursing have been influenced by a nurse acquaintance. Nurses themselves are the best source of positive information and influence out there, and nurses must appreciate this responsibility. It may seem difficult to find passion and joy in nursing during these tumultuous times (Albaugh, 2005). However, it is essential to build and retain satisfaction, not only for the personal and professional energy that comes from passion and joy, but also as an indirect means for resolving the nursing shortage.

- *Management: Support the messengers.* Management and organizational structure can support the RN messenger and influence morale. Many companies, offering a variety of goods and services, tout models for the twenty-first-century organization that treats its people with respect, gives them unprecedented responsibility, holds them strictly accountable, and delivers essential rewards and recognition that allow for heightened satisfaction. Health care facilities that employ nurses need to follow this example and emphasize the value, leadership opportunities, and rewards of their nursing workforce. It is the right thing to do, and it just makes good sense; positive people make positive messengers.
- *Provide accurate information.* Increase dissemination of attractive and accurate information regarding nursing as a career, including an "instant career" upon graduation, the wide variety of settings and schedule options, and desire for both males and females in the nursing workforce.
- *Link career attractors to the attraction of nursing.* We know what matters to youth in career consideration, and many desirable career characteristics are found in nursing. Encourage the development of programs to expose students to the benefits of a career in nursing, starting in grade school, peaking in middle school, and throughout K–12 education.
- *Enhance the attraction to eldercare.* Each state could be encouraged to prepare a detailed plan for addressing long-term care RN shortages in each state, including the long-term plan for attracting youth to nursing. The plan could be based on the collaboration of all stakeholders, identifying current shortages at the state level and setting goals for meeting needs with a 5-year action plan, perhaps tied to funding at the state and federal levels.
- *Attract students from diverse backgrounds.* From 2000 to 2050, the U.S. non-Hispanic, white population is projected to lose population and to make up just 50.1% of the total population in 2050. People of Hispanic origin are expected to increase their proportion of the U.S. population to 24.4% in 2050; the black population is projected to be at 14.6%; the Asian American population is expected to grow at an even faster rate to 8% of our total population by 2050; and the nation's American Indian, Eskimo, and Aleut population is projected to grow steadily, for a proportion of 1.1% by 2050 (U.S. Department of State, 2004). Minorities could well be the majority, but the nation's nursing workforce currently has

a white face (Seago & Spetz, 2005). Recruitment and retention of minority nursing students is a long-standing issue; if the nursing profession is to thrive in the coming years, we need to embrace potential nurses from diverse ethnicities and cultures.

■ *Expand nursing programs and address faculty issues.* Across the nation, schools of nursing have been responsive to the challenge of increasing nursing student numbers. Yet current and looming faculty shortages are of concern in all states. The role of a faculty member can be very demanding and come with high expectations. For potential nurse educators, the appeal to become faculty in higher education is reportedly lessening. Serious solutions need to be implemented for the published deterrents to the academic role, such as salary disparities, role stress, non-teaching requirements, and general demands.

CONCLUSION

The nursing shortage is deepening in the United States. The decision to become a nurse is obviously complex; it involves many factors and influences throughout the life of a young person. Strategies that will best reach potential students and increase student interest are essential, as well as developing strategies to increase the educational capacity of schools of nursing. Targeting elementary and particularly middle school students can result in a long-term investment for the future of nursing. Nurses can play a keen role in recruitment by emphasizing the real rewards and satisfaction of nursing, rather than the stressors and challenges of their education and the work. Nurse researchers and other workforce researchers may use the evidence from these findings to form the basis for new, innovative research, recruitment strategies, and policy changes.

> *A society grows great when old men and women plant trees under whose shade they know they will never sit.*
>
> —Greek proverb

REFERENCES

Albaugh, J. (2005). Resolving the nursing shortage: Finding passion and joy in nursing. *Urologic Nursing, 25*(1), 53–54.

Alexander, C., & Fraser, J. (2001). The promotion of health careers to high school students in the New England health area: The views of high school careers advisers. *Australian Journal of Rural Health, 9,* 145–149.

American Hospital Association. (2006, April). *The state of America's hospitals.* Retrieved February 10, 2007, from www.aha.org/aha/research-and-trends/health-and-hospital-trends/2006.html

American Nurses Association. (1965). *A position paper.* New York: Author.

Amundson, M., Moulton, P., Wakefield, M., Beattie, S., & Gibbens, B. (2007). *North Dakota health care workforce: Planning together to meet future health care needs.* Policy Brief Part 2 of 2. Retrieved April 15, 2008, from http://ruralhealth.und.edu/projects/nursing/pdf/HealthCareWorkforcePolicyBrief2.pdf

Bandura, A., Barbaranelli, C., Caprara, G., & Pastorelli, C. (2001). Self-efficacy beliefs as shapers of children's aspirations and career trajectories. *Child Development, 72,* 187–206.

Beck, C. T. (2000). The experience of choosing nursing as a career. *Journal of Nursing Education, 39*(7), 320–324.

Benz, C. (1996). School to work: Beginning the journey in middle school. *Clearing House, 70*(2), 90–94.

Blasdell, A. L., & Hudgins-Brewer, S. (1999). High school counselors' perceptions of the academic and personality attributes important for a career in nursing. *Journal of Nursing Education, 38*(4), 176–179.

Bloomer, M., & Hodkinson, P. (1997). *Moving into FE: The voice of the learner.* London: Further Education Development Agency.

Boughn, S., & Lentini, A. (1999). Why do women choose nursing? *Journal of Nursing Education, 38*(4), 156–161.

Buerhaus, P., Donelan, K., Norman, L., & Dittus, R. (2005). Nursing students' perception of a career in nursing: Impact of a national campaign designed to attract people into the nursing profession. *Journal of Professional Nursing, 21*(2), 75–83.

Buerhaus, P., Donelan, K., Ulrich, B., DesRoches, C., Norman, L., & Dittus, R. (2007). Impact of the nursing shortage on hospital patient care: Comparative perspectives. *Health Affairs, 26*(3), 227–235.

Cabrera, A., & La Nasa, S. (2000). Understanding the college-choice process. In A. Cabrera & S. La Nasa (Eds.), *Understanding the college choice of disadvantaged students: New directions for institutional research* (pp. 5–22). San Francisco: Jossey-Bass.

Christie, H., Munro, M., & Fisher, T. (2004). Leaving university early: Exploring the difference between continuing and non-continuing students. *Studies in Higher Education, 29*(5), 617–636.

Coffey-Love, M. (2001). Said another way: The nursing shortage: What is your role? *Nursing Forum, 36*(2), 29–36.

Cohen, J., Palumbo, M., Rambur, B., & Mongeon, J. (2004). Middle school students' perceptions of an ideal career and a career in nursing. *Journal of Professional Nursing, 20*(3), 202–210.

Costello, M. A. (2002). Nursing coalition aims to interest children in healthcare careers. *AHA News, 37*(16), 5. Item 4580588.

Ditommaso, E., Rheaume, A., Woodside, R., &. Gautreau, G. (2003). Why students choose nursing: A decade ago, most nursing students said that they chose nursing because they wanted to care for people and help others. Are those desires still true today? *The Canadian Nurse, 99*(5), 25–29.

Friedland, R. (2004). *Caregivers and long-term care needs in the 21st century: Will public policy meet the challenge?* Washington, DC: Long-Term Care Financing Project, Georgetown University.

Goldmark, J. (1922). *Nursing and nursing education in the United States: Report of the committee for the study of nursing education and report of a survey by Josephine Goldmark.* New York: Garland.

Grossman, D., Arnold, L., Sullivan, J., Cameron, M. E., & Munro, B. (1989). High school students' perceptions of nursing as a career: A pilot study. *Journal of Nursing Education, 28*(1), 21.

Grossman, D., & Northrop, C. (1993). What high school students think of a nursing career: A survey of Dade county senior high schools. *Journal of Nursing Education, 32,* 157–162.

Grunwald, P. (2003). *Key technology trends: Excerpts from new survey research findings.* Exploring the Digital Generation. Washington, DC: Educational Technology, U.S. Department of Education.

Haagenson, D. (1995, March 7). *Testimony on SB2192 before the Senate Human Service Committee.* Bismarck, ND: North Dakota Legislative Council.

Harker, D., Slade, P., & Harker, M. (2001). Exploring the decision process of "school leavers" and "mature students" in university choice. *Journal of Marketing for Higher Education, 11*(2) 1–20.

Hemsley-Brown, J., & Foskett, N. H. (1999). Career desirability: Young people's perceptions of nursing as a career. *Journal of Advanced Nursing, 29*(6), 1342–1350.

Institute for the Future of Aging Services. (2007). *The long-term care workforce: Can the crisis be fixed?* (Prepared for National Commission for Quality Long-Term Care). Washington, DC: Author.

Kingdon, J. W. (1995). *Agendas, alternatives, and public policies.* New York: Harper Collins College.

Larsen, P., McGill, J., & Palmer, S. (2003). Factors influencing career decisions: Perspectives of nursing students in three types of programs. *Journal of Nursing Education, 42*(4), 168–173.

Leach, L., & Zepke, N. (2005). *Student decision making by prospective tertiary students. A review of existing New Zealand and overseas literature.* Retrieved April 15, 2008, from http://www.educationcounts.govt.nz/publications/tertiary_education/ student_decision_making_by_prospective_tertiary_students,_a_review_of_existing_ new_zealand_and_overseas_literature

Leonard, D., & Iannone, J. (2000). Recruiting future nurses: A collaborative project. *Nursing Connections, 13*(3), 55–61.

Levy, C., Epstein, A., Landry, L., Kramer, A., Harvell, J., & Liggings, C. (2005). *Literature review and synthesis of physician practices in nursing homes* (Report prepared for Office of the Assistant Secretary for Planning and Evaluation). Washington, DC: U.S. Department of Health and Human Services.

Lewis, E. P. (1985). Taking care of business: The ANA house of delegates, 1985. *Nursing Outlook, 33*(5), 239–243.

Lozada, M. (2001). Job shadowing: Career exploration at work. *Techniques, 76*(8), 30–33.

May, F., Champion, V., & Austin, J. (1991). Public values and beliefs toward nursing as a career. *Journal of Nursing Education, 30,* 303–310.

Mignor, D., Cadenhead, G., & McKee, A. (2002). High school counselor's knowledge of professional nursing as a career option. *Nursing Education Perspectives, 23*(2), 86–89.

Moulton, P. (2006). *Rural health facts. North Dakota health professions: Nursing supply student survey results.* Grand Forks, ND: Center for Rural Health, University of North Dakota School of Medicine and Health Sciences. Retrieved August 20, 2007, from http://www.med.und.nodak.edu/depts/rural/pdf/fs_nursingsupply.pdf

Moulton, P., & Speaker, K. (2004). *North Dakota nursing needs study: Student survey results.* Report part of the North Dakota Center for Health Workforce Data. Retrieved May 24, 2007, from http://ruralhealth.und.edu/projects/nursing/pdf/year2 studentsurveyresults.pdf

National League for Nursing. (2005). *Nurse faculty shortage fact sheet.* Retrieved March 19, 2007, http://www.nln.org/governmentaffairs/pdf/NurseFacultyShortage.pdf

Nevidjon, B., & Erickson, J. (2001). The nursing shortage: Solutions for the short and long term. *Online Journal of Issues in Nursing, 6*(1), Manuscript 4.

North Dakota Healthcare Association. (2002). *Healthcare career perceptions.* Bismarck, ND: Author.

Nurse Practices Act, NDCC 43-12.1-09 (2003). Retrieved March 10, 2004, from http://www.legis.nd.gov/cencode/t43c121.pdf

Pellman, K., & Meyer, C. (2000, May). C.A.R.E.: A recruitment concept shaping tomorrow's nursing supply. *Kansas Nurse, 75*(5), 1–2.

Perna, L. W. (2000) Racial/ethnic group differences in college enrollment decisions. In A. Cabrera & S. La Nasa (Eds.), *Understanding college choice among disadvantaged students: New directions for institutional research* (pp. 65–83). San Francisco: Jossey-Bass.

Peters, M., & Marshall, J. (1996). *Individualism and community: Education and social policy in the postmodern condition.* London: Falmer Press.

Reiskin, H., & Haussler, S. (1994). Multicultural students' perceptions of nursing as a career. *Image: Journal of Nursing Scholarship, 26*(1), 61–64.

Rognstad, M. K., Aasland, O., & Granu, V. (2004). How do nursing students regard their future career? Career preferences in the post-modern society. *Nurse Education Today, 24*(7), 493–500.

Rose, W. (2006). *HB1245: A case study of the process that rescinded North Dakota's nursing education requirements.* Unpublished doctoral dissertation, University of North Dakota.

Seago, J., & Spetz, J. (2005). California's minority majority and the white face of nursing. *Journal of Nursing Education, 44*(12), 555–62.

Stevens, K., & Walker, E. (1993). Choosing a career: Why not nursing for more high school seniors? *Journal of Nursing Education, 32*, 13–17.

Toepfer, C. (1994). Vocational/career/occupational education at the middle level. *Middle School Journal 25*(3), 59–65.

Tomey, A., Schwier, B., Marticke, N., & May, F. (1996). Students' perceptions of ideal and nursing career choices. *Nursing Outlook, 44*, 27–30.

Tyler, D. (1998). Vocational pathways and the decline of the linear model. In *Vocational Knowledge and Institutions: Changing Relationships. Proceedings of the 6th International Conference on Post-compulsory Training,* Gold Coast, Queensland, pp. 77–87.

U.S. Bureau of Labor Statistics. (2006–2007). Registered nurses. In *Occupational outlook handbook.* Washington, DC: U.S. Department of Labor. Retrieved April 10, 2007, from http://www.bls.gov/oco/ocos083.htm#outlook

U.S. Department of State, Bureau of International Information Programs. (2004). *Increasing diversity predicted in U.S. population.* Washington, DC: Author. Retrieved May 30, 2007, from http://www.america.gov/st/washfile-english/2004/March/2004 0318124311CMretroP0.4814264.html

Williams, B., Wertenberger, D. H., & Gushuliak, T. (1997). Why students choose nursing. *Journal of Nursing Education. 36*(7), 346–348.

Wright, S. (2001). In middle school career and technical education programs, the name of the game is "exploration." *Techniques, 76*(8), 26–29.

10

The Looming Crisis of an Inadequate Pipeline for Nursing Faculty

BRENDA CLEARY, JAMES W. BEVILL JR., LINDA M. LACEY, AND JENNIFER G. NOONEY

In the academic year 2005–2006, 137,000 qualified applicants were turned away from schools of nursing across the country, principally because of an inability to fill faculty positions (National League for Nursing, 2006). North Carolina alone denied admission to 8,116 (over 50%) qualified applicants who applied for admission to entry-level RN programs (North Carolina Center for Nursing, 2006a). The situation will likely worsen in light of a shortage of new nursing faculty and the aging of current faculty.

In 2006 the North Carolina Center for Nursing (NCCN) examined the projected supply of nursing faculty in the state in relation to growing demand. Coupled with a longitudinal educational mobility study of the state's registered nurses, the forecast showed that the growing faculty shortage is real and that its root cause is a growing shortfall in the pipeline of RNs prepared educationally to assume faculty roles (Bevill, Cleary, Lacey, & Nooney, 2007; Cleary, Bevill, Lacey, & Nooney, 2007). The purpose of this chapter is to present these findings regarding the faculty shortage and to discuss their implications for public and other policy changes.

FACULTY SUPPLY AND DEMAND

A recent forecast of nurse faculty supply and demand in North Carolina (North Carolina Center for Nursing, 2006b) projects that the state may have less than half of the faculty needed to prepare new nurses by 2020. The demand forecasting model assumed a 25% increase in enrollments in RN education programs and an 8% increase in enrollments in LPN education programs, as recommended by the North Carolina Institute of Medicine's (NCIOM, 2004) Task Force on the North Carolina Nursing Workforce. The NCCN was a collaborating partner on the NCIOM. Projected supply took into account current faculty members' average age, trends in educational mobility among North Carolina nurses, preferences for positions in education versus practice, and expected retirement patterns.

The demand estimates in Figure 10.1 not only assume achievement of the increases recommended by the NCIOM over a 5-year period, from 2004 to 2009, but also assume that enrollments will remain

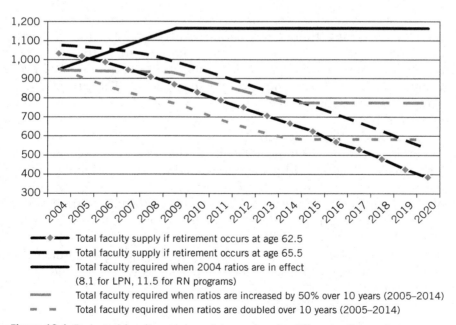

Figure 10.1 Projected faculty supply and demand under different retirement thresholds and student-to-faculty ratios

steady through 2020. The demand for nursing faculty was further con-figured as a product of the number of students enrolled in nursing education programs and the ratio between students and faculty. Al-though the North Carolina Board of Nursing requires all pre-licensure nursing programs to maintain a student–faculty ratio of 10 to 1 or less in clinical settings, overall student–faculty ratios are higher and vary by program type. In 2004 the ratio in North Carolina's LPN programs was 8.1 students for each faculty member, and in RN programs the ratio varied by program type: 13.5:1 in associate degree programs, 8.9:1 in hospital diploma programs, and 10:1 in pre-licensure baccalaureate programs for an average (RN) student-to-faculty ratio of 11.54:1. The three estimates of demand in Figure 10.1 differ because of changing assumptions about those ratios:

- No change (2004 ratios are maintained)
- A 50% increase above 2004 levels in the number of students for each faculty member, implemented gradually over a 10-year period
- A 100% increase (or doubling) in the number of students per faculty, also implemented gradually over a 10-year period.

Changes in the student-to-faculty ratio produce significant shifts in the expected demand for nursing faculty over time. However, consequences of the various scenarios, such as increased compensation requirements, increased burnout, or earlier rates of retirement because of changes in workload, are not taken into account in the forecasting model. Further, neither was the potential impact on the clinical sites explored, if there were larger clinical groups.

Supply projections in this analysis were constructed from two ele-ments: the number of faculty expected to retire, given age demograph-ics and assumptions about retirement age, and the number of RNs with master's or doctoral degrees expected to assume a faculty position. The latter element in the supply projection was derived from a historical analysis of RN education and work patterns in North Carolina from 1995 through 2004, based on information in the RN license renewal forms compiled by the North Carolina Board of Nursing. These patterns re-vealed that even though the number of licensed RNs holding a master's or doctoral degree almost doubled between 1995 and 2004, the percent-age as a total of the RN workforce remained small, and proportionately fewer were employed in nursing education programs each year.

In 1995, 15% of all RNs with master's degrees or doctorates were nurse educators; by 2004, the percentage had dropped to 11%. Using that trend, and extrapolating over time, the predicted proportion is about 8.7% in 2020. An estimate of the expected number of faculty likely to be added to the faculty workforce each year was derived by identifying all RNs who elevated their highest degree status to the master's level each year relative to the previous year, and then applying the annual percentage of all master's and higher-degree RNs employed in schools of nursing. The period 1995–2004 used actual counts. Future estimates were extrapolated from those historical trends.

An age profile of master's and doctorally prepared RNs employed in schools of nursing in 2004 was created from the RN license file database and "aged out" by identifying how many passed the age of 62 or 65 in any given year. The number reaching these retirement thresholds was subtracted from the faculty supply count, and the number of RNs with new master's degrees expected to choose faculty roles was then added. The result is two supply lines in the chart, one assuming that all faculty will leave the workforce between the ages of 62 and 63 and another that assumes they will leave between the ages of 65 and 66. Regardless of which supply line is most accurate, both drop rapidly from 2004 levels, revealing an insufficient number of new faculty coming in each year to replace those being lost to retirement (see Figure 10.1).

THE PIPELINE FOR FACULTY ROLES

The nursing profession has a long history of lack of consensus regarding the educational preparation of registered nurses. Multiple paths exist for pre-licensure educational preparation, and divisiveness around this issue continues despite recent evidence of the impact of a more highly educated workforce on such patient outcomes as mortality (National Quality Forum, 2006). The percentage of RNs holding an associate degree as their highest degree has risen steadily. Despite admirable attempts at strengthening articulation between levels of nursing education across the country, the vast majority of nurses never complete additional degrees in nursing beyond entry, and those who do rarely complete more than one additional degree (North Carolina Center for Nursing, 2006a). We find ourselves faced with an unintended but serious consequence that lies at the very center of the profession's looming crisis: we do not have anywhere near an adequate pipeline for future nursing faculty.

The NCCN, as the first state-level agency dedicated to nurse work-force planning, has compiled 20 years of longitudinal data, including educational information, on the state's nursing workforce. This extensive database places us in an optimal position to understand how patterns of educational preparation led to this current crisis and allows us to develop some insight into how to address it. Although these analyses employ state-level data, they reflect a growing problem throughout the nation.

Method for Examining Issues Related to the Faculty Pipeline

Through information collected as part of the license renewal process in North Carolina over the past 20 years, two cohorts of newly graduated RN licensees were followed over time to determine the extent, nature, and timing of educational mobility beyond their entry-to-practice de-gree. Every RN with an active license to practice in 1984 who graduated from an entry-level program in 1983 or 1984 was selected. A second study cohort was selected from the 1994 licensees who graduated from entry-level programs in 1993 or 1994.

RNs in the 1983/1984 cohort were tracked through 2003 if they maintained an active North Carolina license throughout the 20-year pe-riod. In 1983 and 1984, 3,726 nurses were identified as new graduates, and 2,418 (64.9%) of the original group remained in 2003. RNs in the 1993/1994 cohort were followed for the first 10 years of their careers, until 2003. At the beginning of the analysis, in 1994, there were 5,654 new graduates with active licenses to practice in North Carolina. At the end of their first 10 years in practice, in 2003, 4,211 (74.5%) of the origi-nal group still held active licenses in the state.

Findings

New graduates in 1983 or 1984 were relatively young, with about half of the cohort members under the age of 25. That cohort was predomi-nantly female (95.4%) and white (91.8%). Their initial nursing degrees reflect the expansion of associate degree programs in nursing (ADNs) during the 1970s: nearly 60% of this cohort began practice with an ADN. About 30% began with a bachelor's of science in nursing (BSN), and nearly 11% began in a hospital diploma program.

The 1993/1994 cohort of new graduates in North Carolina was sig-nificantly older: only 30% were under age 25, and 17% were age 40 or older when they graduated from their entry-level programs. Although still a small percentage, there were proportionately more men in this later cohort, but the racial composition of the 1993/1994 cohort remained comparable to the 1983/1984 group. Finally, there was a 10% increase in the proportion of new graduates coming out of ADN programs and a concomitant decrease in representation from hospital diploma programs and BSN programs.

By 2003, 14.6 % of the final 1983/1984 cohort of RNs (n = 2,418) whose pre-licensure education occurred at the associate degree level (n = 1,420) had obtained BSNs, and another 3.4% had obtained a master's of science in nursing (MSN) as their highest nursing degree. None had obtained doctoral degrees. Among the 255 nurses initially receiving diplomas (n = 255), 16.1 % went on to earn BSNs and 3.5% MSNs as their highest nursing degree. As with the associate degree group, none in this group obtained doctoral degrees in the 20-year period of study. Among nurses with BSNs as their pre-licensure educational credential (n = 743), 17.5% earned MSNs, and 0.8% earned doctorates. The timing of advances in education varied widely; some nurses in this cohort advanced just a few years after initial licensure, whereas many others advanced during the second decade of their careers.

The pattern continued in the final 1993/1994 cohort in 2003 (N = 4,211), with 11.7% (n = 298) of RNs initially prepared in North Carolina's hospital diploma programs compared with 8.5% of AD graduates (n = 2,849) pursuing BSNs. Overall results were similar to the earlier cohort—that is, the vast majority who pursued graduate education by 2003 to become prepared at or above the master's level originally had entered nursing with a BSN.

DISCUSSION

As indicated by the composite findings in Table 10.1, the likelihood of eventually attaining a master's or doctoral degree is unquestionably linked to entry-level starting points. Nurses entering the profession through a BSN program require only one additional degree to reach the master's level, whereas traditional articulation pathways require diploma program and ADN graduates to obtain baccalaureate degrees before entering a master's degree program. Policy changes that allow more master's degree programs to accept students without prerequisite baccalaureate degrees may change this historical pattern and thus increase the pool of RNs with master's degrees or higher education.

Table 10.1

PERCENTAGE OF COHORT MEMBERS ACHIEVING MASTER'S AND DOCTORAL PREPARATION

MOBILITY TYPE AND TIMELINE	ENTERED WITH HOSPITAL DIPLOMA		ENTERED WITH ASSOCIATE DEGREE		ENTERED WITH BSN		ALL RN ENTRY DEGREES	
	83/84 cohort	93/94 cohort	83/84 cohort	93/94 cohort	83/84 cohort	93/94 cohort	83/84 cohort	93/94 cohort
After 10 years	n = 304	n = 298	n = 1,664	n = 2,849	n = 882	n = 1,064	n = 2,850	n = 4,211
% MSN	0.3	1.3	0.4	0.9	6.8	14.3	2.4	4.3
% MA/MS	0.3	1.7	1.1	0.7	4.9	3.1	2.2	1.4
% doctorate	0	0	0.0	0.1	0.2	0.3	0.1	0.1
Total %	0.6	3.0	1.6	1.7	11.9	17.7	4.7	5.8
Total #	2	9	26	49	105	188	133	246
After 20 years	n = 255	NA	n = 1,420	NA	n = 743	NA	n = 2,418	NA
% MSN	3.5		3.4		17.5		7.7	
% MA/MS	0.8		1.7		6.6		3.1	
% doctorate	0		0		0.8		0.3	
Total %	4.3		5.1		24.9		11.1	
Total #	11		72		185		268	

Further, a focus on increasing enrollments in pre-licensure BSN programs should increase significantly the faculty pipeline. The initial preparation of 79% of the 133 RNs from the 1983/1984 cohort and 188 (76%) of the 246 RNs from the 1993/1994 cohort who held a master's degree or higher at the end of 10 years was a BSN. Nevertheless, even among BSN graduates, the number of nurses pursuing graduate education is woefully inadequate. Moreover, for the most part, academic sector salaries remain noncompetitive with those in health care delivery, further dramatically decreasing the subset of graduate-prepared nurses pursuing faculty positions. Faculty salaries are another policy area ripe for change.

In addition to the faculty pipeline findings described here in detail, we also discovered interesting effects of age, gender, and race/ethnicity, with younger nurses, male nurses, and nurses of color more likely to further their education. These findings suggest that keeping nursing in front of young people as a desirable career option and the profession's other attempts to increase ethnic and gender diversify may yield benefits beyond what they were originally intended to produce.

Policy Implications

The perfect storm is building owing to the shrinking percentage of RNs in the pipeline for pursuing graduate degrees and interested in faculty positions. The need for a large influx of new faculty members prepared at the master's and doctoral levels is a critical component of nursing's ability to address the foreboding shortage that will occur as a result of the aging of the baby boom generation. Unfortunately, it is doubtful that, given current trends as depicted in this study, we will produce adequate numbers of nursing faculty to meet the increased demand for faculty while at the same time replacing retiring faculty. Based on the evidence reported here, it is also time to be creative and strategic in planning and policy development related to the future of nursing education—to embrace new paradigms in advanced nursing education. The situation calls for forging new partnerships between nursing education and practice, as well as between educational institutions. Further, in order for any increase in faculty-to-student ratios to be successful, it would have to include the cooperation of the clinical sites and their staff in the design of such changes in clinical policies.

Changes in nursing education and practice may require regulatory, professional, or institutional shifts in policy. The last resort would be a legislative mandatory change. Several examples of policy change derived from this study include the following:

- Obtaining additional financial resources directed at increasing enrollments in baccalaureate and higher-degree nursing programs.
- Expanding programs that offer the opportunity for nurses currently prepared at the associate degree level to pursue directly a master's degree.
- Continuing the development of new partnerships between community colleges and 4-year colleges and universities specifically designed to increase the number of BSN graduates. In addition to the hundreds of articulation agreements currently in place between the two types of schools, more innovative and strategic initiatives that produce stronger outcomes are needed, such as the partnership prototype launched through the Oregon Consortium for Nursing Education (2007).
- Furthering the development of partnerships between nursing education and nursing service and the use of clinical simulation to augment clinical instruction.

These are just a few of an impressive array of strategies being developed to address the evolving shortage of nursing faculty, but one thing is for sure—the time to act is now.

REFERENCES

Bevill, J. W., Cleary, B. L., Lacey, L. M., & Nooney, J. G. (2007). Educational mobility of RNs in North Carolina: Who will teach tomorrow's nurses? *American Journal of Nursing, 107,* 60–70.

Cleary, B. L., Bevill, J. W., Lacey, L. M., & Nooney, J. G. (2007). Evidence and root causes of an inadequate pipeline for nursing faculty. *Nursing Administration Quarterly, 31*(2), 124–128.

National League for Nursing. (2006, August). *Data reveal slowdown in nursing school admission growth.* Retrieved August 15, 2007, from http://www.nln.org/newsreleases/databook_08_06.pdf

National Quality Forum. (2006). *Nurses' educational preparation and patient outcomes in acute care: A case for quality.* Retrieved August 15, 2007, from http://www.qualityforum.org/pdf/nursing-quality/FinalNursesEdPreparation.pdf

North Carolina Center for Nursing. (2006a). *North Carolina trends in nursing education: 2003–2005.* Retrieved August 15, 2007, from http://www.nursenc.org/research/Trends2006/Final%20Report%20Schools%202005.pdf

North Carolina Center for Nursing. (2006b). *Forecasting the supply of and demand for nursing faculty in North Carolina: 2004–2020.* Retrieved August 15, 2007, from http://www.ga.unc.edu/NCCN//research/Forecasting%20the%20Supply%20and%20Demand%20of%20Nursing%20Faculty%20in%20North%20Carolina%202004-2020.pdf

North Carolina Institute of Medicine. (2004). *North Carolina nursing workforce report.* Retrieved June 1, 2007, from http://www.nciom.org/projects/nursingworkforce/nursingreport.html

Oregon Consortium for Nursing Education. (2007). *OCNE model.* Retrieved June 1, 2007, from http://www.ocne.org/about.php

Clinical Simulation and the Need for Evidence-Based Policy

FELISSA R. LASHLEY AND WENDY NEHRING

There are many reasons for using simulation for teaching in the health professions. Patients today expect their treatment and care to be delivered by expert, highly qualified personnel, not a novice learner (Murphy, Torsher, & Dunn, 2007). However, many clinical sites can provide only a limited number of placements for students, thus restricting the number of qualified nurses available to provide quality patient care. Still other clinical sites charge for clinical placements and may restrict the type of procedures students are authorized to perform, even when accompanied by their instructors. Emphasis has been placed on preventing patient injuries and reducing medical errors, as highlighted by various national reports, including most notably *To Err Is Human,* which originated from the Institute of Medicine (Kohn, Corrigan, & Donaldson, 2000).

Utilizing simulation is one way in which the students' knowledge, skills, and attitudes can be developed while at the same time patients are protected from unnecessary risk (Ziv, Wolpe, Small, & Glick, 2003). It provides a nonthreatening environment to practice without practitioners being concerned about their responsibility to a patient or worrying about harming the patient (Morgan, Cleave-Hogg, McIlroy, & Devitt, 2002). Simulation may be used across the continuum from novice to expert. Those who have more expertise may take advantage of the simulation approach for such activities as continuing professional education and recertification in a specialty area, thus allowing a systematic career-long approach for acquiring and practicing speed, agility, accuracy (Freeman et al., 2001), and other skills.

The impetuses for incorporating simulation in the health care professions include the following:

- Public demand for fewer patient complications (Ahlberg et al., 2002)
- Less acceptance of the use of animals or human cadavers for surgical or other types of practice or experimentation (Ahlberg et al.)
- A greater need for improvement of clinical competence; need for improvement of clinical expertise
- The need for competency assessment before patient care (Grenvik & Schaefer, 2004)
- Increased enhancement of the quality of patient care (Issenberg, 2006)
- Enhancement of the safety of patient care (Issenberg, 2006)
- Provision of the best possible education for students

In addition, mistakes made while using simulation do not harm actual patients, so they are more easily exposed, discussed, and reviewed without concerns of liability, guilt, or blame. Making mistakes while using simulation allows for the breaking of the culture of silence and avoids denial regarding mistakes made or the questioning of competence (Ziv et al., 2006). Additionally, it allows for a comprehensive evaluation by the instructor of the student's knowledge and skills in clinical practice.

Simulation may refer to various learning modalities and can be defined in many ways. Smith and Gaba (2001) define simulation as the "artificial replication of sufficient elements of a real-world domain to achieve a specified goal" (p. 26). Lammers (2007) defines simulation as "the artificial representation of a situation, environment or event that provides an experience for the purposes of learning, evaluation, or research" (p. 506). Using this definition, we may think of methods of simulation in a very broad sense in regard to utilization in health care. Among the options available for use are full-body and body-part mannequins, high-fidelity patient simulators, standardized patients, virtual human actors, virtual reality, and various computerized and Web-based programs. In this chapter, each of these is discussed briefly along with an in-depth discussion of high-fidelity patient simulation. Last, policy is discussed in relation to the use of simulation in nursing education.

TYPES OF SIMULATION

The earliest used simulators were mannequins, both full-body models and models of parts, such as limbs or organ systems. Names given to the partial mannequins included partial task trainers or low-tech simulators (Ziv et al., 2003). Among the early full-body types of mannequins was the well-known M. Chase doll, which became known as Mrs. Chase. The M. J. Chase doll company manufactured these from 1889 to the 1970s. The potential for use of these mannequins in health care, and particularly nursing education, was realized early on. To fulfill this potential, Mrs. Chase models were manufactured to be waterproof, so that bed baths could be practiced, and advancements in design evolved. These included joints, injection sites, anatomical accuracy, and orifices to facilitate practicing invasive procedures such as the placement of rectal tubes. Models representative of various age groups, such as infants and the elderly, and various ethnic backgrounds were available (Herrmann, 1981; Nehring & Lashley, 2004b).

In the early 1960s, Asmund Laerdal, with others, developed Resusci-Anne, which allowed cardiopulmonary resuscitation training using simulation (Grenvik & Schaefer, 2004). In 1967 Sim One was introduced, a simulated, computerized patient that could breathe; was able to be ventilated; had carotid, apical, and temporal pulses; and responded to medication administration. Sim One was developed and used mainly for tracheal intubation and anesthesia induction by medical students and residents (Abrahamson, 1997; Denson & Abrahamson, 1969). Another development was the Harvey model, which was a partial body mannequin with software for various cardiovascular diseases that allowed the student to assess general appearance, arterial and venous pulses, heart sounds, and chest wall movements (Gordon, 1974).

As evolutions in the sophistication of simulation advanced, eventually a high-fidelity patient simulator was developed. Fidelity refers to the degree to which the method of simulation is realistic or lifelike (Aggarwal & Darzi, 2006). Smith and Gaba (2001, p. 26) define fidelity as the "accuracy with which the simulation reproduces the domain.... and in the faithfulness of those data streams to their real-world behavior." These high-fidelity patient simulators consist of full-body mannequins that are anatomically correct and lifelike, along with having computer software and hardware and displays for physiologic and pharmacologic parameters. These allow for the programming of clinical scenarios for various disease and physiologic states that can be adjusted for a given patient in regard to age, sex, certain health conditions, and so on. Medications, in certain models, are administered via barcode choices.

Current full-body models are made by Laerdal (Sim Man) and by Medical Education Technologies, Inc. (METI, the human patient simulator™ or HPS). These high-fidelity patient simulators have pupils that can dilate and constrict; have a pulse at multiple sites; have heart, lung, and bowel sounds; and allow certain invasive procedures. There are creative ways to incorporate speech into the scenarios so that the simulator has more of a human-to-human bonding connection. The HPS can be adjusted to bleed, to show conditions such as evisceration and others, and to be made up. Such aspects are used to give health professionals practice in facing severe trauma and mass casualty situations and in acting appropriately. High-fidelity patient simulation has also been used to enhance morbidity and mortality conferences (Vozenilek, Wang, Kharasch, Anderson, & Kalaria, 2006). Practice with the high-fidelity simulator also allows the learner to experience the emotional component of a given clinical scenario or simulation.

High-Fidelity Patient Simulators

Among the health professions, medicine has most fully embraced the high-fidelity patient simulators, particularly in anesthesiology, emergency medicine, surgery, and various other high-acuity areas, including disaster and mass casualty training. In nursing, the greatest use has been in nurse anesthesia education programs, nurse practitioner programs, and emergency care, as well as some pre-licensure nursing programs. However, for all of the health professions, integration into the pre-licensure programs has become usual. In nursing, the associate degree nursing programs were the earliest to purchase high-fidelity patient simulators. As we remodeled our learning laboratories at the Southern Illinois University School of Nursing in Edwardsville, we became the first baccalaureate nursing program to purchase and use a human patient simulator.™

Various educators have proposed learning theories to guide simulator use, but most of these proposals have not been research-based. We have proposed the use of critical-incident nursing management, in which the HPS is used to instruct students about the nursing management of critical incidents through the development of scenarios based on an identified critical incident. This is described in more detail in Nehring and Lashley (2004a) and Nehring, Ellis, and Lashley (2001).

High-fidelity patient simulators are used for assessment and evaluation that includes practicing technical skills, repetitive practice without harm, experimentation for student learning without patient consequence, developing patient-care skills, developing the ability to test decision-making skills, and sharpening critical thinking skills (Parr & Sweeney, 2006). High-fidelity patient simulators also are used to improve student confidence by repetitive practice and reflection, to evaluate the total performance or a specific aspect (Takayesu et al., 2006), to identify the role of communication and dynamics of novice learners in team environments (Morgan, Cleave-Hogg, Desousa, & Lam McCulloch, 2006), and to allow free and open communication among team members without concern about the effect on actual patients or others.

One advantage of these simulators is exposure to many types of conditions and illness through the scenarios, some of which are rare and might not be encountered in the typical clinical practice environment. In addition, it is possible to use real time that closely mimics the actual situation and to practice techniques and interventions in a safe and controlled environment, experimenting with various interventions to see physiologic responses. For example, students can say "what if?" and administer varying doses of a certain drug and see the physiologic and pharmacologic results, without concerns about patient or clinician consequences if an error is made. Additionally, an error can be allowed to continue to its natural conclusion without patient risk (Ziv et al., 2006). Further, there is the ability to practice different orders of priorities, and the integrated high-fidelity mannequins can be used to test leadership and decision- making skills and allow for self-reflection during emergencies (Srinivasan, Hwang, West, & Yellowlees, 2006). Other advantages include the ability to recreate patient encounters by presenting a specific cases and the opportunity to collect clinical impressions even by such means as via audience response systems (Vozenilek et al., 2006). These systems also allow the participants the opportunity to watch the virtual patient deteriorate or stabilize as result of decision making, allowing students to be active participants instead of passive learners (Issenberg, McGaghie, Petrusa, Lee Gordon, & Scalese, 2005). Further, simulation allows for the ability to do self-study and reflection and can provide a reduction in patient inconvenience or discomfort by allowing frequent enough practice so that skills can be maintained or mastered (Freeman et al., 2001; Issenberg et al., 2005; Treloar, Hawayek, Montgomery, Russell, & Medical Readiness Trainer Team, 2001).

Disadvantages to using simulation also exist. These include the following: the initial expense and maintenance expenses; the time for faculty to develop scenarios (note that this is changing because of the development of standardized scenarios as part of various curricular projects that may be used across programs and types of simulators); the extensive initial training time for faculty and staff; the need for maintenance of faculty/staff skills in using the simulator; and if videotaping/transmission is not used, a limit on the number of students who can use the high-fidelity patient simulator at a given time (Henrichs, Rule, Grady, & Ellis, 2002; Monti, Wren, Hass, & Lupien, 1998).

Another possible negative can be the knowledge that the simulator is not real and that the simulation environment may not reflect clinical environment restraints, which could affect the students' performance (Smith & Gaba, 2001). Additionally, there is the risk of the student incorrectly learning a procedure or technique because of a defect in the simulation. It is becoming increasingly common for these simulators to be grouped in simulation centers where various health professions can use them in interdisciplinary scenarios or share expensive resources in various models of education.

Computer Screen Simulation

Computer screen simulations, including Web-based and virtual reality, have taken various forms. PLATO (Programmed Logic for Automated Teaching Operations) was developed at the University of Illinois. This computer-based learning environment was launched and further developed in the 1960s, before the Internet. Described by Brian Dear as "the first major social computing environment" (*PLATO*, n.d.), it allowed users to use graphic display terminals connected to a central mainframe. The system continued to evolve through the 1970s and 1980s, allowing online chat, bulletin board notes, and the ability for multiple users to log on. By the mid-1980s, newer generations of PLATO were used globally (*PLATO*). One program on PLATO, for example, allowed the student to visualize a Giemsa-stained and banded human chromosome spread and, by using the computer technology, to arrange the chromosomes into a karyotype. The student received feedback about the accuracy of the student's work, including instructional content. Other programs followed the consequences of the student's choice to a patient outcome that could become terminal.

Many other computer-based and computer-assisted instruction programs appeared in subsequent years as virtual classrooms and distance education became increasingly popular. Various specific computer software programs guide the acquisition of specific skills and help students to use their tools, for example, to develop haptic or touch sensitivity for pressure when performing surgical procedures. CathSim™ is used in some nursing programs to assist in teaching the procedure for intravenous catheter insertion.

The term *virtual world* can be defined as "an electronic environment that visually mimics complex physical spaces, where people can interact with each other and with virtual objects" (Bainbridge, 2007, p. 472). These virtual worlds can be extremely diverse. Virtual reality software models can incorporate specific patient data such as data from MRIs to allow students to visualize virtual models. These models serve as a basis for practicing virtual procedures. Virtual operations may be practiced by interfacing robotic simulation software with preoperative images and data, as has been used in practicing laparoscopic surgery (Hedican & Nakada, 2007).

STANDARDIZED PATIENTS

Simulated patient encounters may occur through the use of standardized patients. *Standardized patients* is the term given to actors or others who are trained to portray a patient with a specific set of symptoms, medical history, and responses to certain anticipated questions. The standardized patient may be a layperson who is or is not an actor or acting student or may be a health care professional or fellow medical or nursing student. Simulated patients may or may not consistently respond in the same way during every student encounter (Bosek, Li, & Hicks, 2007; Makoul, 2006). Simulated patients may be used to help students do the following:

- Practice physical examination techniques
- Hone interview and communication skills
- Make decisions about follow-up care and procedures after eliciting information

Discussion after the encounter may include the use of videotape review of the session and a debriefing that may be structured and placed on a computer screen or that may be informal and in person individually or with a teaching/learning group.

Digital virtual human actors can be used in virtual instructional simulations in various ways. For example, DIANA, a Digital Animated Avatar (an electronic image manipulated by the computer user), is the image of a 19-year-old female in a physician's office that has been developed at the University of Florida. Software has been developed for such virtual characters as the CyberPatient from the Centre of Excellence for Surgical Education and Innovation in Vancouver, Canada. It is expected that eventually the digital virtual characters will be as effective as standardized patients. Roles for these virtual characters can include the following:

- Demonstrating how to do a procedure
- Providing guidance, feedback, information, and encouragement to students
- Allowing practice of tasks that require more than one person working together, which requires communication and coordination
- Serving in an interactive role similar to a standardized patient, but not yet with that degree of sophistication

SIMULATION AND POLICY

The confluence of policy and simulation is relatively recent. The major use of simulation has been as a means of certification of the proficiency of skills, mostly technical, but also some skills that rely on judgment and critical thinking. Thus, competency-based practice can measure expertise and provide a uniform standard against which to measure the performance of the student. This may include comparing the performance of the student with specifically identified criteria or skills, as well as allowing for the identification of both key elements and less critical ones. The use of standardized technology allows students to be compared with each other. Health disciplines are considering the use of simulation as a way to demonstrate skills (especially clinical skills) as part of licensure and re-licensure as well as certification.

In medicine, several groups are recommending or mandating the use of simulation. The American Council on Graduate Medical Education for Graduate Medical Education in Surgery (2007) specifically cites that adequate resources for resident education should include simulation and skills laboratories. In the assessment of resident performance, they discuss focused evaluation that involves the observation of resident performance either live or via videotaping, with an actual patient or a clinical simulation. The clinical simulation could involve realistic mannequins, standardized patients, or animal models. The oral board examination of the American Board of Emergency Medicine uses simulated patient encounters via the verbalization of the examiner painting a picture of a patient situation (Lammers, 2007). However, this method could be updated with newer simulation methods. The U.S. Food and Drug Administration (FDA) is requiring simulation-based training for physicians desiring to use a certain carotid stent (Gaba & Raemer, 2007). Simulation training is one of the mandatory components for certification in anesthesiology for those who receive initial certification beginning in 2007, and this certification must be renewed every 10 years (Gaba & Raemer). The Surgical Council on Resident Education is examining the role of simulation in surgical education (Bell, 2007).

In nursing, there has been some movement toward incorporating simulation as part of either laboratory time or clinical practice time. Because clinical placements for students have become less available nationwide, simulation is seen as a means to practice clinical skills without having to use the resources of a health care agency. Simulation can guarantee a cardiac patient when the didactic content focuses on cardiac disease, and it eliminates the aspect of a hit-or-miss approach to finding a particular type of clinical patient experience for the student. A critical issue is the question of how much clinical time can, or should, be replaced by simulation methods. These are issues for which evidence-based recommendations can be made to change regulations, a form of policy.

Various national nursing bodies have begun to dialogue about the use of simulation in nursing education programs. In speaking to the potential and actual shortage of qualified nursing faculty, the American Association of Colleges of Nursing (AACN, 2005) stated that nursing clinical instruction is resource intensive. Among the solutions they propose are those that "offer effective learning and that require fewer clinical faculty." This includes the increased use of "simulations in the clinical laboratory in lieu of patient care assignments" (p. 19). Among the strategies proposed is to explore the "use of virtual reality/simulated clinical experiences in supervised learning resource centers to reduce demands on clinical faculty" (p. 20). The AACN (2005) has prepared a draft revision of *The Essentials of Baccalaureate Nursing Education.* Under the essential element of role development, under the section of integrative strategies for learning, one of the items listed is "Engage in interprofessional care in simulation labs" (2007, p. 21).

In pre-licensure professional nursing programs, approval for operating the program is granted by the appropriate state agency, usually through a state board of nursing. This board protects the health of the public through regulation of safe nursing practice. The National Council of State Boards of Nursing (NCSBN) is the body of U.S. state and territory member boards. In the position paper developed by its Practice, Regulation and Education Committee, *Clinical Instruction in Pre-licensure Nursing Programs* (2005), the NCSBN addressed the issue of simulation by gathering data from various sources, including a survey of state boards of nursing. This survey received responses from 36 of the 60 boards of nursing and LPN and RN nursing educational organizations to whom the survey was sent. Of the 31 boards responding to whether students should practice on actual patients, 28 responded affirmatively. However, the partial use of simulation was not examined. When this group of respondents was asked about the future of nursing education, the respondents predicted that there would be more clinical education using simulation as well as clinical laboratories and online learning and that they expected there would be sharing of sophisticated simulation centers. The conclusions in this position paper mention that "deliberate controlled practice with simulators is an important asset for clinical learning, but that it cannot take the place of learning in the authentic setting" (NCSBN, 2005, p. 9).

Among the NCSBN recommendations was one that stated pre-licensure nursing education programs might also "include innovative teaching strategies that complement clinical experiences for entry into practice competency" (NCSBN, 2005, p. 9). In July 2006, this same committee spoke to evidence-based nursing education for regulation. In that document the organization states that "research strongly supports using simulation" and goes on to say that it is studying the role of simulation in nursing education (NCSBN, 2006, p. 3).

In a recent research study, Nehring (2008) examined the status of approval for the use of high-fidelity patient simulation in nursing programs, including the status of any regulation changes. A survey was mailed to the executive director of each board of nursing, and the response rate was 88.5%. In response to whether state boards of nursing gave permission for the use of high-fidelity patient simulators for the replacement of clinical hours, 16 states responded that they did. Many states dealt with the percentage of time allotted by stating that this could be done on a case-by-case basis. Most states stated that clinical hour requirements are not specified in the regulations.

Rather than dictating the number or percentage of clinical hours, the regulations are written so that graduates meet objectives of the courses and programs. An exception was Florida, which reported a specific use of simulation for 10% of clinical time. Seventeen states said they would or might consider stipulation of the use of simulators for clinical hours in future regulation changes (Nehring, 2008).

CONCLUSION

It is clear that the use of simulation in health professional education continues to advance both in the types of uses and in frequency of use. However, there is a relative paucity of rigorous research examining the efficacy of this type of learning. Such studies will not only inform the use of simulation and various types of simulators as teaching/learning tools but will also provide the necessary evidence to assist policy makers in making appropriate decisions regarding its use, particularly when it might replace actual clinical practice. Therefore, research with the appropriate sample sizes, randomization, control groups, and all of the requirements of rigorous study is essential in the immediate future. Experts in simulation have discussed how to approach such research across disciplines. For the future, policy makers may well extend regulation of simulation and simulator use beyond replacement of clinical hours and into the accreditation of simulation centers, and perhaps to the certification of the faculty who are primarily engaged in running such centers.

REFERENCES

Abrahamson, S. (1997). Sim One: A patient simulator ahead of its time. *Caduceus, 13*(2), 29–41.

Aggarwal, R., & Darzi, A. (2006). Technical-skills training in the 21st century. *New England Journal of Medicine, 355,* 2695–2696.

Ahlberg, G., Heikkinen, T., Iselius, L., Leijonmarck, C. E., Rutqvist, J., & Arvidsson, D. (2002). Does training in a virtual reality simulator improve surgical performance? *Surgical Endoscopy, 16,* 126–129.

American Association of Colleges of Nursing. (2007). *Draft revision of "The essentials of baccalaureate nursing education."* Retrieved August 1, 2007, from http://www.aacn.nche.edu.

American Association of Colleges of Nursing. (2005, June). *Faculty shortages in baccalaureate and graduate nursing programs. Scope of the problem and strategies for expanding the supply.* Retrieved September 4, 2007, from http://www.aacn.nche.edu/publications/pdf/05FacShortage.pdf

American Council on Graduate Medical Education. (2007). *ACGME Program requirements for graduate medical education in surgery.* Effective July 1, 2008. Retrieved September 4, 2007, from http://www.acgme.org/acWebsite/downloads/RRC_progReq/440generalsurgery01012008.pdf

Bainbridge, W. S. (2007). The scientific research potential of virtual worlds. *Science, 317,* 472–476.

Bell, R. H. (2007). Surgical council on resident education: A new organization devoted to graduate surgical education. *Journal of the American College of Surgeons, 204,* 341–346.

Bosek, M. S., Li, S., & Hicks, F. D. (2007). Working with standardized patients: A primer. *International Journal of Nursing Education Scholarship, 4.* Retrieved May 30, 2008, from http://www.bcpress.com/ijnes/vol4/iss2/art16

Denson, J. S., & Abrahamson, S. (1969). A computer-controlled patient simulator. *Journal of the American Medical Association, 208,* 504–508.

Freeman, K. M., Thompson, S. F., Allely, E. B., Sobel, A. L., Stansfield, S. A., & Pugh, W. M. (2001). A virtual reality patient simulation system for teaching emergency response skills to U.S. Navy medical providers. *Prehospital Disaster Medicine, 16,* 3–8.

Gaba, D. M., & Raemer, D. (2007). The tide is turning: Organizational structures to embed simulation in the fabric of healthcare. *Simulation in Healthcare, 2,* 1–3.

Gordon, M. S. (1974). Cardiology patient simulator. Development of an animated manikin to teach cardiovascular disease. *American Journal of Cardiology, 34,* 350–355.

Grenvik, A., & Schaefer, J. (2004). From Resusci-Anne to Sim-Man: The evolution of simulators in medicine. *Critical Care Medicine, 32,* S56–S57.

Hedican, S. P., & Nakada, S. Y. (2007). Videotape mentoring and surgical simulation in laparoscopic courses. *Journal of Endourology, 21,* 288–293.

Henrichs, B., Rule, A., Grady, M., & Ellis, W. (2002). Nurse anesthesia students' perceptions of the anesthesia patient simulator: A qualitative study. *AANA Journal, 70,* 219–225.

Herrmann, E. K. (1981). Mrs. Chase: A noble and enduring figure. *American Journal of Nursing, 81,* 1836.

Issenberg, S. B. (2006). The scope of simulation-based healthcare education. *Simulation in Healthcare, 1,* 203–208.

Issenberg, S. B., McGaghie, W. C., Petrusa, E. R., Lee Gordon, D., & Scalese, R. J. (2005). Features and uses of high-fidelity medical simulations that lead to effective learning: A BEME systematic review. *Medical Teacher, 27,* 10–28.

Kohn, L. T., Corrigan, J. M., & Donaldson, M. S. (Eds.). (2000). *To err is human: Building a safer health system.* Washington, DC: National Academy of Sciences.

Lammers, R. L. (2007). Simulation: The new teaching tool. *Annals of Emergency Medicine, 49,* 505–507.

Makoul, G. (2006). Commentary: Communication skills: How simulation training supplements experiential and humanist learning. *Academic Medicine, 81,* 271–274.

Monti, E. J., Wren, K., Hass, R., & Lupien, A. E. (1998). The use of an anesthesia simulator in graduate and undergraduate education. *CRNA: The Clinical Forum for Nurse Anesthestists, 9*(2), 59–66.

Morgan, P. J., Cleave-Hogg, D., Desousa, S., & Lam McCulloch, J. (2006). Applying theory to practice in undergraduate education using high fidelity simulation. *Medical Teacher, 28,* e10–e15.

Morgan, P. J., Cleave-Hogg, D., McIlroy, J., & Devitt, J. H. (2002). Simulation technology: A comparison of experiential and visual learning for undergraduate medical students. *Anesthesiology, 96,* 10–16.

Murphy, J. G., Torsher, L. C., & Dunn, W. F. (2007). Simulation medicine in intensive care and coronary care education. *Journal of Critical Care, 22,* 51–55.

Murray, D. (2006). Clinical skills in acute care: A role for simulation training. *Critical Care Medicine, 34,* 252–253.

NCSBN. (2005, August). *Clinical instruction in prelicensure nursing programs.* Retrieved September 4, 2007, from https://www.ncsbn.org/pdfs/Final_Clinical_Instr_Pre_Nsg_programs.pdf

NCSBN. (2006, July). *Evidence-based nursing education for regulation (EBNER).* Retrieved September 4, 2007, from https://www.ncsbn.org/Final_06EBNER_Report.pdf

Nehring, W. M. (2008). U.S. boards of nursing and the use of high-fidelity patient simulation in nursing education. *Journal of Professional Nursing, 24,* 109–117.

Nehring, W. M., Ellis, W. E., & Lashley, F. R. (2001). Human patient simulators in nursing education: An overview. *Simulation and Gaming, 32,* 194–204.

Nehring, W. M., & Lashley, F. R. (2004a). Current use and opinions regarding human patient simulators in nursing education: An international survey. *Nursing Education Perspectives, 25,* 244–248.

Nehring, W. M. & Lashley, F. R. (2004b). Using the human patient simulator™ in nursing education. *Annual Review of Nursing Education, 2,* 163–181.

Parr, M. B., & Sweeney, N. M. (2006). Use of human patient simulation in an undergraduate critical care course. *Critical Care Nursing Quarterly, 29,* 188–198.

PLATO. (n.d.). Retrieved July 13, 2007, from the Department of Physics, University of Illinois, Urbana-Champaign, Web site: http://physics.uiuc.edu/history/PLATO.htm

Smith, B. E., & Gaba, D. M. (2001). Simulators. In C. L. Lake, R. L. Hines, & C. D. Blitt (Eds.), *Clinical monitoring: Practical applications for anesthesia and critical care* (pp. 26–44). Philadelphia: W. B. Saunders.

Srinivasan, M., Hwang, J. C., West, D., & Yellowlees, P. M. (2006). Assessment of clinical skills using simulator technologies. *Academic Psychiatry, 30,* 505–515.

Takayesu, J. K., Farrell, S. E., Evans, A. J., Sullivan, J. E., Pawlowski, J. B., & Gordon, J. A. (2006). How do clinical clerkship students experience simulator-based teaching? A qualitative analysis. Empirical investigations. *Simulation in Healthcare, 1,* 215–219.

Treloar, D., Hawayek, J., Montgomery, J. R., Russell, W., & Medical Readiness Trainer Team. (2001). On-site and distance education of emergency medicine personnel with a human patient simulator. *Military Medicine, 166,* 1003–1006.

Vozenilek, J., Wang, E., Kharasch, M., Anderson, B., & Kalaria, A. (2006). Simulation-based morbidity and mortality conference: New technologies augmenting traditional case-based presentations. *Academy of Emergency Medicine, 13,* 48–53.

Ziv, A., Erez, D., Munz, Y., Vardi, A., Barsuk, D., Levine, I., Benita, S., Rubin, O., & Berkenstadt, H. (2006). The Israel Center for Medical Simulation: A paradigm for cultural change in medical education. *Academic Medicine, 81,* 1091–1097.

Ziv, A., Wolpe, P. R., Small, S. D., & Glick, S. (2003). Simulation-based medical education: An ethical imperative. *Academic Medicine, 78,* 783–788.

SECTION IV. RESEARCH AND EDUCATIONAL POLICY: LESSONS LEARNED

Geri L. Dickson

A sufficient number of students and faculty is crucial to increasing the supply of nurses, which in turn, will assist in addressing the projected gap between the supply and demand of nurses. Although nursing education is an important component of solving the nurse shortage, it is essential that we also close the backdoor through which many nurses leave, especially within their early years of practice. In the previous section, we learned some lessons from the workplace research and some evidence-based policy recommendations. This section is focused on nursing education and policy.

Aiken and colleagues' (2003) seminal research documented the relationship and impact of staffing and baccalaureate-prepared nurses on patient outcomes, such as mortality and failure to rescue. What was particularly unsettling to many nurses was the skilled researchers' report of the impact on patients of having at least 60% of the RNs in hospitals prepared at the baccalaureate level in order to improve patient outcomes, such as mortality or failure to rescue in surgical patients. Estabrooks and colleagues (2005) also reported similar positive gains in patient outcomes when the direct care staff had a greater percentage of baccalaureate-prepared nurses. Both articles were published in prestigious, peer-reviewed journals. Yet today we find that the vast majority of new graduates are not prepared at the baccalaureate level, and small percentages, about 15%–20%, of RNs prepared at the associate or diploma level go on to earn a nursing baccalaureate degree. The varying routes to enter the discipline of nursing have been a double-edged sword: first, it provides upward mobility for students who may not have the financial or other means to enter a generic baccalaureate program, and second, overall, nurses remain the least educated of professional health care providers in the health care system. Generally, patients and others are not aware of this situation, but it remains an issue among nurses, and the following chapters demonstrate the tacit unrest in the nursing profession regarding our entry-into-practice issues in today's complex healthcare system.

In Section IV, researchers reported on some of the prime nursing education issues today, focusing on (a) the attraction of high school students to nursing when choosing a career, (b) the looming crisis of a faculty shortage, and (c) the use of clinical simulation to extend the practice of faculty. So what have we learned about research and policy from these three chapters? Read on.

LESSON 1. BE A POSITIVE MESSENGER

In chapter 9, Rudel and Moulton provided evidence that we, as nurses, play a major role in attracting new recruits into the profession. The vast majority of high school students in this study who were interested in nursing knew someone who was in the field (87%), and another vast majority of high school students who did not want to go into nursing (86%) had a personal relationship with someone who works in the field. This seems to indicate that some students walked away with a positive impression of nursing, but almost the same percentage were left with a negative image of the profession.

So lesson 1 reminds us that how we present ourselves as nurses does make a difference—both positive and negative. We do have a responsibility to help to replenish the field, as well as to make it a desirable profession for young people to enter.

LESSON 2. POSITIVE PEOPLE MAKE POSITIVE MESSENGERS

Rudel and Moulton suggested that health care facilities that employ nurses emphasize the value, leadership opportunities, and rewards of being a nurse. The researchers also reminded us that positive people make positive messengers.

Along with that, consider how our internal battles have led to divisiveness and negative images of nurses, whether the battles are overt or tacit. For the future of the profession, now is the time for all of us to pull together and present a positive image of the profession.

LESSON 3. LINK CAREER ATTRACTORS TO THE ATTRACTION OF NURSING

The researchers identified for us the career attractors that matter to youth when they are considering a career, and many of those attributes can be found in nursing. Developing programs that outline the benefits of a nursing career, starting in grade school, will bear fruit if nurtured properly and will replenish the field. A long-term goal, then, becomes a change in the image of nursing through the positive actions of each and every nurse!

LESSON 4. ACTION NEEDS TO BE TAKEN TO INCREASE THE FACULTY POOL

Although Rudel and Moulton recommended this, Cleary and her team also identified and provided evidence for this recommendation. Such actions necessary to meet this lesson include expanding programs that offer the opportunity for nurses currently prepared at the associate degree level to pursue directly a master's degree, which would enable them to become faculty members. Continued partnerships between community colleges and 4-year colleges and universities to facilitate articulation between programs, as well as programs specifically designed to increase the number of baccalaureate-prepared graduates, serve as some approaches to meet this lesson learned.

LESSON 5. INCREASE INCREMENTALLY OVER TIME THE RATIO OF STUDENTS TO FACULTY

Cleary and team provided differing scenarios demonstrating the significant effect of a 50% increase in students per faculty member from the current requirement of about 10:1 over the next 10 years and a 100% increase in, or doubling of, the ratios incrementally over the next 10 years. Although these increases would result in a major positive shift in faculty distribution, the researchers stopped short of making this a recommendation. However, they do cite this as a recommendation offered by the North Carolina Institute of Medicine. This lesson certainly provides food for thought.

LESSON 6. PARTNERSHIP DEVELOPMENT BETWEEN NURSING EDUCATION AND SERVICE TO SHARE SIMULATION MODELS

All three of these chapters identified partnerships that could develop between education and service to establish regional simulation model centers, some interdisciplinary, to assist in the preparation of students and new graduates in the field. However, Cleary and team stopped short of recommending simulation as a replacement for clinical, whereas Lashley and Nehring suggested simulation could be used in lieu of some clinical practice time. All three suggested that simulation model instruction and evaluation would result in better-prepared nurses entering the practice settings, as well as serve to evaluate and maintain the continued competency of practicing nurses.

In sum, the documented shortage in nurse faculty certainly contributes to the overall current and projected shortage of nurses, as well as the face of nursing and how we present it as a body. To address these issues, some states—for example, Virginia, Pennsylvania, Arizona, and Illinois—have invested state monies into increasing the capacity of nursing education. Others are still dragging their feet and may suffer severe consequences in the future. Let us not forget the following Greek proverb:

> *A society grows great when old men and women plant trees*
> *Under whose shade they know they will never sit.*

REFERENCES

Aiken, L. H., Clarke, S. P., Cheung, R. B, Sloarne, D. M., & Silber, J. H. (2003). Educational levels of hospital nurses and surgical patient mortality. *Journal of the American Medical Association, 290,* 1617–1623.

Estabrooks, C. A., Midodzi, W. K., Cummings, G. G., Ricker, K. L., & Giovannetti, P. (2005). The impact of hospital nursing characteristics on 30-day mortality. *Nursing Research, 54*(2), 74–84.

Funding the Research to Policy Connection

SECTION V

INTRODUCTION

Linda Flynn

Emphasizing the research to policy connection, contributors in previous chapters have described nursing outcomes research and its influence on policy makers, reviewed strategies for collecting and managing policy-influencing data, and presented findings that have the potential to affect nursing pipeline, education, and practice environment initiatives. It is important to realize, however, that none of these important research activities could occur without adequate funding.

In this section, we focus on a key aspect of the research enterprise—getting money to fund your study! The popular motto "no money, no mission" is as applicable to research as it is to health care delivery. We may have a critical research question and a burning mission to inform evidence-based decisions that will impact nurses and their work. But without money to support item development, data collection, analyses, and demonstration projects, well, our best ideas and intentions will never see the light of day.

Research funding can come from a variety of sources, and each source has unique quirks, priorities, and processes to which you, as the researcher, must adapt. In the following chapters you will learn to "dance" in the halls of Congress, "plant" with foundations, and "translate" to the user-worlds of federal funding agencies. Although, at times, the language may seem unfamiliar, and the landscape may seem strange, expert contributors to this section serve as your translators and guides through the mazes within funding organizations. Importantly, I think you will conclude that despite differences in lexicon and milieu, funding sources and researchers share a common goal—to improve the access, safety, and quality of health care for all persons.

12 Of Horses and Ponies: Taking Your Show to Washington

CLAUDIA L. MCDONALD

WHY SHOULD I LEARN TO DANCE?

Obtaining research funding through congressional earmark legislation is probably not for everyone and certainly not for the faint of heart, but funding is scarce for research projects in public and private nursing education. Perhaps learning to dance in the halls of Congress may become a cultivated taste for more nursing academics in the future.

Academicians in the field of nursing are more accustomed to applying for grants than having the instruments of political power strummed by experts on their behalf. Nursing academics are not accustomed to the rules of this game, the steps of the dance, which are more akin to the law of the jungle than due process. Pluck and luck—being in the right place at the right time with the right people and the right idea—contribute as much to success as do the abstract merits of any given project. There are no guarantees, not even for the best of ideas or the most critical of funding needs. There is nothing fair about it. Politics rules the halls of Congress. You can learn your steps and perform flawlessly only to fail through no fault of your own.

Acknowledgment: Ron George, technical writer in the Office of Special Projects at Texas A&M University–Corpus Christi, contributed to this chapter.

239

Indeed, it is unlikely that you will succeed the first time you approach Congress for research money. Persistence is an essential personal and professional virtue in any kind of fund-raising, and certainly in the legislative dance. This author spent 2 fruitless years making inquiries before one dime was appropriated to Texas A&M University–Corpus Christi for Pulse!! The Virtual Clinical Learning Lab; moreover, as Woodrow Wilson wrote in 1885, "Once you begin the dance of legislation, and you must struggle through its mazes as best you can to the breathless end—if any end there be" (1901, p. 297). The dance never seems to end, either, because earmark legislation is renewed annually.

The derogatory term for earmark funding is "pork," but money is money, and wherever two or three are gathered, there is politics, which is how this democratic society distributes some public revenue for the common good. On Capitol Hill, this type of funding is called "plus-up," and members of Congress (MCs) are entitled by long-established custom to sponsor such pet projects that benefit their home districts. Such projects are usually small by federal-budget standards—"budget dust," in the Capitol Hill lexicon—but they have enormous impact and value at the district level, and in the case of academic research, they are likely to have impact and value at the national level as well. (The Pulse!! program received $9.85 million over 3 fiscal years, slightly more than two-thirds of one ten-thousandth of a percentage point of the overall Department of Defense budget of more than $1.4 *trillion* for the same period.)

In 2005, $1.4 billion in earmark funding was appropriated to higher education institutions through federal government research accounts, according to the Office of Management and Budget (2007). Overall that year, the Office of Management and Budget (OMB) estimated appropriated earmarks at $18.9 billion. Higher education research, in other words, drew about 7% of all appropriated earmark funding in 2005. The primary question for those of us who need not just hundreds of thousands but millions of dollars for our projects is whether we have the stamina to cut ourselves a piece of that pie. (Nursing programs received about $54.5 million in 2005 earmarks for construction and non-construction projects. Six projects billed as research received about $14.8 million total.)

This chapter presents the congressional budget process from the perspective of one seeking earmark funds for academic research. There is lingo to learn, and there are pitfalls to avoid and arcane procedures to understand, none of which guarantees success but without which failure is virtually assured.

Sir Geoffrey Palmer (1987) boiled the legislative process down to an essence when he wrote that the dance in the halls of New Zealand's parliament "requires perseverance, stamina and a large degree of eso-teric knowledge" (p. 241). Not a word of this chapter examines how to know whether one has the heart for this type of fund-raising, but per-haps we will shed some light on some of the esoteric knowledge.

Questions Philosophical and Practical

The first question is obvious, but the operative word in it is "federal": What do you want *federal* money for? The implication in this and all other questions you will be asked on Capitol Hill is that there may be other sources of money available for your project. Why does it require $139,000 in *federal* funding, for example, "to recruit and retain minority students in nursing and allied health professions" (OMB, 2007, p. 1750) at Bloomfield College in Bloomfield, New Jersey? There may be many an-swers to that question, but chief among them is that Congress, in 2005, decided to appropriate $146.4 million under Title VII of the Higher Education Act for that very purpose. One way to answer the question, then, comes from doing the same kind of research you would do for any other funding source. You can find out what government may provide in the future by seeing what it has provided in the past. The OMB began publishing an earmark database on the Internet in March 2007. It was a controversial move designed to curb the practice of earmarking, and crit-ics said it was incomplete regarding some politically sensitive recipients. However, there is no reason to suspect the numbers, which are verifiable through the federal budget, and plenty of recipients were forthcoming about how the money was used. The OMB database is a handy tool, but the agency also publishes a number of budget documents on its Web site (http://www.whitehouse.gov/omb/budget/fy2007).

The next question, related to the first, is this: Why should your con-gressional representative step in with an earmark? There are other ways of applying for federal funds. Here is a rule of thumb: MCs want to ben-efit their districts, but they also want to reap political capital for them-selves and their party by benefiting the nation as well. For example, an MC whose district has several military installations might be more in-clined to support a plus-up benefiting the military medicine than one benefiting nursing education, whereas an MC whose district includes a prestigious medical center might support nursing education over mili-tary medicine. (Both funding issues are national in scope, but politics is *always* local, even when there is a significant national issue at stake.)

Next question: Is your project sufficiently urgent to compel Congress to act now rather than wait for the federal bureaucracy to lumber into action? "No" shoves your project down the priority list. "Yes" requires that you make a strong case, and these days that may mean, for example, spinning your research off national defense, homeland security, global warming, or pandemics such as avian flu.

Practical questions are no less important: When do you need the money? (Have a realistic timeline ready to show.) How will you use the money? (Have a realistic budget.) How will the money get to you? (Have an agency and a budget account in mind.) Finally—and this is the killer—how do you plan to make this program self-supporting? It is important from the outset to think of congressional earmark funding as seed money to get you started and *not* to think of it as a steady source of revenue. From the beginning, your project plan must anticipate that earmark funding will end; indeed, your institution will be as interested as the government is in the answer to this question. It is conceivable, of course, that a project simply will end, but that is not the kind of project MCs generally supports with earmarks—because, with all the other reasons MCs support earmarks (for the good of the district *and* the nation in the face of an urgent issue), they also want to invest hard-earned political capital in their legacy—how they will be remembered by the public after they have left office. Legacies may take the shape of buildings named after them or even something less tangible; but in any case, it would not be a research program with a *terminus ad quem.* You want to be able to say of your project that, although federal funding was essential to getting started, it was of sufficient magnitude to take on a life of its own.

THE DANCE: ONE STEP AT A TIME

Educational institutions must decide well before the beginning of each fall semester which projects they will promote for funding directly from Congress. The Texas A&M University System, for example, solicits federal initiatives in January from each of its nine member universities, its Health Science Center, and seven state agencies. These documents put each project in a nutshell, including its funding request and source. A&M–Corpus Christi's Associate Vice President for Research and Scholarly Activities solicits and vets federal initiatives locally and then sends them up the line to system officials to let them know which initiatives will be pursued.

It is crucial that institutions limit the number of federal initiatives— three or four a year at a campus the size of Texas A&M–Corpus Christi

(8,500 students)—because too many proposals dilute institutional effectiveness in pursuing the funds that come directly from Congress via earmark. Once the list has been pared to a workable number, the local institution contacts its congressional office and makes a formal request for federal funds based on the brief federal initiatives. It also notifies its lobbyist—earmark funding proposals simply will not succeed without one—as well as the agency from which or through which federal funds will be sought.

The Dance Has Officially Begun

A word about MCs: They are extraordinarily busy because the dance revolves around them. They are continuously in the company of colleagues and staff, constituents, contributors, and lobbyists, all of whom have a claim or want to stake a claim on legislators' time or talents or federal treasure. You have an idea, but legislative ideas are a dime a dozen on Capitol Hill. You may have a *good* idea, but good ideas are as common as pelicans on Corpus Christi Bay. Great ideas are few and far between, but even these are not shoo-in legislative projects. What matters is whether your idea captures an MC's imagination. Without that, even a great idea will languish like a wallflower.

About lobbyists: They are essential to obtaining earmark funding. Lobbyists operate symbiotically in Washington as catalysts for legislation. They represent the interests of their clients to the legislative and executive branches of government—members of Congress and federal agencies, from the White House to the military and the host of departments and numerous layers of bureaucracy that bring federal programs (i.e., money) to the local level. Lobbyists also inform and advise their clients about the ways and means of official Washington, and this often means letting you know what is possible and what is not—or, in Washingtonese, what has "traction" and what does not.

It may take a knowledgeable lobbyist to help you find a "champion," a member of Congress whose legislative interests coincide with your project and funding needs. A lobbyist may help you sculpt a nonstarter idea into one with traction that actually will make it through the budget process. A lobbyist can help you sell an idea to Congress by letting you know whom to see, where to see them, and how to keep your idea fresh in the minds of MCs and their staffs.

We have all heard horror stories about corrupt lobbyists, but they are exceptions. The overwhelming majority of more than 35,000 registered lobbyists in Washington, DC, are honorable women and men performing an essential function in a large, complex representative government. They are not exactly where the rubber meets the road—that is back home, where the money is spent—but they are essential in making the tires.

You have a lobbyist so that you do not have to become one yourself, and that has legal implications: If you spend more than 20% of your professional time over a 6-month period on Capitol Hill, *you* are a lobbyist and will have to register as such. You are *not* a lobbyist, however, when you are providing information, preferably in writing on the public record, rather than soliciting a political support (Congressional Research Service, 2006, pp. 3–4; Disclosure of Lobbying Activities, 2007). The best practice is to let your lobbyist escort you through the halls of Congress. Let the lobbyist do most of the talking until it is time to *inform* the MC. That is your job. Be prepared. Do not beat around the bush. Leave a one-page summary. Ask for questions.

About travel: If you do not have a travel budget, get one because you are going to be in Washington, DC, several times before the federal budget is passed prior to Congress's summer recess in August. Federal budgets cover a fiscal year from October 1 through September 30.

Plan to visit Washington no later than the end of February with your institutional president, whose company will make it more likely that you and your lobbyist will get a meeting with your MC. This must not be a cold call, and setting it up may be the first indication of whether your idea has traction. Members' level of interest in this or that piece of legislation is reflected clearly in their meeting schedules. They do not have time to waste on funding ideas without traction. Your president will get you in the door as a matter of courtesy. Do not assume that your money is all but in the bank just because you have gotten in the door. You have important work to do during that courtesy call. You will have about 15 minutes to make your case, so try not to open the door to small talk. Do not be rude, but be sure you and your president are on the same page before you arrive. This is the confirmation visit: Let your MC know what you want, why, and how much it costs. Make it *clear*—the whole thing should fit on a single page with pictures and wide margins. Make it *concise*—you have just 15 minutes. Make it *cogent*—that is how you inspire the lawmaker's imagination. Remember, too, that you can get it all right to this point and still not get your money. Better luck next year.

If you are having a hard time scheduling face time with your MC, it may mean your idea is far down the list of the MC's legislative priorities.

You have reached a critical point: without a congressional champion, a member of Congress willing to sponsor and defend your project, it goes nowhere. It may be time for what politicians and their minions call a "gut check."

It is of the ethos of this type of fund-raising that you believe in your idea, not just that it is a good idea but that it is a great idea, not just that it deserves to be publicly funded but that it is a better way to spend public funds than thousands of other proposals on Capitol Hill. It is called a gut check because you must have the stomach for taking money from someone else in order to obtain funds for your project. There is a finite amount of money available, so in order to succeed, you must be prepared to defend your idea with every tool at your disposal, from research data and expert opinions to ethical and moral persuasion, and to sell it as the best project among many. It is called a gut check because it takes courage to promote an idea through the congressional budget process. Your idea will be attacked, especially by committee staff whose job it is to cull and vet MCs' local projects for powerful appropriations committee chairs. You will be grilled. You may be ignored. Your project may simply disappear from the radar screen. It is called a gut check because success goes to the insistent and persistent, those able and willing to bounce back again and again. Success goes to those who keep in mind the Yogi Berra principle: "It ain't over 'til it's over." Do not give up until the *experts* tell you there is no hope—and even then, always ask about next year. Your lobbyist is a key expert in all of this—a stabilizer in times of storm and stress, a buffer from the political rough and tumble, an encourager when there is hope, and a truth-teller when there is not.

It is worth remembering that asking does not mean getting in Washington. Asking is only the beginning, and even that can be a complex process because it may mean modifying your project, tailoring it to meet a need that did not occur to you before your lobbyist or a congressional staffer suggested it.

Assuming your idea has traction, it is smart to make the rounds while you are in the nation's capital, so be sure to touch base with your lobbyist and your contact at the agency through which you hope to receive federal funds, someone you probably have met by introduction through your MC. Federal funds are channeled through a myriad of federal agencies. One of the more notable skills in Washington is knowing who knows which channels are currently open and which are not. These are the essential legs on a three-legged stool—your MC, your lobbyist, and your agency contact. Take one away, and the stool falls over. Your role in the dance—and it is more of a square dance than a waltz—is to be responsive to the key offices of your MC, lobbyist, and agency contact. They will be asking you for information of all kinds to demonstrate the need for and efficacy of your project. They will keep you posted on the status of your legislation. They will be bearers of good news and bad, advances, and setbacks. It is of the nature of the dance of legislation that information will be required as soon as possible and that news good and bad will come suddenly, often without warning.

This process can be exasperating and demanding: "Didn't we answer those questions just last week?" Well, yes, but this form is different and goes to a different committee. "You want it *when?*" Yesterday. "Our proposal was *cut?*" The chairman is on the warpath, but we are working on getting it back into the conference bill. Always remember that you are in charge of your own morale and that of your institutional staff, if you have one. Do not take it personally. Do not hold grudges. Do not lose your composure.

THE FEDERAL BUDGET PROCESS

Slicing and dicing the federal budget begins soon after the president submits his budget proposal on or before the first Monday in February. Congress responds to the president's proposal by April 15 with a budget resolution that serves as a guideline for its deliberations over the coming months. The congressional budget process, however, can begin without a budget resolution, which does not have the force of law and is not signed by the president.

Your earmark funding will come from the discretionary spending portion of the federal budget (about $450 billion for fiscal 2007), which is roughly a third of the entire budget, including almost all defense spending, K–12 education, health research, and housing programs, to mention a few. All other federal spending, roughly two-thirds, is nondiscretionary—Social Security, Medicare, Medicaid, entitlement programs, and interest on the national debt.

Each chamber of Congress—the U.S. House of Representatives and the U.S. Senate—considers its disposition of the federal budget through a complex committee structure that runs along two main tracks: authorization and appropriation.

Authorization bills, which ultimately may be collected into omnibus budget reconciliation legislation, set federal spending policy not only for the coming fiscal year but also for the next 5 to 10 years, especially with regard to nondiscretionary federal spending such as Social Security and Medicare. These bills, drafted by congressional committees with jurisdiction over federal agencies, affect changes in federal law that govern how money is spent, and they are conditioned by provisions in the congressional budget resolution. Committees with legislative jurisdiction over, say, Social Security pensions and family policy (Senate Committee on Finance) or income security and family support (House Committee on Ways and Means) craft legislation that will determine how nondiscretionary government programs are managed by changing benefit eligibility requirements, for example, or changing provisions in the federal tax code.

Thirteen appropriations bills related to discretionary spending are channeled through the appropriations committees and subcommittees of the House and Senate. The appropriations committees and conference committees of both houses produce legislation that must be approved by both houses before it is submitted to the president to be signed into law or vetoed. Figure 12.1 shows a broad view of the path of federal budget legislation, from the president's proposal to the submission of authorization and appropriation bills to the White House for signature or veto. Figure 12.2 gives a slightly more detailed account of the authorization and appropriation tracks.

Your earmark legislation must find its way into both tracks of the congressional budget process—that is up to your congressional champion—and it must survive attempts to have it removed in favor of other earmark projects.

Earmarks are said to be "the trading currency" of Congress because they are traded by members for favorable votes on each other's pet projects. In its simplest form, the transaction goes something like this: "I supported project X in your district, so now please support project Y in mine." In practice, these negotiations can be enormously complex because the calculus includes not only tit for tat and dollars and cents, but also philosophical and political alliances and allegiances. The heart of the congressional seniority system lies within this particular aspect of Congress's political ecology—the more votes members have cast, the more votes they are owed by others; the longer they have served in Congress, the more favors they have done, and the more favors they are owed. Congressional leadership is in the hands of those who have served the longest and who are perceived as having done the most for the most people, from supporting legislation to helping junior members

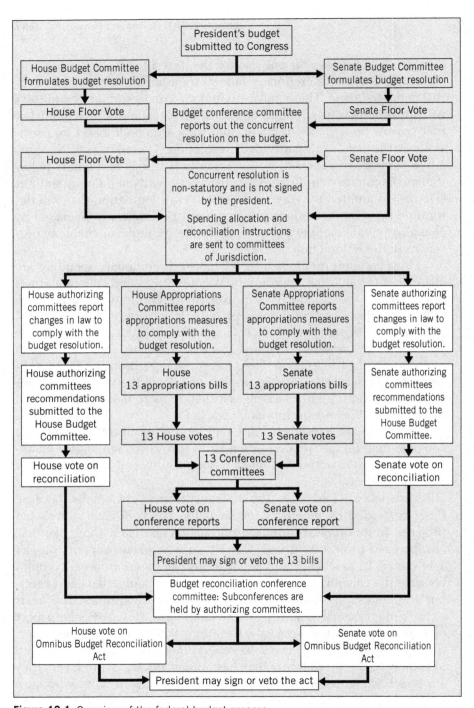

Figure 12.1 Overview of the federal budget process

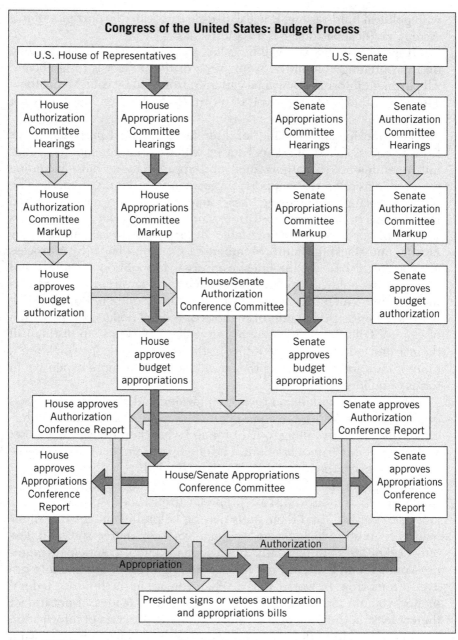

Figure 12.2 Focus on the congressional budget process

with political fund-raising. If legislative earmarks are the currency of this system, political patronage is its culture.

It is unlikely that you will be called to testify before an authorizing or appropriating committee. Your piece of the budget is insignificant. All pertinent information will be gathered from you by your MC's office. There are other reasons for you to return to Washington, but this is not one of them.

The "racking and stacking" of discretionary budget proposals stems from a process called "markup," during which committee members submit amendments to authorization and appropriations bills, including earmark legislation that supports projects in their home districts. (The phrase "racking and stacking" has found its way into many contexts, but it seems to have originated from gambling jargon for what happens when a player leaves a gaming table and prepares to cash in chips by racking and stacking them.) Members of Congress know by a process of what might be called political osmosis—via tradition, seniority, and party caucus politics—roughly how much they can send home as earmarks. Junior members have less than senior members do, and such figures are measured in tens of millions of federal dollars. In the jargon of Capitol Hill, these amendments are called "plus-ups" to distinguish them from "adds," new line items in the federal budget, which are a more secure form of funding than earmarks and far more expensive in terms of political capital.

MCs and their staffs do their own racking and stacking—a process of prioritizing—before the committee markup process begins to determine what they are willing to fight for and what they are willing to lose, all within the MC's earmark limit. The closer your project is to the top of this earmark list, the more likely it will be funded.

Throughout the process, your job is to provide information, promptly, which means you also must be *prepared* to provide it promptly. Your lobbyist, your MC, and their staffs may be helpful in anticipating information requests, which usually originate with committee staff and, less often, other MCs or their staffs. It is a good idea, too, to anticipate inquiries yourself and to secure the information before you are asked to deliver it tomorrow, or worse, today. When you are in the hunt for federal money, you are constantly making the case for your idea, if not in fact then at least in the back of your mind. Your case consists of information you must be able to deliver in 5 minutes or less while walking down a noisy hall or while jammed into an elevator. You will seldom have an opportunity to make it at your leisure because there simply is not time enough on Capitol Hill.

You may, however, from time to time, have an opportunity to showcase your idea at industry or professional conferences attended by representatives of government agencies. Such confabs are veritable beehives of networking for industry and government reps, academics, consultants, and entrepreneurs, any one of whose connections may turn the key for you in getting federal funds. Be selective, though, because you will probably hear about more conferences than you can possibly attend. Avoid squandering your time and travel budget on conferences that do not help you in some specific way. Read deeply into the program. Make some calls to get some feedback on previous meetings from colleagues and legislative partners. If key government people are going to be there, make some appointments with them; do not rely solely on chance meetings in the exhibit hall. If you are an exhibitor or are making a presentation, be sure the appearance of your materials bespeaks a project operating at a high professional level. It does not hurt, as a matter of policy and practice, to deliver some sizzle with your message. Slapdash materials deliver no sizzle.

It is unlikely that the final House and Senate versions of the bills that include your earmark funding will be identical, which means they must be reconciled by a conference committee. House and Senate conferees are appointed by the presiding officers of each house. Conference committee members have a lot of seniority—and a lot of power, all of which may be exercised behind closed doors. A bill reported out of a conference committee is virtually ironclad. Your earmark funding may simply disappear behind those closed doors, and you will not know why or by whose hand, unless your MC or his or her staff has a reliable pipeline into the conference deliberations. Rarely, funding cut in conference may be restored on the floor of the House or Senate, but that is so unlikely that it is not even polite to ask an MC to expend political capital by rehearsing in public what was done in private by senior MCs. Better luck next time. Now is a good time again to remember that "no" on Capitol Hill—especially given that your project has gotten this far—usually means, "Not now. Come back next year."

Then again, you just may have landed your big fish. If so, it is unlikely that you have received all you asked for, which means you may have to return for more earmark funding, year after year, until your project is fully funded. Returning for more funding gives you additional leverage with Congress: Why squander what has already been spent by cutting off funding in subsequent years? Clearly, you must be able to demonstrate three things: (1) that you have something to show for the funding you received, (2) that you have not misspent any federal funds, and (c) that further funding will take your project to its next watershed.

Now that you have your funding, prepare to wait awhile to start spending it. Typically, you will be required to apply for it from the agency handling your money, and that can take months. It is not uncommon for earmark funds passed by Congress in September—the federal fiscal year begins October 1—actually to arrive the following April or May, but by then, you will be well under way to storm the Hill for the next round of funding.

Care to dance?

REFERENCES

Congressional Research Service. (2006). *Lobbying Congress: An overview of legal provisions and congressional ethics rules* (J. Maskell, Ed.). Retrieved from the U.S. Senate Web site: http://156.33.195.33/reference/resources/pdf/RL31126.pdf

Disclosure of Lobbying Activities, 2 U.S.C. 26, Sec. 1602(8)(B)(i–xix) (2007).

Office of Management and Budget. (2007). *FY 2005 Authorization Earmarks.* [Data file]. Retrieved from the Office of Management and Budget Web site: http://earmarks.omb.gov/authorizations_home.html

Palmer, G. (1987). The New Zealand legislative machine. *Victoria University of Wellington Law Review, 17,* 285.

Wilson, W. (1901). *Congressional government: A study in American politics* (15th ed.). Boston: Houghton Mifflin.

13

AHRQ Funding Opportunities for Nurse Researchers

KATHLEEN KENDRICK, GAIL S. MAKULOWICH, AND MARY L. GRADY

Innovations in health care are emerging every day. Some of these innovations involve direct patient care, including new medications, new surgical techniques, and more effective treatments for chronic conditions, to name a few. Other innovations focus on new ways to organize and pay for care, strategies to improve the quality of care and reduce medical errors, public health strategies to address natural disasters and potential bioterrorist events, and evidence to assist policy makers as they formulate health care legislation, rules, and regulations. Innovations such as these hold great promise for better, more accessible, and more affordable health care for all Americans. However, effective innovations that are not disseminated and adopted on the front lines of health care delivery or innovations that never arrive at the testing phase represent missed opportunities to improve care and wasted research dollars.

The Agency for Health Care Research and Quality (AHRQ) is an agency of the U.S. Department of Health and Human Services, whose mission is to improve the quality, safety, efficiency, and effectiveness of

AHRQ has begun its transition to electronic receipt of grant applications. In conjunction with the change from paper to electronic filing, the current PHS 398 application will be replaced by the Standard Form (SF) 424 Research and Related (R&R) application. These changes are being phased in gradually; they began in December 2005 and are expected to be complete by mid-2008. Go to http://www.ahrq.gov/path/egrants.htm for more information about this change.

health care for all Americans. The agency's challenge is to ensure that the findings from AHRQ-supported research make their way into everyday clinical practice and policy making at all levels. We believe that nurses play a pivotal role in implementing evidence-based care and in researching ways to improve care. Nurse researchers are critical to the future development of health services research. Findings from nurse research can influence policy and decision making at both the local care-delivery systems level and the state and federal levels.

This chapter provides nurses with an overview of AHRQ's funding priorities, as well as tips on how to be successful in obtaining funding. Individual sections address AHRQ's changing mission, health services research priorities, nurse funding opportunities and examples of grants given to nurses, training and development programs, and finally, tips on how nurses can get an AHRQ grant.

AHRQ'S CHANGING MISSION

AHRQ's mission continues to focus on safer, more effective, and more cost-effective health care for all Americans. Although this has been our core mission for some time, we are in the midst of a strategic redirection. We need to accelerate the pace of innovation and implementation of new knowledge in order to ensure value through more informed choices, assess innovation faster to prove its worth and utility, and implement effective interventions more quickly. This means that we need to do a better job of ensuring that innovations are evaluated and then disseminated to frontline users in a timely manner. Our goal is to quickly reach people and organizations that use the findings from AHRQ-supported research to make a difference in people's lives.

Implications for Researchers and Clinicians

The implications of this strategic redirection for AHRQ's mission include an emphasis on the production and use of evidence in policy making and health care decision making. We are also more focused on a value-added approach in awarding research grants and increasing synergy between intramural and extramural research within portfolios—that is, broad areas of research interest such as prevention and long-term care. We have also placed more emphasis on real-world problem solving, including obtaining user input in deliberations about the relevance of research ideas.

To get the most out of our research dollars, AHRQ is working as a science partner with like-minded agencies and organizations. This helps us to leverage our resources and achieve buy-in from stakeholders, policy makers, health system leaders, clinicians, and consumers. We are focusing on issues that are important to decision makers. Our goal is to close the gap between evidence and practice. Finally, we must nurture the next generation of health services researchers so that we continue to have the capacity and expertise needed to continue this important work.

As we identify research topics and make funding decisions, we are balancing two priorities: (1) the need to create new knowledge about clinical and organizational effectiveness and what works in quality improvement and (2) the need to bring about improvements in clinical practice.

AHRQ'S RESEARCH PRIORITIES

Balancing Priorities: A Framework for Decision Making

AHRQ's focus on creating and disseminating new knowledge that can enhance clinical practice pays dividends in several ways. This focus transforms research findings into practice, improves outcomes through research, promotes the use of evidence to improve health care, and improves health care quality for all Americans.

Areas of Emphasis

AHRQ's focus is on health services research, which often builds on and extends biomedical research. As outlined in Figure 13.1, health-related research often begins with biomedical research, which includes the basic sciences and controlled clinical trials. This research then transitions to health-services research, which involves analysis of cost-effectiveness, quality and outcomes research, syntheses and meta-analyses, and finally, organization, financing, and delivery research.

AHRQ encourages and supports health services research that falls within 10 areas of emphasis. We call these research areas cross-cutting portfolios. The first 5 areas include (1) prevention, to increase the adoption, delivery, and use of evidence-based clinical preventive services in the United States; (2) health information technology, to increase the development, diffusion, and adoption of health information technology;

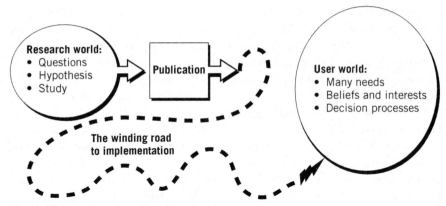

Figure 13.1 Supply-side research paradigm
Source: "Beyond the Dusty Shelf: Shifting Paradigms and Effecting Change," by D. McNeil, H. Holland, & K. Henriksen, 2005, in K. Henriksen, J. B. Battles, E. S. Marks, & D. I. lewin (Eds.), *Advance in Patient Safety: From Research to Implementation: Vol. 3. Implementation,* p. 384. Rockville, MD: Agency for Research and Quality. Reprinted with permission from AHRQ.

(3) quality and safety of patient care, to decrease errors, risks, or hazards in health care and their harmful impact on patients; (4) care management, to promote the receipt of effective, evidence-based, and patient-centered care for acute and chronic conditions; and (5) development of tools, to measure health care quality, efficiency, and effectiveness that will facilitate data use and translation into usable information by external and internal stakeholders. The other 5 include (6) system capacity and emergency preparedness, to empower communities and health care systems to support all people prepare for urgent and emergent demands and needs; (7) long-term care, to improve outcomes, quality, and evidence-based information focused on long-term care (e.g., assistance with mobility, homemaker services, etc.); (8) pharmaceutical outcomes, to improve health outcomes through the safe and effective use of pharmaceuticals; (9) cost, organization, and socioeconomics, to improve quality, efficiency, and effectiveness of health care by providing public and private decision makers with the information, tools, and assistance they need to make improved decisions; and (10) training, to continue to foster the growth, dissemination, and translation of the field and science of health services research.

Research findings must make it from the research world—which comprises questions, hypotheses, and studies—to the user world, which features many needs, multiple benefits and interests, and varying decision processes. As outlined in Figure 13.1, we can think of this as a supply-side research paradigm, in which ideas travel along a winding road from the research world, where they are transformed into findings, to the publication interface in the scientific literature, and finally to the user world, where findings are put into practice.

However, only a fraction of original research makes it all the way to implementation in the hospital, doctor's office, or other health care setting. Indeed, it can take as long as 17 years to translate just 14% of the original research submitted to AHRQ to the benefit of patient care as outlined in the supply-side research paradigm (see Figure 13.1).

RESEARCH FUNDING OPPORTUNITIES

Research funding opportunities at AHRQ include support for research projects, conference grants, and training and career development grants. The agency has funded numerous grants to nurse researchers over the years. Topics of funded research projects have ranged from analyzing the prescribing practices of nurse practitioners to measuring the impact of nurse staffing on adverse patient outcomes to researching mammography access for older women of color. AHRQ funding opportunities are announced online at http://www.grants.gov and in the *NIH Guide for Grants and Contracts*. The various funding opportunities available from AHRQ are described briefly here. More information on current funding opportunities at AHRQ (see http://www.ahrq.gov/fund/) and detailed instructions on how to apply for an AHRQ-supported grant may be found at http://grants.nih.gov/grants/guide and at http://www.grants.gov.

Investigator-Initiated Research Funding

Many of the research projects supported by AHRQ are funded through investigator-initiated grant applications. Applications in this category are submitted by investigators who develop an idea for a research project that fits within AHRQ's areas of interest. Opportunities in this area include large (R01) research grants, research demonstration (R18) projects, small research (R03) grants, and large and small (R13) conference grants. In order to be considered for funding, applications must be responsive to AHRQ's priorities and program objectives.

Large Research (R01) Grants

An R01 research grant provides support for a discrete, specified, and circumscribed project that addresses areas of interest to AHRQ. The project is to be performed by the applicant in an area representing his or her specific interests and competencies, and it must be in line with AHRQ priorities and research objectives. Applications are reviewed for scientific and technical merit. Funding decisions are based on a priority score, the availability of funds, and program balance among research areas.

This type of research grant may be funded up to $300,000 a year; application receipt dates are February 5, June 5, and October 5 of each year. Several years ago, AHRQ awarded an R01 research grant to Dr. Marie Cowan of the University of California, Los Angeles, to compare the effectiveness of care management by a hospitalist MD/acute care nurse practitioner team with conventional approaches to hospital care delivery for acutely ill general medical inpatients. This approach reduced the average length of hospital stay from 6 to 5 days. Through reduction of the number of hospital days after the first 4 days, which are the most profitable ones, hospital profits increased by $1,591 per day for each patient without increasing hospital readmission or mortality rates (Cowan, 2006). This study addressed improvement in care management, a research priority for AHRQ. Findings from this study have the potential to improve traditional delivery of services at the hospital and systems level.

Research Demonstration and Dissemination (R18) Grants

Research demonstration and dissemination (R18) grants provide support for the development, testing, and evaluation of health service activities and foster the application of existing knowledge for the control of categorical diseases. Criteria for an R18 research demonstration and dissemination grant are similar to those for an R01 grant. As with all other investigator-initiated applications, applications for R18 grants must demonstrate applicability to AHRQ's priorities and program objectives. The application dates for R18 grants are January 25, May 25, and September 25 of each year.

In 2000, AHRQ funded an R18 grant led by nurse researcher Joann Congdon of the University of Colorado. The goal of this 4-year project was to develop and evaluate ways to assist consumers in using quality factors in choosing a nursing home. The nurse investigators examined the most useful indicators of nursing home quality to aid in the development of nursing home report cards. As a result, the Centers for Medicare and Medicaid Services began publishing quality report cards for all U.S. nursing homes in 2002. These report cards have prompted many nursing homes, especially those with poor scores, to take actions to improve care (Mukamel, Spector, Zinn, Huang, Weimer, et al., 2007). Thus, the development of the report cards had a significant impact on federal policy aimed at improving the quality of nursing home care.

Small Research (R03) Grants

AHRQ also provides support for small research projects that are more limited in time and amount for research in particular program areas that are germane to AHRQ's research agenda. These small grants provide flexibility for initiating studies and generally are for preliminary short-term studies and are not renewable. Small grants may be funded up to $100,000 in total costs; application receipt dates are February 16, June 16, and October 16 of each year.

In 2002, AHRQ funded an R03 grant for 1 year to nurse researcher Dr. Regina Cunningham of the University of Pennsylvania. The goal of the research was to examine the impact of post-prostatectomy care by advanced practice nurses (APNs) on the clinical outcomes of men who had undergone prostatectomy. Cunningham found that APNs consistently followed guidelines to alleviate post-prostatectomy symptoms such as depression, incontinence, and impotence. She concluded that APNs might be a valuable resource to help generalist nurses interpret and implement these guidelines and improve overall quality of post-prostatectomy care delivery (Cunningham, 2006).

Conference (R13) Grants

Through our conference grant program, AHRQ provides support for large and small meetings, including national and regional meetings, conferences, and workshops. Small conference grants are funded for 1 year, and applicants may request up to $50,000 in direct costs. Application receipt dates for small conference grants are February 20, April 20, June 20, August 20, October 20, and December 20 of each year. Large conference grants are funded for up to 3 years, with a maximum of $100,000 per year. Application receipt dates are April 12, August 12, and December 12 of each year.

In 2002, AHRQ awarded a small conference grant to Kathleen Stevens of the University of Texas Health Science Center, San Antonio.

This grant provided partial support for a national conference focused on preparing nurses for an increasingly active role in evidence-based practice (EBP), to improve patient care outcomes through translation of research into practice. One conference goal was for participants to develop an action plan for implementing EPB in their own health care organizations. Ideally, EBP will reduce practice variation, improve effective practices, and achieve better outcomes consistent with the Healthy People 2010 and Institute of Medicine priorities.

In 2005, AHRQ awarded another small conference grant to Ms. Mary Johnson of the North Carolina Board of Nursing, Dr. Brenda Cleary of the North Carolina Center for Nursing, and Dr. Gail Mazzocco of the School of Nursing, University of North Carolina–Chapel Hill. The conference examined the problems faced by newly licensed nurses when they transition into the clinical workforce. For example, many do not know when and how to call a physician or do not understand the pharmacological implications of medications. The conference also addressed concerns about the ability of newly licensed nurses to avoid and catch medical errors before they harm patients. One result of the conference was a tool kit to measure 14 areas of competency for new nurses. The ability to assess the competencies of newly licensed nurses can inform policy on nurse education and has the potential to reduce medical errors and increase retention of newly licensed nurses. This will become even more important over the next 20 years, as large portions of the nursing workforce (up to 50% in some areas) reach retirement age.

Solicited Research Funding

AHRQ uses two mechanisms to announce funding opportunities for solicited research: the request for applications (RFA) and the program announcement (PA). The RFA is used most often to announce these funding opportunities. More information and a listing of current RFAs and PAs may be found at http://www.ahrq.gov/fund/grantix.htm.

Requests for Applications (RFAs)

RFAs are issued to invite grant applications in a single, well-defined area with specific objectives. RFAs have a single receipt date and specific funding levels. Special emphasis panels review applications received in response to an RFA.

Program Announcements

PAs are formal statements that describe continuing, new, or expanded program interests for which grant or cooperative agreement applications are invited. Applications in response to PAs are reviewed by peer review committees of the AHRQ Initial Review Group (IRG). Some PAs are sponsored solely by AHRQ, and others are cosponsored by AHRQ and one or more other federal agencies. There is no set funding level for these projects.

Examples of Solicited Nursing Research Projects Funded by AHRQ

Several years ago, AHRQ funded a number of research projects related to nursing under an RFA focused on the impact of working conditions on quality of care. It was hoped that the results of these studies would suggest ways to improve the staffing, organization, and delivery of care to ensure better patient safety and quality of care. It was also expected that the research findings would better inform policy on organization and staffing. Examples of these projects include a project on staff nursing fatigue and patient safety conducted by Dr. Ann Rogers from the University of Pennsylvania. Rogers examined the impact of hours worked by nurses on fatigue and medical errors. For example, the research team found that the risk of making an error nearly doubled when critical care nurses worked 12.5 or more consecutive hours. Yet, 67% of nurse work shifts were longer than 12 hours. In addition, the risk of falling asleep doubled on shifts longer than 8 hours. The study's findings support the Institute of Medicine's recommendation to minimize use of 12-hour shifts. These findings also raise questions about the need to limit work hours for nurses, as has been done for resident physicians. In addition, the second part of the project examined strategies to minimize the adverse effects of fatigue on nurse performance.

Another study by Nancy Donaldson from the University of California, San Francisco, investigated the impact of nurse staffing and workload at the hospital-unit level on indicators of patient safety and quality, such as falls and pressure ulcers. Studies such as this have had a major impact on shaping policies for nurses' work conditions, most notably the implementation of staffing ratios in California.

Other projects included analysis of nursing home working conditions and quality of care by Dr. Jill Scott from the University of Colorado.

Dr. Scott analyzed the impact of the work culture and environment, staff interaction, and staffing on patient quality of care in nursing homes (Scott, Rogers, Hwang, & Zhang, 2006). In addition, Dr. Chris Kovner from New York University led a project that looked at patient safety in home care. This project focused on the care provided by nurses and its relationship to patient safety in home care. The safety of home health care has been less widely studied than patient safety in hospitals and nursing homes.

In 2005, AHRQ funded a 3-year project on discharge management of low-income, frail elderly individuals, which is being led by Dr. Kyle Allen of Summa Health System. For this project, researchers are testing the effectiveness of a comprehensive care management strategy, including care coordination by a nurse care manager, for elderly patients with chronic illness and functional impairment who are discharged from an acute care hospital.

In 2003, AHRQ awarded a grant to Dr. Josie Williams from Texas A&M University to examine the role of public health nurses in bioterrorism preparedness. Williams's study revealed the importance of public health nurses' strong network of informal communications in the community in obtaining critical disease surveillance information (Akins, Williams, Silenas, & Edwards, 2005). However, they found that nurses face many barriers to becoming active participants during bioterrorism emergencies. The study findings can inform federal and state policy makers about the potentially critical role that public health nurses can play during bioterrorism and other public health emergencies, as well as ways to facilitate their help.

Notices of Special Emphasis

From time to time, AHRQ issues special emphasis notices to alert researchers that the agency plans to place special emphasis on a certain area in the agency's grants portfolio. These special emphasis notices are posted in the Funding Opportunities section of the agency's Web site at http://www.ahrq.gov, and they are published in the *NIH Guide for Grants and Contracts* as well.

In fiscal year 2006, AHRQ issued a special emphasis notice to announce the agency's interest in research on the care of sicker patients. Many studies have focused on disease-specific interventions, such as the optimal procedures or medications for heart disease. However, there has been limited work addressing the unique needs of sicker patients who typically suffer from multiple chronic diseases and risk factors. AHRQ encouraged potential applicants to propose projects that examined the research gaps in patient-centered care for such complicated patients. For example, the agency encouraged research on topics that ranged from effective methods for managing polypharmacy in individuals suffering from multiple coexisting conditions to strategies to reduce racial, ethnic, and social disparities in the care of these vulnerable individuals.

In fiscal year 2007, AHRQ issued a special emphasis notice to announce research priorities in the area of systems and organizational interventions for improving health care quality for low-income people served in under-resourced settings and communities. A second special emphasis notice with a focus on research implementation for small grants was also issued in fiscal year 2007.

These notices of special interest are particularly useful to investigators as they are developing their research plans in advance of submitting an application to AHRQ.

TRAINING AND CAREER DEVELOPMENT PROGRAMS

AHRQ has a variety of intramural and extramural training programs in health services research. They include predoctoral and postdoctoral educational programs and career development grants, support for health services research at the institutional level, and other opportunities. AHRQ's training and education programs are briefly described here. More detailed information is available from AHRQ's Web site at http://www.ahrq.gov/fund/training/trainix.htm.

Training Goals and Opportunities

AHRQ is committed to activities and programs that further the educational development of the next generation of health services researchers, including nurse researchers. Our goals are to foster the growth of the next generation of researchers and knowledgeable users of research findings and to nurture the careers of budding researchers who are just embarking on their career development. We also strive to promote institutional and individual diversity in the field of health services research and to provide support for the planning and development of health services research in traditionally minority-serving institutions and institutions in states that traditionally do not receive significant health services research funding. Finally, we work to encourage and support the development of an integrated science of health services research and to refine its foundation in order to be responsive to agency and Health and Human Services departmental priorities.

We know that our best hope for ensuring a continuing and strong health services research effort depends on a continuing commitment to training and infrastructure development and support.

Predoctoral and Postdoctoral Training Grants

Successful applicants for AHRQ training grants will focus on methodological and research topics that are in line with the agency's mission and research interests. Receipt dates, application materials, and instructions for applicants are different for these training programs than for other types of grants (see the AHRQ Web site at http://www.ahrq.gov/fund/training/trainix.htm for more information).

The agency supports pre- and postdoctoral training of individuals who are interested in pursuing a career in health services research. Support is provided through National Research Service Award (NRSA) fellowships, including both individual and institutional programs. NRSA predoctoral fellowships provide up to 5 years of support and are intended to promote diversity in health-related research. Postdoctoral fellowships provide opportunities for 1 to 3 years of academic training or supervised experience. Three examples of research projects funded to nurses through AHRQ fellowships include strategies used by intensive care unit nurses to develop nurse–family relationships, the use of computers to identify nursing resources for the elderly, and the use of mental health services by Asian and Pacific Islander Americans.

Dissertation Grants

In addition to these NRSA fellowships, AHRQ also has a dissertation grant program that supports research undertaken as part of an academic program to qualify for a doctorate. Nurses and nursing research have figured prominently in this program. Over the past few years, 20% of the dissertation grants funded by AHRQ either went to nurses or were focused on topics closely related to nursing. Some recently funded dissertation research topics have included the following: categorizing nursing homes based on quality performance, intensive care unit nursing workload, ways to increase the supply of certified nursing assistants, the use of incident reports to assess falls in nursing homes, hospital patterns of nursing personnel substitution, patient outcomes related to hospital discharge planning collaboration, and the use of physical restraints in at-risk elderly patients.

Career Development Awards

Grants for career development are also available. They include mentored clinical scientist (K08) development awards and independent investigator (K02) awards. Awards for both programs are for 3 to 5 years and are nonrenewable.

The mentored clinical scientist program targets individuals with clinical doctorates, including those in patient-oriented research, who need mentoring and have the potential to develop into independent investigators. AHRQ recently granted an award to a nurse researcher to measure the quality of care for homeless adolescents.

Independent investigator awards are aimed at promising new clinical and nonclinical investigators who are out of training 5 years or less and have a demonstrated need for intensive research focus. AHRQ recently granted an award to a nurse researcher to examine the effects of Medicaid policy on access to dental care.

RESEARCH INFRASTRUCTURE SUPPORT PROGRAMS

AHRQ funds projects under two initiatives that focus on research infrastructure support: the Minority Research Infrastructure Support Program (M-RISP) and the Building Research Infrastructure and Capacity (BRIC) programs.

The objective of the M-RISP initiative is to increase the health services research capacity of academic institutions that predominantly or substantially serve racial and ethnic minority populations. Institutions funded through this program, including their faculty members, receive grants to improve their ability to conduct health services research that is suitable for dissemination, implementation, and translation into practice and policy. AHRQ's goal is to strengthen the research environment in minority institutions by developing or expanding their existing capacity for conducting health-related research.

The goal of AHRQ's BRIC initiative is to enhance competitiveness for research funding among institutions located in states where successful applications for funding have been historically low. In fiscal year 2006, AHRQ funded five 2-year BRIC projects at institutions in Arkansas, Maine, Nebraska, North Dakota, and West Virginia.

GETTING AN AHRQ RESEARCH GRANT

Getting funding support from AHRQ for research begins with a grant application. Before you prepare your application, however, you need to do your homework. That is, you need an understanding of the agency, its priorities, and how it operates. Given AHRQ's policy emphasis, focusing on the policy relevance of your research proposal will strengthen your application. You also need to familiarize yourself with the application SF 424 (R&R). You will find this form, as well as related resources, on AHRQ's Web site at http://www.ahrq.gov/fund/sf424.htm.

Initial Steps in Developing the Research Proposal

A critical first step in formulating any research proposal for submission to AHRQ is to communicate with an appropriate AHRQ project officer. A project officer is an AHRQ staff member who has general knowledge about research practices, specific knowledge about a substantive area of interest to AHRQ, and a thorough understanding of AHRQ's research processes and priorities. The project officer can provide a valuable perspective about the suitability of a particular research idea in light of AHRQ's priorities.

To identify an appropriate project officer, go to the key contacts page on the agency's Web site (http://www.ahrq.gov/about/contacts.htm) and look for a staff member who is working in your area of interest and expertise. Alternatively, you may decide to submit a brief concept paper outlining a potential research idea before you begin to prepare a formal research application. This can be a mechanism for establishing contact with AHRQ and beginning a dialogue with an AHRQ project officer who has expertise in your area of interest.

There is a special interest section on the AHRQ Web site that is devoted to nursing research (http://www.ahrq.gov/about/nursing). There you will find information on conferences and workshops of interest to nurses and nurse researchers, a listing of funded grants submitted by nurses, and information about nurses who are on staff at AHRQ.

Tips for Completing the Grant Application

Meanwhile, here are a few tips to help you get started in the grant application process; you will find many more suggestions on the AHRQ Web site at http://www.ahrq.gov/fund/apptips.htm:

- First, give yourself plenty of time to write the grant application— at least 3 to 6 months.
- Before you begin writing your grant application, read the application instructions carefully and become familiar with all requirements.
- Whether you are responding to an AHRQ PA or to an RFA, be sure to read the announcement and all instructions carefully.
- Contact an AHRQ staff member to answer any questions you may have.
- If possible, contact someone in your institution (e.g., in the research administration office) who can assist you in understanding and completing application materials.
- Determine human subjects requirements.
- Develop a detailed budget with full justification.
- Contact AHRQ program staff to present your research plan and solicit feedback.
- Have an outside reader review the application to provide objective comments before you submit your proposal to AHRQ.
- Use clear writing, try to avoid jargon, and follow application format requirements.

OVERVIEW OF THE GRANT APPLICATION SUBMISSION, REVIEW, AND AWARD PROCESS

Once your application is routed to AHRQ, it is logged in and assigned to a project officer and to a peer review group (study section committee) or to a special emphasis panel. You will receive written notification of your review assignment within 6 weeks. Your application will be sent to the reviewers, and subsequently it will undergo initial peer review at AHRQ.

After the application review has been completed, you will receive a summary statement with the review results within 3 months. As noted previously, funding decisions are made by AHRQ based on scientific and technical merit, the agency's research priorities, and the availability of grant funds.

If your application is approved for funding, an AHRQ grants management staff member will contact your institution to negotiate the terms of the grant award. A notice of grant award will then be sent electronically to the applicant institution, usually within 6 weeks of the funding decision. If your application is not funded, you may discuss options with your AHRQ project officer, including the potential for revising and resubmitting the application.

Getting Technical Assistance

AHRQ staff members are available to provide technical assistance to you during the grant application process. They can discuss agency priorities, explain the scope and intent of PAs and RFAs issued by AHRQ, and answer questions you may have about the grant application process. Contact information for appropriate AHRQ staff is provided in all PAs and RFAs, as well as on the AHRQ Web site at http://www.ahrq.gov/about/contacts.htm.

In addition, as noted previously, your project officer can assist you in understanding and addressing any deficiencies or problems that may have emerged during the peer review process. Exhibit 13.1 presents some common problems identified during peer review, which may result in your application being scored as noncompetitive.

To keep researchers and other constituents abreast of agency news and research findings on key topics, the AHRQ publishes an electronic newsletter several times each month. Subscriptions to the electronic newsletter are free. The latest issue and subscription information are available at http://www.ahrq.gov/news/ahrqlist.htm.

Exhibit 13.1 Common Problems

- Uncertainty about whether research will produce significant information
- No apparent translatability of research into practice or policy
- Overly ambitious research plan; volume of proposed work unrealistic
- Proposed methods not appropriate to answer research questions
- Too little detail in the research plan
- An inadequate literature review
- Lack of investigator or study team expertise in needed areas
- Lack of study controls
- Lack of adequate preliminary data
- Insufficient consideration of statistical needs
- Inadequate attention to protection of human subjects or population representation

CONCLUSION

As described in this chapter, AHRQ is first and foremost a research agency. However, we know that research is only a beginning and not an end in itself. On a daily basis, this means doing everything we can to ensure that providers use evidence-based research findings to deliver high-quality health care and to work with their patients as partners.

Evidence garnered from research helps patients to become more informed consumers and to play an active role in decisions about their own care. AHRQ's research findings play a very important role in informing policy makers at all levels—federal, state, and local—as they formulate and debate legislation, rules, and regulations that affect America's system and the ways in which consumers access, use, and pay for care.

Accomplishing these goals requires a strategic approach to ensure that research findings are ready to be used, widely available, and actionable. It also means working at the grassroots level to help local policy makers understand what they can do to improve the quality of health care for their constituents and ensuring that local public health officials have the latest information to help them coordinate their resources and be prepared in the event of a public health emergency.

These steps are critical components of AHRQ's new vision, which is to foster and support research that helps America's health care system provide access to high-quality, cost-effective services and to be accountable and responsive to consumers and purchasers.

America's rapidly evolving system poses challenges to all of us: providers, purchasers, policy makers, researchers, and the public. The recent increase in public attention to such issues as patient safety, quality, and disparities in health care highlights the importance of research that can both identify problems and develop viable solutions. AHRQ's goal and commitment is to provide support for the production, translation, and dissemination of research findings geared toward transforming and improving our health care system. Ultimately, the goal is to improve health status and quality of life across the nation.

REFERENCES

Akins, R. B., Williams, J. R, Silenas, R., & Edwards, J. C. (2005). The role of public health nurses in bioterrorism preparedness. *Disease Management—Response, 3*(4), 98–105.

Cowan, M. J. (2006). The effect of a multidisciplinary hospitalist/physician and advanced practice nurse collaboration on hospital costs. *Journal of Nursing Administration, 36*(2), 79–85.

Cunningham, R. S. (2006). Clinical practice guideline use by oncology advanced practice nurses. *Applied Nursing Research, 19,* 126–133.

McNeil, D., Holland, H., & Henriksen, K. (2005). Beyond the dusty shelf: Shifting paradigms and effecting change. In K. Henriksen, J. B. Battles, E. S. Marks, & D. I. Iewin (Eds.), *Advance in patient safety: From research to implementation: Vol. 3. Implementation* (pp. 383–393). Rockville, MD: Agency for Research and Quality.

Mukamel, D. B., Spector, W. D., Zinn, J. S., Huang, L., Weimer, D. L., & Dozier, A. (2007). Nursing homes' response to the nursing home compare report card. *Journal of Gerontology: Social Sciences, 62B*(4), S218–S225.

Scott, L. D., Rogers, A. E., Hwang, W-T., & Zhang, Y. (2006). Effects of critical care nurses' work hours on vigilance and patients' safety. *American Journal of Critical Care, 15*(1), 30–37.

14

From Issues to Action: How the Robert Wood Johnson Foundation Influences Health Policy

LORI MELICHAR AND SUSAN B. HASSMILLER

The Robert Wood Johnson Foundation (RWJF) seeks to improve the health and health care of Americans through social change. To change society and the lives of American citizens for the better and alter the trajectory of entire neighborhoods and communities, the foundation is committed to addressing health and health care issues on the broadest level. To attack problems at their deepest roots and to help make a difference on the widest scale—particularly for the most vulnerable among Americans—the foundation engages a wide range of individuals, including providers, patients, private organizations, purchasers, and insurers, all of whom together produce the outcomes of the U.S. public and private health care system.

Policy changes on both the governmental and the organizational level are important to the foundation's efforts to achieve social change. In addition to the fact that even RWJF's assets pale relative to federal budgets, it is impossible without the tools of the law to erect barriers to harmful health behaviors, to remove legislative barriers to improvement, and to restructure government financing systems to align incentives for quality. In this chapter, we describe how the nation's largest foundation devoted exclusively to health and health care seeks to influence policy at both the governmental and the organizational level.

Specific examples of the process used by the foundation to influence policy are found in this chapter. The process begins with identification of the problem and continues to the implementation and evaluation of projects designed to build evidence for change through fostering collaboration, conducting research, educating policy makers, and convening stakeholder groups. This chapter provides useful information for nurses considering funding for evidence-producing strategies to underlie policy changes.

GOVERNMENTAL POLICY: RWJF'S ROLE IN ADVANCING THE NURSE PRACTITIONER ROLE

In 1972, while searching for ways to increase Americans' access to high-quality health care, RWJF recognized the potential for a new nursing role, the "nurse practitioner," to expand primary care. Nurse practitioners (NPs), able to treat both acute and chronic conditions, as well as prescribe medications and therapies for patients, provided much of the same basic, non-emergent care as was provided by physicians. To many physicians, the concept of the new professionals meant authorizing unprepared and unlicensed medical practice. To many nurses, the concept meant that the nurses would become "physician extenders" and that the profession would lose ground in its struggle to escape subordination to medicine. This professional resistance prevented the federal government and the states from engaging in debates around the issue until the late 1970s. To explore the validity of these fears and to capture potential benefits of the innovation, the foundation initiated a series of regional demonstrations focused on the training and deployment of nurse practitioners. Evaluations of five multisite networks provided evidence that nurse practitioners could play a vital role in the nation's health care, and the foundation proceeded to promote this role. Although necessary evidence alone is not always sufficient to influence the political process, the goal was that the findings from these evaluations would facilitate evidence-based policy changes at the organizational and governmental levels that would support this new nursing role.

In spite of evidence suggesting nurse practitioners were a cost-effective way to expand access without sacrificing quality and hospital cost-cutting, the hostility of academic nursing toward NP programs impeded progress toward widespread deployment of the profession in the health care labor market. Realizing that without an educational infrastructure to promote these professions, they were doomed to fail, RWJF sought to engage strategic partners in academic nursing—especially nursing deans. Most of them responded negatively, but a handful of leaders of graduate nursing faculties who had been trained as NPs and who were emerging as leaders in this evolving area came together to support each other's efforts to demonstrate the value of the program and to advocate for federal support.

In addition to identifying and bringing recognition to academic leaders in the nurse practitioner movement, the RWJF demonstration project fostered the development of leaders in this emerging field by imparting advocacy skills and establishing a network to facilitate promotion of the profession both within the field and with policy makers. Additionally, RWJF helped create a science-based curriculum that could be a standard for curriculum nationwide.

Overall, the foundation invested in developing the role of the NP by funding demonstration projects that produced evidence to support that the new role was effective, by developing the advocacy skills of emerging nurse leaders, and by facilitating the development of a standardized, science-based curriculum for NP education. Due in large part to the foundation's early investments in the nurse practitioner movement, the federal government and the states have subsequently encouraged and funded the nurse practitioner profession, a role that has transformed the face of health care delivery in both acute and outpatient primary care settings. The U.S. Bureau of Health Professions has played, and continues to play, a pivotal role in financing the educational infrastructure of nurse practitioners. The strength of the role has withstood time, and many of the health care reform plans recommended by policy makers call for the inclusion of NPs in efforts to increase access to high-quality care for all Americans (Keenan, 1998).

The example of the nurse practitioner movement illustrates one of the ways Robert Wood Johnson Foundation investments have influenced health policy to increase the capacity of the U.S. health care system. As a result of these investments, there are 115,000 NPs practicing in the United States today—providing care to patients who might not have received care at all (American Academy of Nurse Practitioners, 2007).

ORGANIZATIONAL POLICY: TRANSFORMING CARE AT THE BEDSIDE

Improvements in the policies of health care *organizations* are also an important part of the foundation's strategy to improve health and health care. In organizations, the "policy makers" are those who have the authority to set rules about how work is organized or conducted and to make decisions about how to allocate resources to alternative activities within an organization. Examples of improvements in organizational policy include improvements to human resource practices that result in healthier, happier, more productive employees; allocation of funding within organizational budgets to adequately equip workers to carry out their work efficiently; and the provision of training for workers that allows them to contribute more effectively to the mission of the organization.

In 2003 the foundation sought solutions to the problem of high turnover rates for nurses working in hospitals. Through a partnership with the Institute for Healthcare Improvement, the foundation developed a program called Transforming Care at the Bedside (TCAB). This program engaged nurses and other staff on hospital units across the country in work to diagnose key quality deficiencies, suggest innovative changes to combat quality problems, test innovations developed to improve quality, assess progress toward quality goals, and share ideas and processes with nurses and other staff within and across hospital settings. Anecdotal evidence from the nurses who participated in this program revealed increases in morale, improvements in doctor–nurse relationships, reductions in adverse events such as bed sores and falls, and reduced turnover. Communications experts worked with representatives from each hospital to help them tell these compelling stories to others who might be convinced the program could improve quality of care in their hospital as well.

The foundation, recognizing the potential of this innovative program to transform the quality of care delivered at the bedside, sought to spread TCAB to other organizations across the country. After funding a study to determine how hospital administrators made decisions about budget allocation, the foundation realized that in order to convince other administrators to allocate financial resources to the TCAB program for innovations and staff time, as well as to reallocate authority from senior nurse executives to frontline nurses, it would need to produce evidence of the program's impact, cost, and information to guide implementation.

A major evaluation that documented reductions in turnover and increases in quality accompanied the second phase of the program. Qualitative information from the evaluation was valuable to help the foundation understand what elements were crucial to the program's success and what elements could be dropped. This information guided the foundation's development of a less resource-intensive version of the program that, theoretically, could be spread more easily to more hospitals across the country. The results of the impact of "TCAB-lite," a strategic partnership between RWJF and the American Hospital Association's Organization of Nurse Executives, are yet to be determined. An evaluation of the effort will inform future foundation investments in the area as well as inform the policy decisions of hospital leaders seeking ways to decrease cost and increase quality of care.

THE PROCESS OF INFLUENCING POLICY

In the preceding examples, the people who guide, manage, and work for RWJF engaged in a multistep, multi-investment strategy to influence policy. First, the foundation *identified the problems* of access and the nursing shortage to be priorities for the foundation. The foundation next *identified promising solutions to these problems* and then designed *demonstration projects* to examine the potential of these solutions to improve health or health care and to demonstrate feasibility. *Evaluations of demonstration projects* were conducted to produce evidence of success or failure that would be viewed as rigorous and unbiased and to identify barriers and facilitators to spread of successful innovations. Where individuals, organizations, or existing or pending policies posed barriers to improvement, the foundation *funded research* to understand the opposition or educate detractors. Research results were *translated and communicated* to key decision makers. In addition, the foundation *engaged strategic partners* in convening efforts to align interest toward a common purpose. Along the way, the foundation made investments to build *the capacity of individuals and institutions* in order to sustain gains reaped through improvements in policy.

How RWJF Identifies Priorities

Even a very large health foundation can have little hope of effecting social change unless it focuses on a few well-defined areas in which it seeks to have a meaningful impact.

RWJF's priorities have been determined in different ways over the years. Current priorities are based on an impact framework. These priorities generally meet several criteria. First, RWJF chooses to address problems for which there is a significant need for change and for which solutions are believed to exist. Then the foundation identifies opportunities for grants to bring about significant improvements in the area. Finally,

RWJF seeks to fill a niche by making investments in underfunded areas, or areas for which the foundation has a comparative advantage over another funder interested in improvement and where market forces are unlikely to result in change at the desirable pace. Current priorities of RWJF include the complex issues of improving the quality and equality of care, reducing childhood obesity, bolstering the public health infrastructure, and finding ways to cover the uninsured.

Most issues remain priorities for the Robert Wood Johnson Foundation for years or even decades. Large, persistent problems such as lack of insurance and childhood obesity require long-term investments. The foundation also addresses emerging opportunities such as the current nurse faculty shortage. In addition to its targeted investments, the foundation allows for new ideas and special opportunities by putting funds aside to combat emerging, urgent problems such as the effects of the 2005 tsunami and Hurricane Katrina. For each issue, the foundation sets a specific objective, a time frame, and a plan and then allocates a budget to accomplish the objective. That is, rather than providing grants to address generally the nursing shortage in the United States, the foundation makes informed, staged, coordinated strategic grants to eliminate the problem. Many of these plans include a strategy of changing policy.

Over time, the priorities of the foundation have been influenced by an interdisciplinary staff of nurses, physicians, public health practitioners, economists, engineers, psychologists, health plan administrators, experts in business, and lawyers—each of whom has brought a unique perspective to the problem. In addition, because the foundation's board of directors includes leaders in the health and health care community, as well as leaders in non-health-related fields, including communications, law, business, and finance, they serve as a sounding board to the foundation leadership.

The example presented in Exhibit 14.1 describes how the foundation first identified the nursing shortage to be of high priority. The foundation then examined the nature of the problem, evaluated the possibility of alleviating the problem, determined the promise of investments to achieve policy change, and finally, selected a strategy for increasing retention.

Strategies to influence policy are more appealing when the political climate appears favorable enough to give a reasonable probability of success—that is, when the goals of foundations are aligned with the goals of policy makers. Policy makers whose children have related diseases have allocated funding to research into neurological diseases.

Exhibit 14.1 The Adoption of the Nursing Shortage as a New Priority

In 2002 the board of directors for RWJF gave a message to the staff that reducing the nursing shortage was to be a strategic area of focus for the foundation's investments. Though the foundation had a history of making investments in the field of nursing, these investments had been sporadic and uncoordinated. Although much had been learned, the foundation had not developed a unified strategy to confront the shortage. The charge from the board resulted in the formation of a team of staff convened around a goal of reducing the nursing shortage. First, the team conducted scans of the field to better understand the issue and to consider what area RWJF could most effectively influence. A scan of the nursing shortage problem revealed the root cause of the nursing shortage to be the high turnover of nurses in acute care settings, especially medical-surgical units. A scan of the investments of other funders revealed a niche in improving retention, given that other funders were focused on recruitment and education. From this initial decision, the nursing team created an action plan to research and develop programs that would address retention. The results of a literature review, focus groups, and interviews with key informants suggested that without widespread changes in the policies of organizations, facilitated by changes in governmental policy, retention of nurses was unlikely to improve. Ongoing interaction with a collaborative of organizations that make nursing-related investments ensures that the foundation continues to fill a niche in the area.

A grandparent of an autistic child is likely to consider that issue a high level of priority for federal research dollars. A policy maker who was the victim of domestic abuse may feel a personal responsibility to reduce harm to others. Hospital administrators who are married to nurses may have a more acute understanding of how nurses' work environment influences their professional engagement. Acceptance of nurse practitioners became much more appealing when the government was seeking ways to increase access to care and lower costs of care. In general, issues that present an opportunity for change receive a high ranking in the prioritization activity. Issues that are important to policy makers and their political platforms or administrators' list of priorities, but for which no concrete policy options exist, are ripe for research investments.

Sometimes foundation staffs are hired based on their expertise to make determinations about strategic investments to address particular issues. When individuals employed by a foundation do not have the expertise to suggest strategic investments in an area of focus, foundations collect information from key informants, external experts, and survey firms to inform foundation decisions. Another way foundations collect, organize, and present information to inform strategic investments is by hiring consultants to conduct "scans" of a particular area. These scans can be done many ways but often involve literature reviews, Web searches, and importantly, interviews with known leaders in the field. Additionally, foundations employ pollsters and other political consultants to help identify policy opportunities. Opportunities to influence health care organization policy may be identified through consultation with those who can represent the opinions of key leaders in the organizations. Sometimes this consultation takes place on an individual basis. Other times groups of experts are convened around key issues. In 2005, for example, RWJF convened a group of nurses, measurement developers, and researchers with measurement expertise to set priorities for a research agenda that would produce important, accurate, and useful measures of the quality of nursing care provided in hospitals.

IDENTIFYING PROMISING SOLUTIONS TO IMPROVE HEALTH AND HEALTH CARE

Once the staff of RWJF reach consensus on a strategy to address a priority health or health care issue, they move to seeking innovative processes or policies that, if implemented widely, could result in dramatic improvements in health and health care over a long period of time. Sometimes, that means (a) finding innovative ideas that exist but have not been broadly implemented; (b) finding ideas that exist, but only in the minds of innovative individuals; or (c) generating new ideas with groups of innovative individuals. The process of identifying innovation involves personal conversations, site visits, and focus groups.

Sometimes innovative solutions are generated by those currently engaged in the study and delivery of health and health care. However, many ideas come from other industries as well. For example, the Robert Wood Johnson Foundation engaged a design firm best known for designing products such as toothpaste tubes and shopping carts to explore optimal hospital design. Many ideas that are no longer innovative in a non-health-related field can have new legs when applied to address health and health care issues. Experts in environmental preservation have been funded to think of antibiotic effectiveness as a national resource to be preserved. Concepts developed in the biological sciences such as network analysis are increasingly being applied to health and health care problems as well. Continuous quality improvement—long a concept driving progress in manufacturing—has brought new vigor and impressive results to the movement to improve the quality of health and health care provided in the United States. In the example at the start of this chapter, the foundation, seeking to identify an innovative idea to improve access to health care, found innovation in the field of health care in the form of a new health care professional, the nurse practitioner.

For problems for which there is a dearth of plausible solutions, RWJF often funds research to explore problems and uncover possible policy solutions. By allocating funding to targeted research studies or by funding a group of research proposals submitted in response to a call for proposals around a common theme, RWJF has sought to understand how information technology such as Computerized Physician Order Entry and Barcode Medication systems affect the work of nurses and the quality of care they are able to provide. Separate grants to several teams of researchers explored the potential intended and unintended consequences of implementing minimum nurse staffing ratios in hospitals. Funding allocated through the foundation's Interdisciplinary Nursing Quality Research Initiative (INQRI) is supporting a series of studies to uncover the processes of nursing care that lead to higher-quality patient outcomes.

Because of the time it takes to conduct rigorous research, these types of research-driven idea-generation activities are useful to guide future investments only if the foundation has committed to remain in a given area for an extended period of time. Programs such as the RWJF Investigator in Health Policy Research Award fund research projects intended to uncover policy solutions for problems not yet addressed by the foundation or others. Because this program funded work on nursing quality long before the foundation had identified the nursing shortage to be a strategic priority, the results from that work were available to guide the foundation's nursing investments.

CREATING THE EVIDENCE TO CONVINCE POLICY MAKERS TO IMPROVE HEALTH AND HEALTH CARE POLICY

Before seeking to spread promising solutions to health or health care priorities, RWJF examines the evidence base supporting the idea's potential to improve health and health care. When literature reviews and key informant interviews suggest a proposed solution is likely to be broadly beneficial at a reasonable implementation cost, the foundation seeks simultaneously to make the idea available and to convince policy makers across the country to facilitate its spread across the United States. When the evidence that exists about a given idea is not sufficient to convince key decision makers of either the need for or the value of an innovative policy, the foundation often funds research and demonstration projects to fill this gap.

Research agendas are prioritized according to the maturity of the field, the state of the evidence base, and the information needs of policy makers. In fields where a problem is not commonly understood, general evidence of the existence and magnitude of the problem (e.g., nurses' work environments are not conducive to quality patient outcomes) is more critical to produce than evidence of a policy intervention's ability to address the problem (e.g., demonstrating that mandated "quiet time" contributes to the quality of the nurse's work environment). Consideration of a policy maker's need for information can also help develop priorities in investments to build the appropriate evidence base. Proof that America's hospitals are suffering as a result of the nursing shortage is useful to elevate the issue of nursing quality in a politician's platform. Evidence that a particular policy or practice is likely to improve nurse retention is useful to a policy maker who is already convinced of the problem and is looking for solutions, especially if the solution is one that is likely to save money.

On the flip side of efforts to convince policy makers to implement a particular promising policy or practice, research can also help document the positive and negative intended and unintended outcomes associated with a particular type of policy, to guide the decisions of others. Research that captures negative unintended consequences of a policy that has already been implemented can affect future policies or actions. For example, research into the consequences of California's minimum nurse ratio law may inform California policy makers' decisions to repeal, revise or continue the law and can inform the decisions of policy makers in the states considering implementing the policy.

Research to motivate and guide policy change may be conducted using data that were collected previously for another purpose. Other times, funders build funds into the research grant that allow investigators to collect original data before and after the implementation of a particular policy or practice. When data exist in systems such as billing records or medical charts, RWJF often funds extraction and conversion into data sets that can be quantitatively analyzed. In addition, RWJF has funded a great deal of surveys over the years. Recently the foundation conducted a survey of newly licensed registered nurses to understand how many nurses leave the profession within 2 years of being licensed and the policies of hospitals that lead to a reduction in turnover. This information, which can help the foundation and others address the nursing shortage, does not exist in any of the data sets that are publicly available for research.

Though analysis of past innovations can often shed light on the likelihood that similar initiatives that have not yet been implemented will be successful, this evidence may be insufficient to convince policy makers to make costly investments or pass politically difficult legislation. In cases such as these, demonstration projects are needed. As noted in one of the examples in the beginning of the chapter, the foundation funded a demonstration program called Transforming Care at the Bedside. This demonstration program tested the impact of an initiative that prepares and empowers frontline nurses to engage in continuous quality-improvement projects on nurse retention and patient outcomes. Throughout the years, the foundation has made many other investments to demonstrate the impact of a policy or program on health and health care outcomes. The foundation has a long history of funding demonstration programs to validate the feasibility and potential of an innovative idea to impact health and health care outcomes.

The usefulness of a demonstration program is dependent on the ability to share lessons learned about strategies employed by the foundation, such as why they were or were successful with an eye toward encouraging others to duplicate worthwhile efforts, to refrain from duplicating wasteful efforts, and to facilitate their implementation of successful solutions. For these purposes, qualitative data often supplement quantitative information. Qualitative data are especially important to allow teams of evaluators to distinguish between a failed strategy and failed implementation of a valid strategy. Most often, lessons are collected and shared through the funding of program evaluations conducted by researchers external to the program team. Some programs conduct self-evaluations, which, depending on the nature of the data, can provide as objective an assessment as an evaluation conducted by an "unbiased" individual. Evaluations constitute a significant portion of funds expended by RWJF for improvement—often as much as 10% of a program's total authorization.

Translating and Synthesizing Information to Influence Policy Makers

After adjusting for patient and hospital characteristics (size, teaching status, and technology), each additional patient per nurse was associated with a 7% (odds ratio [OR], 1.07; 95% confidence interval [CI], 1.03–1.12) increase in the likelihood of dying within 30 days of admission and a 7% (OR, 1.07; 95%CI, 1.02–1.11) increase in the odds of failure-to-rescue. After adjusting for nurse and hospital characteristics, each additional patient per nurse was associated with a 23% (OR, 1.23; 95% CI,1.13–1.34) increase in the odds of burnout and a 15% (OR, 1.15; 95% CI, 1.07–1.25) increase in the odds of job dissatisfaction. (Aiken, Clarke, Sloane, Sochalski, & Silber, 2002, p. 1987)

The preceding excerpt from an abstract of an article published in an academic journal suggests that hospitals with a higher nurse–patient staffing ratio have been found to have more satisfied nurses and better patient outcomes. The policy implications of this work, which derived from work funded through an RWJF Investigator in Health Policy Award, might have been overlooked had this finding remained obscured by technical language in a journal read only by those with the technical expertise to interpret the results. In fact, the policy implications of this work have been widely debated thanks to work by the investigators, consultants, journalists, and others to translate the information into language that policy makers can understand and to disseminate widely the information. Translation, the converting of technical language to language understandable by a key audience for the information, is a key ingredient in the recipe for policy impact through research. Unless evidence produced by academics is translated into information that policy makers can understand and use, important evidence contributes little to health policy debates and is unlikely to result in policy change.

The Robert Wood Johnson Foundation commonly pays consultants to provide one-on-one technical assistance to researchers to help them turn information into messages. Additionally, staffs create research and policy briefs that present RWJF research findings in concise terms meant to be accessible and understandable by policy makers. Because many messages are delivered to policy makers through the media, rather than by the researchers or advocates themselves, many of the foundation's funded programs that produce information intended to influence policy also provide assistance to grantees to help them develop messages the media can and will pick up and spread.

A project funded by RWJF found that policy makers and their legislative assistants are more likely to use a research result when defending or challenging policy prescriptions when they understand the context of the result as well as the nature of the evidence that exists in the literature—including the literature that appears contrary to the preferred policy prescription (Emont & Emont, 2005). When information that can convince a policy maker to work to effect change in a particular area is located in more than one article, RWJF has found that synthesizing the information from several sources can greatly enhance understanding of, and therefore increase discussion of, possible policy solutions. In some cases, policy debates can be greatly improved through syntheses of existing work, without the funding of any additional research. Synthesis briefs such as the foundation's "Charting Nursing's Future" policy brief series bring together research findings and best practices on subjects such as nurse–patient ratios and the faculty shortage.

How Foundations Use Strategic Communications to Improve Health Policy

The best evidence, translated and synthesized, can influence policy only if it reaches the eyes and ears of policy makers at the right time and is understood. RWJF has long invested in strategic communications activities to influence policy, and foundation funding often includes substantial budgets to fund promotional products and outreach. Over the years, the foundation has shifted from providing assistance to grantees seeking to promote their own work to our current strategy of working with grantees to create messages that put their findings in the context of a much broader set of information. For example, a researcher able to document the extent of the current and future nursing shortage can have more of an impact on policy when his or her results are put in the context of how a nurse shortage may affect health care quality. When these messages are packaged with information about how to measure accurately nurses' contributions to care quality and information about how to improve performance on such nursing-sensitive measures, hospital administrators are more likely to act on these messages.

The foundation employs a large communications staff and engages in contracts with external communications firms. Communications staffs engage in several activities to convey accurately the right information to the right audience at the right time. First, staff and consultants seek to know the audience and then to develop messages to influence behavior. To develop messages, it is helpful to understand how members of a key audience receive and process the information that drives their actions. History has shown that policy makers often act when a particular issue affects them or someone close to them.

Similarly, efforts to influence hospital policy can be successful only if one understands what motivates the leader of the organization and to whom or what that leader turns for information to guide his or her decisions. For example, efforts to convince hospital administrators to allocate resources to improve the nurses' work environment must be guided by information about the administrators' relative value of reputation versus profitability. Hospital administrators who care more about profits may respond better to a message that demonstrates how a particular policy can minimize or save costs for a hospital. Administrators who care about reputation may be more convinced by a message about how a policy can improve quality in their hospital.

Some policy makers may be more inclined to take an issue that sets them apart from their colleagues. Others may want to support a policy to be one of the crowd and on the bandwagon. Knowledge of these such tendencies can also play into message development. Communicating to a governor that including nurses prominently in his or her health reform plans could make the state an innovative model for other states can be an effective motivation for change. A message to "be a pioneer for quality" may lead a hospital administrator to take some gambles on improving nursing care in his or her hospital.

Once messages are developed, communications staff engage in additional activities to test the messages and materials through focus groups, surveys, and market research. Finally, messages are delivered to the public, to policy makers, and to other health care leaders. Often, communications firms employed by the foundation use a strategy of a campaign to alert the public to a problem and encourage them to advocate for solutions to the problem. The media is a key partner in campaigns and other efforts to reach the public and, through the public, the legislators. In addition to inspiring public advocates, the foundation may engage professional advocates whose primary job is to advocate for change. Advocates can also be individuals from local communities who are inexperienced with the role of convincing decision makers to act. Through training and other technical assistance, the foundation arms advocates with messages that allow them to present information in a way that aligns findings with policy makers' interests or organizations' missions and with appeals to their heart and their gut. Often personal stories and anecdotes are used to bring a generalized result to the individual level. Advocacy messages developed by consultants to the foundation are often accompanied by training to help advocates deliver these messages to policy makers. A Robert Wood Johnson Foundation program called Project Connect teaches those grantees who are seeking to influence policy around a particular issue how to talk about their issue with policy makers and get results.

Often, a multipronged communication strategy is the most effective at influencing policy. In RWJF's work to address the nurse faculty shortage, we are working at the community, state, and national levels to bring the message to policy makers. At the community level, the foundation is funding local coalitions composed of leaders from the areas of nursing, health care, education, and workforce development to work collaboratively on solutions that are right for their community. Best practices are highlighted in the local press and used as examples nationally as we promote solutions in this area. The previously mentioned policy brief series, "Charting Nursing's Future," devoted an entire issue to the complexities of the faculty shortage and solutions that are either ready for adoption or in need further development.

Information is a funder's currency for policy change. Protecting the value of that information is paramount to funders' power and credibility. That means great care must be taken to protect a foundation's reputation for being an unbiased broker of information. For example, the message that "results show that hospitals employing more baccalaureate-educated nurses will experience better outcomes" may be a powerful motivator for change. However, if research results only demonstrate that hospitals employing a higher percentage of baccalaureate-educated nurses have better *patient* outcomes, then a foundation must be able to understand the difference in these two messages and communicate only what it knows from the research finding without reading more into the finding than the evidence can support. The careful communication of research findings is essential if foundations are to preserve their reputation for unbiased, accurate information. This also means communicating results of studies that did not turn out the way the foundation expected. A foundation that tells the world when it was wrong is more likely to be believed when it tells the world it is right.

RESTRICTIONS ON LOBBYING: A DELICATE BALANCE

Because private foundations receive special tax treatment, foundation funds cannot be allocated to activities that constitute lobbying—communication with a *legislator* reflecting a view on specific legislation. Specific legislation includes bills, repeals, amendments, renewals/budgets, appropriations, and earmarks or proposals for legislation not yet introduced, such as model acts and Senate confirmation.

Foundations are also not allowed to participate in grassroots lobbying, which includes communicating with the public in a way that reflects a view about a specific legislation and accompanying that communication with a call to action. Foundations cannot be perceived as having intervened in an election, and thus, there are limitations on how research can be disseminated.

The restriction on lobbying does not prohibit foundations from producing information that can *inform* policy. Foundations can express view on public policy (even specific legislation) and can conduct and disseminate public policy research. For example, RWJF can commission research to examine the effects of impending legislation and can advocate for general policy change as long as this advocacy does not favor or oppose a particular candidate.

How Foundations Engage Strategic Partners

To accomplish both short-term and long-term goals, the foundation seeks to engage strategic partners, including business, government, families, and communities, to create jointly the social change the foundation promises. Perceived as unbiased and apolitical, foundations can engage individuals, who together might have an impact that collective individual efforts would likely never create. Activities to engage strategic partners, such as convening, can result in agreement or progress toward agreement. They can lead to a clearer understanding of the issues underlying a given problem and a clearer understanding of the range of practical and powerful solutions. By providing incentives for people to work together, foundations can more quickly achieve progress while avoiding opposition from special interest groups.

Some recent examples of ways that RWJF has used effectively the engagement of strategic partners to advance progress on the nursing crisis include (a) bringing end users of nursing quality research together with researchers funded through the foundation's Interdisciplinary Nursing Quality Research Initiative to inform research plans and (b) bringing frontline nurses from hospitals across the country to share best practices.

Currently, RWJF is engaging strategic partners to reduce the nurse faculty shortage in New Jersey. In August 2007, RWJF convened a meeting of business, education, government, and nursing leaders in New Jersey to enable them to plan a strategy for addressing the nursing faculty shortage in this state. By engaging the nursing leaders and representatives of key nursing organizations in the state, the foundation hoped to provide formal and informal networks of individuals and forums for discussion to tackle a problem that has persisted for years—in part because of disagreement among key stakeholders about what should be done. The goal was to create common ground for groups that had somewhat different interests in the nurse faculty shortage. The stakeholders in the effort to address the nursing shortage are numerous and diverse, from the nurses themselves to the CEOs who hire them, to the workforce investment boards interested in the economic well-being of their communities, to community-based organizations looking to increase access to care. Working together on a similar message can increase their power and strengthen the message overall. Being a neutral convener can help disparate groups focus on the similarities of their plight rather than their differences. Despite differences, they came together and decided that having a sufficient supply of nurses in the state was in everyone's best interest.

As in the preceding example, the foundation often convenes other funders around a particular issue. When multiple stakeholders are drawn to an issue, great gains can be derived from coordinating roles and responsibilities. When RWJF geared up to address the latest nursing shortage a number of years ago, the foundation knew it could not fund all the many strategies that might lead to a general solution, such as strategies aimed at better recruitment mechanisms, image, retention, the work environment, and eventually the faculty shortage. So the foundation began to call on other funders to pay attention to strategies related to issues such as recruitment, image, and in the early years, the faculty shortage. Those early discussions led to the Robert Wood Johnson Foundation becoming the coordinator of the National Nurse Funders Collaborative, a group that still convenes around finding solutions for the nursing and nurse faculty shortages.

The Nurse Funders Collaborative led to a partnership between RWJF and the Northwest Health Foundation on a national program effort called Partners Investing in Nursing's Future (PIN). The PIN program is an important example of how the foundation has engaged multiple partners in collaborations that result in improvements in policy. The goal of the program is to provide an incentive for local foundations (provided with a matching grant) to collaborate with their local nursing leaders, workforce investment boards, and others to address local solutions to the nursing shortage. After just 2 years of funding, nearly 50 local foundations are now involved with PIN, investing their own dollars in their own communities. Many of these local foundations have applied because they see the program as aligned with their mission to boost the economic development of their community through nursing jobs. Local foundations and organizations are also charged with serving the underserved and increasing diversity, and PIN grants help them with these goals as well, as many local foundations see nurses as a population interested in serving the underserved (depending on the project) and increasing diversity.

Strategic partnerships can lead to increased efficiency of efforts and can also better foster evidence generation and health policy development. They are, however, costly to establish and maintain. Partnerships must be entered into carefully, with clear expectations of each other's goals for the collaboration.

BUILDING CAPACITY OF INDIVIDUALS AND INSTITUTIONS

To increase future capacity to achieve policy goals and sustain gains reaped through improvements in policy, the RWJF makes investments that will increase the ability of individuals and institutions to partner in the foundation's efforts to improve health and health care. Through programs in its Human Capital Portfolio, the foundation seeks to create the scholars, leaders, providers, and frontline workers who by enhancing their abilities are able to conduct rigorous health policy research, inform key decisions, make wise investments, lead innovative organizations, design productive policies, and provide higher-quality health care.

The foundation has a large portfolio of programs intended to improve the human capital of members of the nursing profession. The foundation's Executive Nurse Fellows program seeks to equip nurse leaders with the skills and network necessary to raise nursing's voice in the discussion and delivery of health care. A new program of the foundation, the Nurse Faculty Scholars program, is intended to create a cadre of leaders in academic nursing. The Interdisciplinary Nursing Quality Initiative (INQRI) has as one of its key goals an increase in the rigor and visibility of nursing research. RWJF's Community Health Leaders program brings recognition to heroes from nursing and other health professions.

Crucial to the ability of the Human Capital Portfolio to increase the capacity of those who will drive future health and health care policy is its goal to increase diversity among the ranks of leaders, scholars, and providers. The foundation believes that individuals from diverse

backgrounds bring important perspectives that enrich health policy debates. Several of the Human Capital Portfolio's programs have explicit
goals to increase the presence of historically underrepresented racial,
ethnic, and socioeconomic groups in the pool of grantees the foundation might engage in its work to influence health policy. Increasing the
diversity of the nursing profession is a particularly difficult task, but one
the foundation is undertaking through targeted recruiting and efforts
such as a diversity ambassador program, wherein alumni of foundation
programs might recruit others of diverse backgrounds to take advantage
of human capital–increasing opportunities.

In addition to investing in the capacity of individuals to improve
policy, the foundation invests in organizations that can own, run, and
sustain the advocacy efforts. Recently, the foundation engaged in a strategic partnership with the American Association of Retired Persons
(AARP), long recognized for its expertise in advocacy, and is making an
investment in that organization's ability to champion the interests of the
nursing profession. Whether seeking to create new organizations or to
add to the capacity of organizations that currently exist, the foundation
takes care to encourage and support the development of plans to sustain
the new efforts of the organization once the foundation's funding has
expired.

CONCLUSION: HOW RWJF INFLUENCES POLICY

Foundations engage in a strategy to influence policy change for many
reasons: (a) when federal support is needed to create or sustain a program determined to be beneficial; (b) when behaviors are unlikely to
change without intervention—whether they are in opposition to business
or individual self-interests; (c) when opportunities exist for new policies
to accelerate change; or (d) when "bad" policies appear to be preventing
improvement. To influence policy in a way that leads to the alleviation of
complex health and health care problems, the foundation uses many important tools—individually and simultaneously—to provide the evidence
that policy makers need to create change. As depicted in this chapter's
examples and reviewed earlier, the people who guide, manage, and work
for RWJF engage in a multistep, multi-investment strategy to influence
policy. First, the foundation identifies priority problems and promising
solutions. Often, the foundation designs demonstration projects and evaluations to examine the potential of these solutions to improve health

or health care and to demonstrate feasibility. Clearly, qualitative and quantitative research facilitates the steps of problem identification and solution testing. Moreover, the foundation funds, translates, and communicates research findings to key decision makers. Where possible, the foundation engages strategic partners to align interest toward a common purpose. Where capacity does not exist, the foundation makes investments to build the capacity of individuals and institutions in order to sustain gains reaped through improvements in policy.

To provide the necessary evidence for policy change, these steps are accomplished by monetary foundation grants to individuals and organizations. In addition, the foundation makes non-financial investments in the form of expertise, connections, staff time, reputation, and neutral space for convening. Expertise gathered through years of grant-making, combined with access, allows the foundation to play the strategic role of connector—identifying and linking individuals and organizations that together can have more impact than they would have if they worked apart. Foundation staff and members of the foundation's National Advisory Committees add value to grants by taking the time to find qualified creative grantees and by managing progress and ensuring deliverables match promises.

This chapter describes the current practices of a single health foundation in the United States, and many of the statements included do not pertain to all foundations. There is much variety, for example, in the amount of funds foundations expend on evaluation. Many foundations work less intensively with grantees to produce and disseminate results. Some foundations work even more intensely to control the products of their grantees—often coauthoring reports. In addition to lending insight into how you might interact with the Robert Wood Johnson Foundation, we hope you will find that RWJF has a lot in common with other large foundations and that the lessons shared here help you influence policy through grants you might receive from other funders.

REFERENCES

Aiken, L., Clarke, S., Sloane, D., Sochalski, J., & Silber, J. (2002). Hospital nurse staffing and patient mortality, nurse burnout, and job dissatisfaction. *The Journal of the American Medical Association, 288*(16), 1987–1993.

Emont, S. L., & Emont, N. C. (2005, April). *Assessing the information needs of the substance abuse policy research program's policy audiences.* Robert Wood Johnson Foundation internal document.

Keenan, T. (1998). Support of nurse-practitioners and physician assistants. In J. Isaacs & J. P. Knickman (Eds.), *To improve health and health care 1998–1999: The Robert Wood Johnson Foundation anthology* (pp. 215–230). San Francisco: Jossey-Bass.

American Academy of Nurse Practitioners. (2007). *Why choose a nurse practitioner as your healthcare provider.* Retrieved December 6, 2007, from http://www.aanp. org/NR/rdonlyres/evwsnlw2366mgchbliqqu4crlfylu7dgwpl7xcg6c35kjsc7dury4bke ehrjcie36mnchdi5jk3ck6ye2juh7aq2rvb/FAQs+-+What+is+an+NP.pdf

15

A Metaphor for Addressing the Nurse Shortage in Oregon

JUDITH L. WOODRUFF

There is currently a multidimensional shortage of registered nurses and allied health professionals in the United States. There has been an abundance of popular media and scholarly attention to the issue, and the causes of this shortage have been well documented and include the following:

- An aging population with more chronic diseases
- Fewer young adults entering the workforce
- An aging nursing workforce moving toward retirement
- A lack of racial, ethnic, and gender diversity in the nursing profession
- More professional career options for women
- A stressed and shortage-impacted work environment
- A lack of respect for nursing as a profession

Each of these factors contributes to the shortage, but the shortage is exacerbated by the input of multiple stakeholders, a lack of resources, and a changing global society. It is not only in the United States that the available nursing workforce is not adequate to meet the demand; the shortage of nurses and other providers is worldwide. Critical nursing shortages in the United States, Great Britain, and other industrialized countries have generated a demand that has spawned a plethora of business opportunities targeting nurses from the less-developed world for recruitment. Bonuses and other financial incentives are being offered, along with relocation coverage or premium benefits packages to lure nurses to work in specific facilities. These efforts have had limited effect because they simply redistribute the supply of nurses, not increase it. These economic incentives also do not address the changing nature of health care, the introduction of new technologies and higher expectations regarding health care treatment. Tomorrow's environment requires nurses with new technical competencies, broader clinical experience, and advanced leadership skills. For the profession of nursing to be prepared for the challenges of the twenty-first century, nurses will have to be more than multitaskers; they will need to be multi-thinkers. Nurses will be working in an era of chronicity—their patients will be experiencing multiple chronic diseases, and the work environment will be experiencing chronic staff shortages.

The solutions to the global crisis must be strategic, be based on the underlying issues driving the shortage, focus on the structural issues, and aim for the long term. Nurses must lead this development of the profession, define the scope of their practice, and reform the system.

Collaborative partnerships among educators, employers, state government, nursing leadership, and regulatory bodies are needed to address these complex issues. National efforts are limited by the diversity and complexity of the nursing profession, state licensing requirements, adequacy of training opportunities, and state education funding. Collaboration among local, regional, and national nursing organizations and funders is, therefore, vital in order to create an adequate workforce for the twenty-first century.

NORTHWEST HEALTH FOUNDATION

The Northwest Health Foundation (NWHF) is a private independent foundation serving the Oregon and southwest Washington region. Since 1998, the mission of the Northwest Health Foundation has been to advance, support, and promote the health of the people of Oregon and southwest Washington. The foundation pursues its goals by funding projects and engaging in issues related to health and through responsive grant making, focused funding initiatives, convening the community to share information and build collaboration, and providing training and technical assistance to organizations dedicated to the improvement of health. One of our goals is to develop adequate and appropriately educated human resources for health, capable of responding to the complex health needs of an increasingly diverse and aging society.

FARMING AND THE RELATIONSHIP TO THE NURSING WORKFORCE CRISIS

In farming, the relationship between people and the earth is the key to a successful operation. Unlike complex issues such as the need for more nurses in the health care system or how to provide adequate health care to the uninsured, in agriculture the nature of the problems and solutions is easily seen and understood. However, farming can provide a useful metaphor for foundations and other funding agencies to consider when addressing the workforce shortage issue. And more important, a sustainable farming operation can be a useful metaphor for creating a stable, skilled nursing workforce capable of meeting the health care needs of the millennium.

The primary aim of agriculture is to cause the land to produce more abundantly while at the same time protecting it from deterioration and misuse ("Agriculture," 2003). Nevertheless, sustainable agriculture requires more than planting seeds and praying for rain. Sustainability rests on the principle that we must meet the needs of the present without compromising the ability of future generations to meet their own needs. We must address the nursing workforce shortage as a long-term investment in the future of a healthy society, not simply create additional nurses to fill available positions by hiring them from other countries or lowering standards of education and training to meet a current shortage of workers.

Growing an abundant crop of health care professionals without creating new problems in the future requires a view of the workforce as a living system. This perspective is essential to understanding sustainability. In farming, this means that to ensure production of crops, the farmer must depend on the soil, water, air, and sunlight to get healthy plants. The farmer may be able to affect parts of the system, but he or she can never be certain whether the outcome will be a bumper crop or a devastating loss, simply because of the many variables involved in agriculture.

Viewed in the broadest sense then, the shortage is the "crop" of a variety of participants, including the educational system (both K–12 and higher education), the regulatory arm of government (boards of nursing), employers (hospitals, long-term care, the government), insurance plans and other payers, state and federal government, policy makers, labor unions, management organizations, and communities affected by the system (both locally and globally), not to mention nurses themselves. Although it is a complex process, using a systems approach to address the nursing workforce issue provides tools to explore the interconnections between nursing and other aspects of our community, including economic and workforce development. It invites and understands the need for interdisciplinary effort and input from various stakeholders. It has the potential for buy-in and support at every level that can ultimately lead to sustainable change. The Northwest Health Foundation has adopted this systems approach in order to ensure positive impact on the nursing crisis in Oregon. We recognize that each decision can make a difference and contribute to the entire system, advancing the work to impact the greater community. The wrong approach or moving forward without understanding the systems affected by the application of our decisions can also lead to negative impact on our communities.

Like farming, addressing fundamental change in the nursing workforce requires a long-term investment of time and financial resources. For the foundation to have major impact, we had to build an awareness of the nursing workforce system that goes beyond the specific activities, tactics, and patterns that make up the existing entities and their relationships to one another. Systems change requires a *commitment* to the process of creating a shared vision for the future and then requires taking the first step. The process, which is ongoing, requires the ability to look at structures and be willing to make changes in them to realize the shared vision. It may also require willingness to let go of long-held beliefs, power, and decision making to achieve the goals.

In 2001 the Northwest Health Foundation decided to use an understanding of systems change to address the nursing shortage in Oregon. As "farmers," we had to get our hands dirty, dig some ditches and divert some water, and learn to collaborate with other farmers to ensure that there will always be an appropriately trained nurse in the right place at the right time.

CULTIVATING THE ENVIRONMENT FOR NURSING

The nursing shortage crisis is much like a root-bound plant. The roots have become entangled and matted together, and the nursing profession has become stunted. One only has to look at a plant removed from a too-small pot to observe how the roots often circle around and around the soil attempting to find more nutrients for the plant. The plant lives but does not grow or bloom, instead existing in a state of inertia. To induce them to once again grow outward and to broaden their thinking beyond their own "pot," the Northwest Health Foundation had to begin cultivation beyond the individual pots of nursing schools, nursing associations, or nurse executives, to cultivate the entire nursing community. Cultivation of a field requires breaking up the soil surface, removing weeds and rocks, and preparing for planting. Cultivating solutions to the nursing shortage required similar activities. To begin, the Northwest Health Foundation (1) gathered information (soil preparation), (2) brought together key stakeholders (taking out the rocks), and (3) consulted nursing leaders for the development of strategy (reading many books by master gardeners).

In 2001 the Northwest Health Foundation commissioned a study to provide information about the nursing workforce in the region and to develop a framework for discussion of potential initiatives that could have a substantial impact on the shortage. That study was presented by the foundation in its first issue brief: *Oregon's Nursing Shortage: A Public Health Crisis in the Making* (Northwest Health Foundation, 2001). Researched by a team of nursing professionals and authored by Dr. Christine Tanner, the report identified causes and a number of opportunities to influence positively both the recruitment and the retention of professional nurses in Oregon and southwest Washington. At that time, the NWHF board chairman, Senator Mark O. Hatfield, said, "This is an opportunity for the Foundation to promote sustainable solutions. By commissioning this report, we are able to bring clear focus on an urgent issue affecting public health" (Northwest Health Foundation, 2001).

The second strategy used by the foundation was to support the convening of the nursing leaders in the state to begin working on developing solutions to the shortage. Fortunately, the leaders had already started gathering around the issue. The Oregon Nursing Leadership Council (ONLC) had formed in 2000 and was represented by leaders of the Oregon Nurses Association, the Northwest Organization of Nurse Executives, the Oregon Council of Associate Degree Programs, the Oregon Council of Deans, and the Oregon State Board of Nursing. These leaders were aware of the pending crisis, having heard anecdotal reports for some time about the shortages. However, the issuance of the report served to galvanize the ONLC and other key stakeholders to work together and to find solutions. Where there previously had been competition between the various leadership groups, the report highlighted the need for bold action from a collaboration of leadership. The Oregon nursing leaders rose to this challenge and came together to forge new understandings and create solutions that benefited the entire region.

In June 2001 the ONLC was successful in developing a 5-year plan that identified the following major goals:

- Double the enrollment in Oregon nursing programs by 2004.
- Redesign nursing education to meet the changing needs of Oregonians.
- Recruit and retain nurses in the profession, particularly men and minorities.
- Develop, implement, and evaluate staffing models that make best use of the available nursing workforce.
- Create Oregon Center for Nursing (OCN) to coordinate implementation and ongoing evaluation of the strategic plan.

In response to the development of this statewide strategic plan, in 2003 the foundation launched a 5-year initiative to provide resources for the nursing leadership to create collaborative solutions to the crisis. Later named "Investing in a Healthy Future: Strategies to Address the Nursing Shortage," the goal of the program was to make a long-term and strategic investment in the health of the region by growing a stable, skilled nursing workforce. This was the foundation's first initiative, requiring a segregation of resources and a commitment to "taking the long view." Because the issues of the shortage are complex, the foundation's system approach meant that the solutions had to be multifaceted and shared among many stakeholders. The foundation appreciated the broad thinking and diverse ideas provided by Oregon and southwest Washington nursing professionals as they grappled with necessary change, and their input has continuously helped to shape the elements of the initiative.

Although the foundation had previously directed specific resources to a focused funding effort in health research, this was the first time since the foundation's inception that resources were being dedicated exclusively to one subject, with program staff assigned to work exclusively on the issue. The NWHF set aside $5 million for this effort. As a young foundation, with limited resources and with a wide geographic area, the NWHF's commitment to reserving these funds (30% of the available funds annually) to the nursing shortage was at the time unprecedented in the field.

Consistent with the NWHF's prior practice within the community, a board of directors committee and foundation staff consulted with the nursing community to identify potential funding and outreach opportunities. The foundation considered the earlier issue brief's findings, the ONLC strategic plan, and interviews with key leaders in nursing, education, and health care to determine the possible grant making activities. Ultimately, the foundation operationalized the initiative in three ways:

- Providing funding to develop and sustain the Oregon Center for Nursing
- Providing funding for collaborative and sustainable solutions to the shortage
- Supporting the development of policy change and advocacy within the nursing community

Potential funding opportunities were identified to include (1) increasing the number of nursing faculty necessary to educate additional nursing students; (2) increasing the ethnic, racial, and gender diversity of the nursing workforce; (3) increasing the breadth, depth, and quality of the preparation of nurses; (4) developing specialty practice areas such as long-term care, public health, and mental health; and (5) providing educational assistance to students through mentoring, scholarships, or other support programs. The foundation was particularly interested in making an investment in the *future* nursing workforce in the region and not just awarding funds for short-term strategies.

The Northwest Health Foundation also made a commitment to collaborative evaluation of the nursing projects and programs. The foundation believes that the purpose of evaluation is internal learning as well as external accountability. Evaluation is also a collaborative process among the funder, grantees, students, evaluation team, and key stakeholders and requires the NWHF to facilitate multiple opportunities for information sharing and group learning. To make evaluation meaningful, we decided to reserve 10% of the initiative's resources for a long-term evaluation of the impact of our involvement in nursing. The NWHF then hired a team from Portland State University led by Dr. Sherril Gelmon. Broadly, Dr. Gelmon and her team are charged with evaluating (a) the funding program, including the experience of grantees, and (b) the initiative's impact on nursing in Oregon and southwest Washington. The foundation supports the work to understand a pivotal question: How do we know that our work makes a difference? Key to the evaluation is the provision of technical assistance and consultation to all the grantees and other nursing entities as determined by the foundation's objectives and interests. This technical assistance is seen as an added value to the grantee, beyond the award itself.

Planting the Seeds for Change

The ONLC strategic plan had a stated goal of doubling the enrollment in nursing programs by 2004. To stimulate new growth in the nursing community—to make the goal attainable—the foundation issued a broad call for proposals that focused on expanding the capacity of nursing education to receive additional students. The initiative's first competitive grant cycle, Expanding Capacity to Prepare Entry-Level Nurses, supported educational institutions to develop plans for building capacity of nursing education centers and programs and to implement strategies to increase the capacity of educational programs to train new nurses. Twenty proposals were received, highlighting the need for funding in multiple areas of nursing education around the state. The foundation made awards totaling over $650,000 to five projects in Oregon:

- Peace Harbor Hospital Foundation to plan for a collaborative distance-based nursing program for Oregon's central and southwest coast
- Chemeketa Community College to create more clinical nursing instructors through intensive mentoring from experienced faculty
- Multnomah County Health Department to recruit and train more nursing students in public health practice and to develop a culturally diverse public health nursing workforce through the support of incumbent workers
- Clackamas Community College to enable foreign-certified nurses residing in Oregon and southwest Washington to become active members of the nursing community through a recertification course
- Oregon Consortium for Nursing Education (OCNE) to help redesign nursing education by developing a cohesive nursing curriculum to be shared statewide, providing for expanded enrollment by maximizing the use of scarce nursing faculty

As these seedlings grew, the foundation sought to plant even more varieties (flowers, vegetables, herbs, and a few weeds), broadening the diversity of the garden. Following up on the first grant-making focus, and to encourage projects that focused on increasing the number of new nursing faculty with advanced skills and interest in teaching, the foundation issued the second round of competitive grant making, Strengthening Capacity to Prepare Entry-Level Nurses. This grant program also sought to increase nursing students' opportunities for clinical practicum outside of hospital settings. The latter goal was particularly important to the Northwest Health Foundation. As a philanthropic organization rooted in the community, the foundation wanted to pay particular attention to the shortage as it would be experienced within community settings such as the long-term care continuum, public health, community health clinics, and schools, not primarily within the acute health care system. In 2004 awards totaling $540,000 went to the following organizations and institutions:

- College of Nursing, Washington State University Vancouver (on the northern border of Oregon), to increase the number of master's-prepared nurse educators by expanding access to coursework through Web-based/distance offerings
- Susannah Maria Gurule (SMG) Foundation to promote the health and wellness of the community and to provide clinical practicum to nursing students by pairing *promotoras*[1] and nursing students in activities to support the prenatal care needs of Latina women
- School of Nursing, Oregon Health and Science University, Southern Campus, to provide a variety of learning experiences for nursing students highlighting the needs of culturally diverse vulnerable populations in the Rogue Valley

Pinching Back, Staking, and Grafting

The third strategy of the NWHF initiative was to recognize the need for long-term investment in programs to ensure sustainability. Contrary to typical practice in philanthropy, in 2005 the foundation did not issue a call for new projects. Instead, the foundation "pinched back."[2] The NWHF made a targeted investment in three of the original nursing grantees, allowing these projects to strengthen the collaborations and to realize some successes without the burden of constantly seeking new funds. The collaborations and synergy between NWHF-funded projects and other projects also began to grow.

This latter effect has been a key feature of the workings of the initiative and is integral to how the Northwest Health Foundation seeks to function within our community. We know that the initiative has provided the framework for multiple organizations to work collectively to address the nursing shortage. For example, support for groups that convene nursing leaders and facilitate collaborations has helped position nursing leaders to take action on nursing education and nursing workforce issues in other arenas, such as with state policy makers. Many of the projects supported through the nursing initiative have strong community connections, which has encouraged health care facilities and other health care providers to participate in this work, providing resources directly to projects in some cases and providing indirect support for the efforts through release time for their nursing leaders to participate.

Another major impact is the creation of what some call "the Oregon Model": a new model for the way that foundations can work collaboratively with grantees on specific issues. This model has been extended nationally via Partners Investing in Nursing's Future, a partnership between the NWHF and the Robert Wood Johnson Foundation to help local foundations invest in nursing issues in their communities nationwide.[3]

Staking is the practice of driving a stake into the ground next to, and as a support for, a plant (without strangling it in the process). The NWHF recognized the projects' need to have additional support over a longer period of time, ensuring a strong base. We leveraged our existing investments in the nursing work by brokering additional funding from other foundations and funding partners. This activity helped to stake these projects, strengthening their collaboratives and increasing their momentum. The foundation also increased emphasis on building the capacity and sustainability of the projects, supporting activities of the grantees around the development of business and operational plans and external fund-development projects.

The NWHF was not interested in growing annuals—we want hardy, native perennial plants to be deep-rooted in Oregon. That requires dedicated staff available for technical assistance and strategy coaching as we seek to involve the broader community in the issue of the nursing shortage. This staff time includes efforts at developing and leveraging funding from diverse sources to ensure both broad stakeholder involvement and adequate resources for sustainability.

For the largest and most ambitious of the projects, the OCNE, and for the OCN, the plans for development and funding security are an essential piece of our strategy to reform nursing education and promote the leadership of the profession. Additional funding for these projects has included support for board development, business planning, and infrastructure.

Grafting is a technique often used to produce a hardier or more disease-resistant plant. For example, to create hybrid roses, you graft newer, weaker, and sometimes more fragile stems of experimental roses to the rootstock of a different, but sturdier rose. For the nursing projects, the NWHF created opportunities for grafting (albeit voluntary) by inviting the project leaders to regular facilitated meetings. Through these required semiannual meetings of nursing grantees, the project leaders shared their challenges and celebrated their successes. This was facilitated in recent years by having one meeting each year off-site with an overnight requirement (paid for by the foundation). The ability of nursing project leaders and evaluators and the foundation staff to meet in a separate and relaxed setting has contributed to the sense of keeping our eyes on the larger goal of having the right nurse, in the right place, at the right time. In the casual atmosphere of the meetings, what at first appeared to be distinct and disparate projects started to appear more like an integrated initiative-supported system. For example, the partners involved in the OCNE, who were pioneering work with high-fidelity simulation laboratories, provided an opportunity for the Clackamas Community College's immigrant nurse reentry program to train their nurses/students in a safe and controlled environment. This enabled the foreign-trained returning nurses to build confidence in their nursing skills and to experience nursing in the real world long before they attempted to work in an actual patient-care setting. Likewise, the SMG Foundation project that provided clinical experiences for nursing students by pairing them with Latina *promotoras* became an opportunity for the OCNE to develop a new clinical placement/internship site with the project. At some point during the initiative, it became difficult to discuss one funded project without describing and including one or more of the others.

The foundation has supported these synergistic relationships that have developed among grantees and all of the various stakeholders of this initiative. We believe that a significant factor in the overwhelming degree of change experienced in Oregon is the ability of the projects and partners to see themselves as part of the larger picture, in support roles to their peers, and not as competitors for funding streams. The grafting process is complete when it is impossible to tell that the branch came from a different rosebush. Oregon's nursing community has begun to resemble more of a rose hedge with hybrid and traditional varieties being represented.

Pruning for Growth

The NWHF has consistently relied on the OCN and the ONLC to develop nursing-led opportunities to change to the system. In 2004, led by the OCN, these leaders revised the strategic plan, incorporating some of the successes of the earlier plan and identifying new areas where resources should be focused. Utilizing unique partnerships between nursing programs and industry and by the creation of two new private college nursing programs in Oregon, they achieved particular success in increasing the capacity of educational programs. Specifically, between 2001 and 2004, the nursing education programs in the state expanded capacity by 45%, and by 2007 the capacity increase had exceeded 76%.

However, much remains to be done. The new plan stressed the development of strategies for the recruitment and retention of nurses in the workplace and the implementation of identified nursing competencies in the practice setting. Reforming nursing education continues to be a focus area, including developing innovative educational methodologies and increasing program capacity, but the OCN is also continuing initiatives to diversify the nursing workforce to promote culturally competent care and to promote leadership development for nurses at all levels and throughout the health care continuum of care settings.

In response to the revised plan, the Northwest Health Foundation pruned back yet again, to focus on key pieces of the plan. Incorporating the lessons learned so far in the initiative, the NWHF developed a third grant-making program. We identified a strategy that focused attention on "hard to recruit/retain sectors," such as long-term care, public health, mental health, and rural nursing. In particular, long-term or elderly care (whether in a facility, at home, or in community settings) was becoming more prominent both in the literature and in national discussions, as a severely neglected nursing issue.

The foundation decided to address this "hard to recruit" nursing practice area with a new competitive RFP. At the beginning of the initiative, the foundation had identified this area as part of the potential funding programs, and it was time to use our experience and resources to support innovative, practice-centered, and collaborative approaches to increasing the number of nurses entering into long-term care. In 2005 the program Caring for Our Future: Strengthening the Long Term Care Workforce was introduced.

Caring for Our Future is intended to create, expand, and strengthen partnerships between nursing education and providers of long-term care services across the continuum of settings. The goals of the program are not simply to create new clinical experiences for nursing students in long-term care settings, but to make systemic change by placing the growing needs of the region's elderly community at the forefront of education and training of current and future nurses, essentially growing an experimental but hardier plant. From the broader systems view of the nursing workforce challenge, the long-term care patch of the garden had its own "pests" to deal with, including a poor nursing image, low pay, and difficult work. These require a different approach to developing human resources, one that includes changing the culture of the long-term care community.

Two projects were selected for funding. The first, Enriching Clinical Learning Environments Through Partnerships in Long-Term Care (ECLEPs), is an outgrowth of the OCNE and is built upon success within the long-term care community of addressing direct care worker turnover through the Oregon Better Jobs Better Care program (BJBC).[4]

This project builds capacity for long-term care facilities to be *excellent* clinical learning sites for nursing students. Through community–academic partnerships, this project will create a model program that provides long-term care staffs with essential knowledge and skills to enhance their practice setting and support students' learning. The project will create four enriched long-term care clinical education sites for nursing students, in a variety of settings, including assisted living and residential care.

The second project is a partnership between the Linfield College Good Samaritan School of Nursing and Marquis Health Services Companies, a partnership that has developed a program with two broad goals:

- Increase the number of baccalaureate-prepared nurses committed to working in long-term care.
- Enhance and expand the knowledge and skills of current Marquis Company nurses in a more defined preceptor role to work with undergraduate nursing students.

The program will provide scholarships to baccalaureate nursing students who commit to entering practice in Marquis Company settings. In addition, registered nurses already practicing in long-term care will be offered an educational opportunity to enhance and further develop their knowledge and skills as preceptors to nursing students. This partnership between an educational institution and a system of care for older adults provides a unique opportunity to increase the number of baccalaureate-prepared nurses working in long-term care settings while strengthening the current nursing workforce, which will benefit the students in clinical placement and, hopefully, retain nurses in the setting because of increased satisfaction with the work.

Maintenance of Our Efforts

In addition to the project support, the foundation has again focused funding efforts on building the capacity of nursing organizations to develop collaborative solutions. In 2007 the NWHF supported the work of Making Oregon Vital for Elders, or MOVE, the Oregon organization affiliated with the national Pioneer Network. MOVE is a coalition of long-term care organizations, public agencies, academia, and others whose mission is to promote person-centered care in Oregon. This effort at "culture change" in long-term care settings is a national movement, focused on the preferences, interests, strengths, and choices of the individual. It recognizes that some individuals are unable to tell us with words what their wishes are but that the key to what will most honor their current wishes lies within their past choices and present behaviors. It also recognizes that the quality of the relationship between resident and caregiver is the most important factor in satisfaction for both residents and staff, and improving the environment for the resident means a better working environment for the nursing personnel. Because long-term care will be such a large part of the nursing profession in the coming decades, developing the setting as a "placement of choice" for both the residents and the nursing staff is of primary importance, and an effort in which nurses are leading the way.

A second organization, the Community Based Care Nurses Association, has received funding to support the development of educational programs, statewide annual conferences, and their Web site. Community-based care is a specialty area of nursing practice with subspecialties by practice setting that encompass the lifespan of the client. It includes adult foster care, ambulatory care clinics, child foster care, community mental health, congregational health, corrections, home health, hospice, schools, and other community settings.

Finally, the NWHF supports the Oregon Chapter of the National Association of Hispanic Nurses (NAHN) to develop the local organization to do the following:

- Provide a forum for nurses to analyze and evaluate the needs of the Hispanic community
- Assess the safety and quality of delivery services to the Hispanic community
- Identify barriers to the delivery of health services to Hispanic consumers and recommend appropriate solutions to local, state, and federal agencies
- Develop, test, and promote culturally sensitive models of intervention that provide effective nursing care for Hispanic communities
- Disseminate research findings and policy perspectives related to Hispanic needs to local, state, and federal agencies in order to affect policy making and the allocation of resources
- Collaborate with, and provide assistance to, other Hispanic professionals
- Identify Hispanic nurses throughout the nation in order to monitor the size and growth of this group of professionals who may provide culturally sensitive nursing care to Hispanic consumers
- Identify barriers to quality education for Hispanic nursing students and recommend appropriate solutions to state, local, and federal agencies
- Work toward recruitment and retention of Hispanic students in nursing education programs, in order to increase the number of bilingual and bicultural nurses who may provide culturally sensitive nursing care to Hispanic consumers

Funds have been used for developing a mentoring relationship with the Los Angeles chapter of NAHN to build the capacity of the local board to meet the needs of Hispanic nurses in Oregon, for attending national and regional conferences, and for providing marketing materials. The NWHF usually hosts the meetings of the group, providing meeting space, parking, and catering services. This type of "soft" money is important to the development of the nursing organizations as they grow into strong, and diverse, voices for the nursing profession.

PLANNING FOR FUTURE CROPS: SUPPORTING A NURSING POLICY AGENDA

Throughout the initiative, the NWHF has participated in other activities around the region, such as efforts to increase the diversity of the nursing workforce and to stimulate community–campus partnerships to address the complex issues of the nursing profession, introducing key projects to other local and regional foundations, and presenting our experiences at conferences. Resources have supported individual leadership development in the nursing community, focusing the public's attention on the shortage issues, and we continue to develop relationships with key policy makers around this subject.

In the fifth year of the initiative, the foundation moved to focus more attention on the development of nursing policy and advocacy strategies. The foundation's major strategy was to support the work of the OCN and to position the OCN as the collaborative leader and expert in nursing workforce issues.

Since 2001, the NWHF has provided core financial and technical assistance support for operations of the OCN. This has enabled the OCN to coordinate statewide activities related to nursing leadership, develop the diversity of the nursing workforce, and direct other task-force or workgroup activities, essentially making the ONLC strategic plan live and breathe. The OCN has also become the source of updated information addressing the Oregon nursing workforce shortage with their recent publication titled *When, Not If…A Report on Oregon's Registered Nurse Workforce*, which provides information using 2004 data (Burton, Morris, & Campbell, 2005).

Some of the OCN's accomplishments include the development and distribution of two nursing recruitment posters: "Are you man enough to be a nurse?" (2002) to recruit men and "Caring knows no boundaries" (2004) to recruit minority students. The first poster has won numerous awards and has been used nationally and internationally to recruit men into nursing.

The OCN also has spearheaded the establishment of programs to introduce nursing to high school students and has developed StudentMAX to support the expansion of nursing education. StudentMAX is a centralized clinical placement software program designed to match available clinical sites with the needs of the schools of nursing student experiences. It is a web-based tool available to schools of nursing, hospital managers, and students. This placement system is now being licensed to other states to address the need for expansion and better use of clinical placement sites. The major reason for the success of the Oregon/Southwest Washington StudentMAX experience has been the collaboration and commitment of the education and clinical partners.

Additionally, the center has created (with funding from the NWHF) a program titled Leadership at the Point of Care: Moving into Action, based on a statewide leadership conference held in 2006. This leadership program focuses on the value of the professional role in nursing and communication as essential facets of clinical nursing leadership development. The program provides 1-day trainings to all nurses in multiple locations in the state. In 2007 the foundation awarded $150,000 to the OCN to further develop the leadership initiative, including broadening opportunities for nurses in the hard specialty areas, such as long-term care, school nursing, and mental health. Again, we have looked at our success with the center and supported it to take the fledgling programs "to scale" and have reinvested when necessary with an eye toward long-term sustainability and impact on the profession.

The Northwest Health Foundation is a strong advocate for the Oregon Center for Nursing. In addition to funding various projects, workgroups, and task force activities, it is important that the NWHF support the development of the infrastructure of the center to ensure long-term impact and sustainability. This includes providing core support for salaries, but also technical assistance regarding board development, fund-raising, and communications. Additional funds were awarded in 2007 specifically for the purpose of these key areas.

Reliable, consistent funding is essential for nursing workforce centers to be agents of change within the system, for project management and developing policy. To that end, in the 2007 legislative session, the NWHF supported the hiring of a governmental relations specialist to lobby for state support for the OCN. Again, this financial support for direct advocacy is a first experience for the Northwest Health Foundation. Previously, there had been support for advocacy efforts at the grassroots level through grants to develop coalitions and constituent support, but there had not been acknowledgement of the need for professional expertise in the legislative arena.

The return on investment was substantial, in that the OCN received $800,000 from the state general fund for the 2007–2009 biennium. Even more important was the technical assistance provided to the OCN by the specialist and the capacity building achieved through this relationship. It has also provided the foundation leadership with the knowledge that our next step, after this legislative period, is to develop a statewide conversation about policy issues and that in addition to a policy agenda from nursing for the next session, we can also create one that has long-term objectives. This is a particularly positive outcome of the funding. Being able to move beyond a policy agenda that is one-dimensional to a slate of goals and objectives for the future will be important to the sustainability of the work that nursing leaders have been doing in Oregon. It will also harness the inherent power in the multitude of nurses in the state to affect all areas of our society, from education to access to affordable, quality health care to transportation to quality-of-life issues.

The bill was also the vehicle by which the OCN was positioned as the leadership entity for nurses in the state. Testimony before the legislative committees was often about the center and its position as the go-to organization for policy makers as they struggle with the issue of health care workforce in the future. The next step will be to involve policy makers before the next session as the issues and agenda become clearer.

The foundation is also dedicated to finding and creating opportunities to prepare nurses to provide policy leadership in a variety of settings, including helping them learn to identify and critically analyze laws, regulations, and policies at the institutional, local, state, and national levels and to devise and use strategies to effectively advocate for policy changes within the health care system. To support that, the foundation will be establishing a statewide policy workgroup of nurses, not only to discuss the obvious nurse-related issues, but also to involve nurses in the work of reforming and improving health care in this country. We seek to have nurses collaboratively participate in influencing Oregon and Washington public policy regarding the issues that are most important to nursing—their ability to provide quality care to their patients and to promote good health for the community. In the future, the foundation anticipates building the power of the nursing community in policy advocacy and other issues. This means supporting nurses to develop more expertise in the field, but it also means reaching out to the nurse at the bedside, at the school, and at the community clinic to become informed and involved in developing and improving the health of our region.

CONCLUSION AND KEY FINDINGS

What have we learned? As "farmers," we have developed a keen understanding of the landscape of the nursing workforce issue. We know that taking the long view may require substantial resources and extreme patience to be effective. A foundation's success in affecting the human resources issues requires that the effort become a major priority, with educated and dedicated staff. Foundations must be able and willing to convene the big-picture thinkers and other stakeholders to discuss and develop a vision and hire personnel who understand the systems and can communicate between the various interested parties.

We learned that we must begin by facing the reality of the nursing workforce shortage and commit to a common future through collaboration and trust. In order to reach the goal of sustainable change, all participants in the system have to take responsibility. Each group has its own part to play, its own unique contribution to make to strengthen the nursing community.

The NWHF has also learned that an initiative to impact the nursing shortage requires a collaborative process, involving collective problem solving and relationship building. We also have to recognize the leaders within the system, whether or not they are designated as such, and support their ability to develop solutions. We have to put in funding both on the small scale (for meeting space, coffee, and mileage costs) and on the large scale (for rolling out a new program). We have to pay nursing leaders to get training in policy advocacy and pay nurses to attend conferences to share their work. We have to help them create and publish multimedia presentations on Web sites and through other media.

In short, we have to be willing to maintain the garden on a constant basis. Of course, it is work; of course it demands exertion and effort and time. However, when every act of garden maintenance is carried out mindfully and with attention to the bigger picture, deep satisfaction and impact are the likely results.

In his book *The Tipping Point,* Malcolm Gladwell (2002) uses the analogy of an infectious disease in explaining a tipping point for social change. An infection may linger among the general population for some time or may be confined to a small subgroup of the population, but then suddenly there is an outbreak and a widespread epidemic of the disease. Gladwell explains that the virtue of an epidemic is that just a little input is enough to get it started, and it can spread very, very quickly. He further suggests that positive social issues, like infectious disease, reach a tipping point, where there are conditions present that explode a contained infection into an epidemic change. Tipping points occur when three conditions are present. The first condition is present when we create fertile ground for change. This occurs when people are searching for new ideas to replace old ones. The second condition is met when people who are effective in spreading ideas to others start sharing the idea. The third condition is present when the idea is "sticky." This is when people express it in a way that makes it impossible to forget or ignore (like a commercial jingle or a whining child). When all three are in place, it is difficult to stop the spread of a good idea. We can believe with certainty that the nursing shortage is a pandemic, reaching all corners of the globe. Using Gladwell's model, the question becomes how to diffuse the positive and innovative solutions in much the same way as the shortage itself has exploded.

In Oregon the fertile ground for change has been laid during the last 5 years, by supporting collaboration and innovative thinking. The foundation has experience and expertise in the field, but it was borne out of listening to nurses first and then putting our resources in places where others had not and letting nurses use their significant critical thinking and collaboration skills to develop collaborative responses to meet the health needs of our communities. We are just beginning to spread the word about how to be effective at changing the nursing workforce system. As the foundation works to build the capacity of nurses in the region to speak for themselves and their communities, the spread of this "positive epidemic" will be made easier and solutions to the challenges of the nursing workforce system will be discovered and multiplied.

NOTES

1. A *promotora* is an outreach worker in a Hispanic community who is responsible for raising awareness of health and educational issues.
2. Utilizing the thumb and forefinger to nip back the very tip of a branch or stem. Pinching promotes branching and a bushier, fuller plant.
3. See http://www.partnersinnursing.org
4. A statewide demonstration project funded in part by the Robert Wood Johnson Foundation to address the workplace culture issues in long-term care.

REFERENCES

Agriculture. (2003). *The Columbia electronic encyclopedia* (6th ed.). Retrieved June 11, 2007, from http://www.answers.com/topic/agriculture

Burton, D. A., Morris, B. A., & Campbell, K. K. (2005). *When, not if...A report on Oregon's registered nurse workforce.* Portland, OR: Oregon Center for Nursing.

Gladwell, M. (2002). *The tipping point.* New York: Little, Brown.

Northwest Health Foundation. (2001, April 26). *Foundation's debut report highlights causes of Oregon's nursing shortage.* Press release.

SECTION V. FUNDING THE RESEARCH TO POLICY CONNECTION: LESSONS LEARNED

Linda Flynn

Crucial to the research to policy connection are the identification of potential funding sources and the successful procurement of funding to support your research. Similar to the other research activities, such as data collection, statistical analyses, or the publication of findings, funding-related activities require researchers to develop specialized knowledge and skill sets.

In this section, contributors have discussed funding resources that may be overlooked by some nurse researchers. Each chapter identified lessons that can be learned when seeking funding for your research.

LESSON 1. YOUR CONGRESSIONAL LEGISLATORS ARE A FUNDING RESOURCE

In chapter 12, Claudia L. McDonald introduced a potential funding resource that might be easily overlooked—your own congressional representative! She described the purpose and availability of earmark funding or plus-ups, known to most of us as "pork-barrel" funds. She explained that despite its derogatory nickname, the purpose of earmark legislation is really to fund projects in the representative's home district that will have an enormous impact nationally, as well as at home. In this way, members of Congress have the opportunity not only to support initiatives that benefit their constituents but also to develop their legacy by contributing to the good of the nation.

We learned in this chapter, however, that before we can successfully seek earmark funds, we must learn the congressional dance of politics and process. First, we start with a gut check by asking ourselves a few key questions. Does your proposed project represent more than a good idea—is it a *great* idea? Is your proposed project sufficiently *urgent* to compel congressional action? Do you honestly believe that funding your project, instead of funding competing projects, is a *better* use of public money? The author then taught us the "steps of the dance" by generously sharing her own experiences and successful tips regarding interactions with (a) members of Congress, (b) lobbyists, and (c) collaborating federal agencies. Although not for the faint-hearted, pursuing an earmark may be a possibility for you, in which case these lessons learned are invaluable.

LESSON 2. KNOW THE FEDERAL HEALTH CARE RESEARCH PRIORITIES

In chapter 13, Kathleen Kendrick, Gail Makulowich, and Mary Grady described the mission and research priorities of the Agency for Healthcare Research and Quality (AHRQ) and the implications of those priorities for policy-influencing research. Explaining that AHRQ primarily funds research that investigates the organization, financing, and delivery of health care, these authors described the work of nurse researchers, funded by AHRQ, that influenced development of organizational and public policies. For example, we learned about the research of Dr. Joann Congdon, a nurse investigator from the University of Colorado, who developed quality indicators or "report cards" to assist consumers in selecting a nursing home. Her findings led the Centers for Medicare and Medicaid Services to a policy of publishing quality report cards for all U.S. nursing homes.

Importantly, in chapter 13 we also gained insights into the application process for AHRQ funding awards. The expert contributors to this chapter described the foundation-building interactions between researchers and program officers that should occur *prior* to the submission of a full proposal. Last, the authors discussed the role of the researcher in translating research findings into actionable recommendations that can be implemented in the user world.

LESSON 3. NATIONAL HEALTH CARE FOUNDATIONS ARE VALUABLE PARTNERS

In chapter 14, we learned of the funding priorities of the nation's largest foundation devoted exclusively to health and health care—the Robert Wood Johnson Foundation (RWJF). Lori Melichar and Susan B. Hassmiller, representatives of the RWJF, also shared specific examples of how the research and evaluation projects that they funded influenced professional, organizational, and public policies. They described the step-by-step process through which the RWJF uses research funding initiatives to (a) identify a problem, (b) develop promising solutions to a problem, (c) design demonstration projects to test promising solutions to a problem, and then (d) evaluate the effectiveness of the solutions in resolving or diminishing the problem.

We also learned how the RWJF (a) develops strategic partnerships to achieve common goals, (b) invests in enhancing the capacity of researchers to shape the message of their findings in ways that resonate with policy makers, and (c) facilitates the efforts of researchers and organizations to translate research findings into practice. Overall, we learned in chapter 14 how researchers might interact with the RWJF to conduct policy-influencing research and subsequently to transform their evidence-based recommendations into evidence-based practices and policies.

LESSON 4. GET TO KNOW YOUR LOCAL PHILANTHROPIC HEALTH FOUNDATION

In chapter 15, Judith Woodruff from the Northwest Health Foundation explained the role of the foundation in addressing nursing education, nursing workforce, and other health care delivery issues. Using an agricultural metaphor, she explained how the foundation has invested its resources to cultivate the soil of ideas, plant seeds of collaboration and change, and stake fledging demonstration projects by committing to continued support. Using Gladwell's concept of the tipping point of an idea, Woodruff related Gladwell's concept to one region of the nation, which led to an innovative redesign of nursing education that not only could be replicated, but that also could dramatically enhance the nurse workforce.

LESSON 5. FUNDING SOURCES INVEST MORE THAN MONEY

Another important lesson so clearly illustrated in this section is that the investments of funding sources, whether they are members of Congress, federal agencies, or private foundations, far exceed the mere monetary contributions to a project. In addition to money, funding sources invest their hopes—hopes that the studies, demonstration projects, and evaluations that they fund will make a difference—an important lesson to remember.

In summary, we learned in this section that before policy-influencing research can be conducted, funding sources willing to sponsor the project must be identified and engaged. This requires researchers to develop a specialized body of knowledge and skills related to the procurement of funding awards. Such skills include identifying appropriate funding mechanisms, aligning your projects' aims with funding priorities, describing the significance and anticipated contributions of your project, establishing pre-proposal relationships, and navigating the complexities of funding organizations, to name a few.

Making the Research to Policy Connection

INTRODUCTION

Geri L. Dickson

As we reach the end of our journey in search of turning evidence-based research into health policy, we have learned how to ask research questions, collect data, analyze secondary databases, and identify key workplace and educational policy issues. Further, we have explored research funding options, and now, in this section we glean important knowledge on what policy making means for advocates of change.

Section VI begins with Lucille Joel challenging us to take seriously our responsibility as citizens in a democracy and to advocate for change. She describes the legislative process, the power of numbers, and the participation in the politics of change at all levels—organizational, professional, and governmental. Further, she identifies the continued role of political advocacy in the governmental rule-making process.

Joel notes three attributes necessary for creating change: a "willingness to participate in change, the tenacity to work toward that end, and knowledge of the work of nursing" or other disciplines. Joel stresses the increased sophistication of nursing with the advent of more RNs with advanced education and roles, which have opened up the profession to a new mechanism, human capital, for creating change—nurse scientists, advanced practice nurses, nurse executives, and educators.

In chapter 17, Mary Val Palumbo outlines the process that nurse leaders in Vermont used to obtain state funding for faculty loan repayments, thereby increasing the potential faculty pool in Vermont. However, most importantly, it was the research presented by the Vermont Office of Nursing Workforce that supplied the foundational evidence on which this public policy change was built.

Moreover, she frames her chapter in light of Kingdon's (2003) framework of a political action theory. The political process that the nurse researchers and leaders engaged in benefited the nursing community by legislative action designed to increase the faculty pool, and they joined forces with other health care disciplines for a much stronger and more successful approach.

Last, Linda Flynn, Charlotte Thomas-Hawkins, and Sandra Bodin demonstrate in chapter 18 the use of evidence, the power of numbers, and the willingness and tenacity to follow through on the legislative process. They were successful in presenting research to the Centers for Medicare and Medicaid Services (CMS) in support of revising existing regulations so that the presence of an RN during dialysis treatments would be mandated. It took not only the evidence they provided to CMS but also the collaboration between the researchers and the professional organization to provide the impetus for CMS to adopt a change in policy for the protection of dialysis patients.

In sum, this is the final section of the book presenting research as evidence for policy change. The research, in and of itself, is not sufficient to create the change for it is the work of translating the research into action that makes policy change come alive—the ultimate research to policy connection!

16

Policy Development and Nursing

LUCILLE A. JOEL

CITIZENSHIP IN A DEMOCRACY

Success is more dependent on great citizens than great leaders (Lamm, 2006). And citizens do not always equate with followers, although when they choose to follow, they are unbeatable. Citizens in a great *democracy* are focused on the future because they believe in something, and they believe that they can make a difference. They feel responsible for the albatrosses that they could unwittingly hang around the necks of their children. The American ethic never has been to let the future take care of itself (Joel, 1998).

To Americans, democracy has always required that citizens fully participate in decisions about their lives, and excuses to avoid this obligation are unacceptable. Democracy often requires the postponement of rights without any relief from duty. Freedom comes only when tempered with self-discipline, and excessive individualism is a liability (Joel, 1998). This may seem contrary to the thinking of many today, but democracy is not an easy choice. It often carries pain and sacrifice.

Tocqueville (1835), the French political philosopher and historian, became so intrigued with citizenship as it played out in American life that he wrote a book about it. Here he made the distinction between citizens and inhabitants. He warned that inhabitants become complacent, accepting things as they are and preferring to be taken care of, usually by the government.

How far have we strayed from the American vision of democracy? Remember that the concepts of democracy and citizenship apply as readily to the nursing profession as they do to the nation or the state or the county or the city or our place of employment. And democracy assumes the development of policy to give structure and predictability to our lives. Whether we are talking of the development of professional, institutional, or public (governmental) policy, prevailing opinion should eventually surface, be debated, and be negotiated. After due consideration, policy will emerge, frequently requiring that most of us relinquish some degree of freedom in favor of the common good as society or the constituency in question sees it. That is democracy, often hard to live with, but impossible to live without if we hope to achieve any sense of community.

NURSES AS PARTICIPANTS IN A DEMOCRATIC COMMUNITY

In the best of all worlds, nurses as nurses should be involved and invested in three dimensions of community: the professional, the organizational, and the governmental. Unfortunately, most nurses find being inhabitants more comfortable than being citizens and additionally have not treated their outspoken and militant colleagues too kindly. For many among us, it has been easier living with the devil we know than the devil we might get with change. Nursing always was and always will be, we think. These attitudes may have been infuriating to many of us in the past. Now they are deceitful and dangerous.

The U.S. population has become exceedingly dependent on government for safety and welfare, most especially the state government. This has not been the heritage of this country, forged on the tradition of freedom, personal autonomy, and responsibility. We have been a humanitarian and generous people, and it remains highly debatable just how much government in our lives is good.

The foundation for social welfare programs in this country was laid in 1935 with the enactment of Social Security. Shortly after, World War II intervened, distracting our attention from more home-front reform until the 1960s. In 1965 we saw the activation of our social conscience in the establishment of Medicare and Medicaid. Almost immediately, there was trepidation over the cost, access, and quality of these programs, and legislation and rule making ensued to institute economies, extend coverage, and monitor value. The benefits available to the privately insured were gradually extended to Medicare and Medicaid recipients, and models of reimbursement used by the government were adopted by the private sector, one influencing the other. However, slowly and incrementally, much of this was accomplished through rule making and institutional policy change as opposed to legislation. "Pass-through" legislation was rare, although where there were federal changes, the states often followed suit of their own accord. Nursing home reform is a good example. Changes initiated at the federal level for Medicare reimbursement to nursing homes were subsequently taken up in more or less exact form by the states for Medicaid.

Pass-through legislation is federal legislation that demands state compliance. This is a difficult and dangerous tact in a society based on states' rights. The only situation in memory where pass-through legislation in health care has occurred was the federal requirement for Medicaid to reimburse pediatric nurse practitioners and midwives. This followed damning evidence of the poor maternal and child health among the poverty-stricken in the United States. Even then, this applied only in states that already recognized these providers, though they were not directly reimbursable.

The presence of states' rights in this country is very strong, as is the power of home rule. Home rule brings the political process and much policy development down to the local level. And quite literally, the health and welfare of the citizens of this country are constitutionally defined as the responsibility of the states. This is a very important understanding as we move forward to consider our options in influencing public policy.

When the federal government picks up the full cost of a program, the federal government can impose its requirements. The state has the option to refuse participation in the program. But if there is cost-sharing between the state and the federal government, the state law prevails. This is the situation with Medicare and Medicaid. Medicare is funded totally with federal dollars, whereas the Medicaid program is funded by a combination of federal and state funds and thereby is driven by state policy. This has created a significant difference in rates. In 2003 Medicaid nursing home reimbursement ranged from a median statewide rate of $83 per day in Louisiana to $323 per day in Alaska (Swan, 2003).

Block grants further reinforced the autonomy of the states, consolidating and handing over the administrative control of select categorical programs to the states with few federal requirements for operations or dispersal of funds. The first of these programs to be disbursed were mental health, substance abuse, and maternal child health. The reasoning behind this strategy was both to streamline federal government and to provide funds more quickly to those who needed them most. There was an assumption that the states would be much better qualified to make decisions about the best use of these funds. Naysayers believed that monies for these critical programs would be jeopardized by state politics absent federal control.

This subtle federal–state relationship is characteristic of U.S. public policy and demands a strong presence of nurses at the state level, the health and welfare of the people being a state constitutional imperative. The progress of state legislation and rule making has also accelerated over the last generations, in regard to both public protections and protections for nurses themselves. Universal precautions, latex protection, mandatory overtime, managed care restrictions, and more have been approached at both the federal and state levels, with homogeneity of some sort eventually being achieved.

THE POWER OF NUMBERS

Everyone claims to be an expert on health care, yet no one is more socialized into the details of the system than the nurse. Further, nurses who have been successful in influencing public policy realize that they must be part of a constituency. Moreover, given that base of a collective, decision makers in government value their opinions.

In every arena where policy is forged, whether legislative, organizational, or professional, success is often a matter of numbers. Though groups may be at odds with one another, they must put aside their differences and come together where there is a mutual agenda. Coalitions and interest groups may be formed on a very short-lived basis, but in the favor of getting things done, these networks are essential. This process of building intricate networks is correctly described as "pluralism." These coalitions penetrate every socioeconomic stratum and include a variety of strange bedfellows who come together around a common agenda. Nursing has been creative in building and joining networks, with success in research and education financing, prevention of HIV-AIDS, civil rights, family leave, pay equity, pension reform, workplace safety, women's health, nursing home reform, and so on. The American Nurses

Association (ANA) has long been the convener of women's groups in Washington, a seemingly disparate but powerful coalition of liberals and conservatives, often pursuing one issue.

The proper question to ask before jumping into coalition building is, "Whose issue is it anyway?" A group may do little more than lend its name in support of an issue when the issue in question is of interest but not the group's priority. In these days of limited resources, such decisions have to be made very carefully and early on. There are many programs that nursing wishes to support but would not do so alone and commit to the full weight of advocacy. Such things as whistle-blowing, patient safety, prescription drug coverage under Medicare, and the format of final directives are nursing's issues, but not nursing's priorities. Mandatory overtime for nurses, staffing ratios, universal precautions, and funding for nursing education are nursing's priorities. Yet even here, our political muscle is diminished if we do not speak with one voice. How unwise it would be to lobby for nursing education reform without representation from all segments of the nursing academic community: associate degree, as well as baccalaureate and higher degree.

The Nursing Organizations Alliance, more commonly known as "the Alliance," is a coalition of 70 nursing organizations. The Tri-Council for Nursing links the ANA, the Association of Nurse Executives, the National League for Nursing, and the American Association of Colleges of Nursing. There are similar coalitions of nurse practitioners and psychiatric nurses. Internationally, the World Health Professions Alliance unites the International Council of Nurses, the World Medical Association, the World Dental Federation, and the International Pharmaceutical Federation. The coalition has drawn attention and has been heard transnationally. An important aspect of these groups' work, though not their only work, is legislative advocacy. These are established groups, but it is just as possible to create your own coalition or interest group around an issue at hand.

POLITICS FOR POLICY

Politics may be defined as the art or science of influencing policy. There is a legitimate tendency to think of politics in the context of government, but effecting policy at the institutional level is often just as important in the work life of a nurse. The term *in-house law* has been used to describe the process of establishing policies and procedures that affect daily work life. Examples abound. There are clinical policies, such as those that state that nurses may (or should or must) develop and implement teaching plans for patients or arrange for referrals to the visiting nurse, which have been blocked by physicians or administrators in some hospitals. There are policies that direct staffing or speak to the adequacy of an acuity system that drives staffing decisions. There are policies that drive decisions on the use or purchase of material resources. Further, there are human resource policies, which are distributed frequently in a manual to new employees and which incidentally have the weight of law. And this list is not all-inclusive.

There has been an increasing recognition that nurses must become involved in policy development at every level or find that someone else has made the decisions on health care and workplace issues that affect their practice, their economic security, and ultimately their patients. Nurses bring important information and sound arguments to any situation that involves the work of nursing. Though anyone would be hard pressed to dispute this statement, nurses are frequently denied a place at the policy table. The reasoning is often that involvement in policy decisions could jeopardize their ability to unionize for collective bargaining. Whether their opinions are binding is not the issue. Nurses bring solutions to problems that are humanistic, sound, and workable. Any employer would be foolish to dismiss such counsel.

Another important component of lawmaking is lobbying, which is generally defined as an attempt to influence a decision of the legislature or other governmental body. Because it is a type of petition for redress of grievances, lobbying is constitutionally guaranteed (Joel, 2006). Lobbying exists in many forms, from a single individual who contacts a legislator about a particular issue of personal importance to the interest groups that carefully (and often expensively) organize systems for monitoring legislation, initiating action, or blocking action on matters that concern them. Lobbying is a subtle dance, often two steps forward and one step back.

Though the concept of lobbying is most often associated with lawmaking, it holds a broader connotation. You can lobby your administrator at your place of employment for changes in administrative policy. You can lobby the professional association for changes in policies and positions. To breathe life into the last statement, let us borrow an example from the history of advanced practice. In years past, the ANA advised that advanced practice not be included in state nursing practice acts or addressed anywhere in the law or regulations. It was the ANA belief that advanced practice nurses, notably the clinical nurse specialist and nurse practitioner, were covered under the provisions of the practice acts as they existed. This proved to create considerable difficulty in reimbursement because if you were not mentioned in law, you did not exist as far as the insurers were concerned. The intense lobbying of advanced practice groups with the ANA reversed this policy and moved states in turn to lobby for inclusion of advanced nurse practitioners in the law.

The important element in lobbying is to be clear on the bottom line of your efforts (Wray, Cohen, & Reinhard, 1998). What are the principles that are nonnegotiable? Many compromises may be necessary to secure enough support for your position, but be careful that as you nibble around the edge of the issue, you do not sacrifice that nonnegotiable principle. An example may help here. The federal Medicare nursing home reforms of 1987 were intended to require the significant presence of registered nurses (RNs) in long-term care facilities, among many other things. During the staging and refinement of this legislation, the word "registered" was replaced by "licensed." This was a result of efforts by the nursing home industry, claiming that an existing nursing shortage would make recruitment of RNs in sufficient numbers impossible. The ANA felt that it was better to accept some gain rather than none and work toward a higher standard in subsequent legislation. Others felt that a principle had been sacrificed and that the legislation should have been stopped from proceeding.

The "half a cup is better than none" philosophy can be strategic, or it can be dangerous and undermining. Over time, the language contained in the nursing home reforms legislation of 1987 filtered down to state Medicaid programs, and the licensed practical nurse became the staffing standard in nursing homes. What other options could have proven useful to both sides of the issue? A provision may have been developed for exceptions to the RN rule if recruitment were impossible. Those exceptions could have been tightened and more rarely justified as the shortage abated. In this way, the RN requirement would have been preserved. Or from another perspective, was the RN presence one of the nonnegotiable principles or an item to be bartered to gain support for other items? The ANA was only one among many associations who came together on behalf of these reforms.

Professional lobbyists must be registered with the clerk of the house or assembly and the secretary of the senate. They spend all or part of their time representing the interests of a particular group or groups.

These people are influential with legislators, but so are special interest groups and most especially the "folks back home," who determine whether the legislator or public official will be returned to a seat in government.

The most effective way to influence governmental policy is to support someone aspiring to hold or keep public office. And the most effective people to wield that influence come from the constituency of the legislator. This is grassroots lobbying and may involve an interest group or an individual. Large contributions to campaign funds are not necessary but appreciated, as is the investment of effort in election campaigns and advocacy on the behalf of a candidate who is a friend to nursing. Looking to the philosophy of Tip O'Neill, the late and great Massachusetts politician, all politics is local (1987).

Grassroots activities may take the form of telephone calls, telegrams, and letter-writing campaigns as well as letters to the editor, press conferences, and various other media activities. A strategic first step is making contact with your legislator, public official, or candidate. Become acquainted, identify yourself as a nurse, and explain nursing's platform and what you could do for each other. You have now become a known quantity before any crisis occurs. Plan periodic revisits and educate and reeducate about nursing's issues. Get to know the legislator's staff. Gaining the ear of staff is often the key to successful lobbying. They are commonly assigned to specific policy areas, are already intimately aware of your issues, and are the major source of advisement to the legislator. The same tactics apply to the executive branch of government. Know the scope of power of your governor. In some states, this chief executive can bring about significant change by executive order alone.

The process of political advocacy does not end when a bill becomes a law. Laws are usually general; too much specificity makes them rapidly obsolete and requires another trip through the legislative process to amend. Therefore, through the process of rule making, the governmental agency or department within whose purview the law falls develops rules and regulations. For instance, rule making to allow enforcement of the Nursing Practice Act is the responsibility of the department under which the state board of nurse examiners falls. On the national level, health legislation is sent to the Department of Health and Human Services. Advisory committees of citizens are usually appointed, as spelled out by the law or the practice of the department. Public notice of hearings for the proposed rules allow interested individuals to monitor progress or testify.

Rules are published in the Federal Register (states have counterparts), and comments are entertained. Regulations have the force of law, but it is illegal to lobby during rule making. However, it is appropriate to educate, provide testimony, and respond to the published rules. Suggestions are taken seriously, and modifications and changes within the limits of the law are very usual. It is possible to influence the interpretation of legislation at this point and to strengthen or weaken the intent of the law. Regulations have been changed after hearings or publication (a first and final publication are usual) because of major protests by interested groups and individuals, the presentation of well thought-out alternative policy, or letters written in response to the proposed rules.

BEYOND BASELINE

Much of what we have detailed can be accomplished by any nurse. Many of the talents detailed do not require higher education, but they do require the willingness to participate in change, the tenacity to work toward that end, and knowledge of the work of nursing. But the profession has moved to a new level of sophistication. We count researchers, nurse executives, educators, and advanced practice nurses among our ranks. We have the competency to marry the science with the policy skills needed for reform. After all, a policy based on evidence of the impact of nurses and their care on patients lives is much more likely to catch an administrator or legislator's ear when we are educating and advocating for policy changes.

Many of the policy gains in past years have been made possible by research and program evaluation, which has been ideally suited to reform. The Teaching Nursing Home Project funded by the Robert Wood Johnson Foundation directly influenced the nursing home reforms of 1987. The Magnet hospital study of 1983 set the stage for the Magnet hospital program offered by the American Nurses Credentialing Center. The faculty practice initiative of the American Academy of Nursing gave credibility to service-education unification efforts that have since become the standard in bringing the best of nursing to both students and patients. We have moved into a new action mode, with the capacity to use the best of every nurse in the work of change. We need the intellectual products of our researchers and program specialists. And we need the interpersonal savvy and numbers that the citizens of this great profession can provide.

REFERENCES

Joel, L. (1998). On citizenship in a great profession. *The American Journal of Nursing*, *98*(4), 7.

Joel, L. (2006). *The nursing experience*. New York: McGraw-Hill.

Kingdon, J. N. (2003). *Agendas, alternatives, and public policy (2nd edition)*. New York: Longman.

Lamm, R. (2006). Great nations need great citizens. *The Social Contract Journal*, *16*(3), 183–186.

O'Neill, T. P. (1987). *Man of the house: The life and political memoirs of Speaker Tip O'Neill*. New York: Random House.

Swan, J. (2003). *Medicaid reimbursement rates*. Wichita, KS: Wichita State University.

de Tocqueville, A. (1835). *Democracy in America*. New York: Signet Classics.

Wray, R., Cohen, S. S., & Reinhard, S. (1998). Lobbying policymakers: Individual and collective strategies. In D. Mason, & J. Leavitt (Eds.), *Policy and politics in nursing and health care* (3rd. ed., pp. 481–489). Philadelphia: Saunders.

17

State Funding for Nurse Faculty Loan Repayment: The Vermont Experience

MARY VAL PALUMBO

Vermont may be best known for its maple syrup and Ben and Jerry's ice cream, but the Green Mountain state is also home to an actively engaged nursing community with a track record of accomplishments. The fact that Vermont has a population of just over half a million, 16 hospitals, 5 nursing programs, and about 5,000 registered nurses currently working in Vermont (although 13,000 RNs are currently licensed here) makes the state a perfect laboratory for testing nursing workforce initiatives and proposing policy changes. Within this setting, most nurse practice areas are represented, and all are governed and regulated; therefore, comparisons may be applied to smaller regions of other states or rural states with similar geographic challenges. The purpose of this chapter is to demonstrate what a small state's nursing community has accomplished to address the nurse faculty shortage, focusing on collaboration and the use of data-driven evidence.

APPLYING KINGDON'S FRAMEWORK

In John W. Kingdon's (1995) theory on agenda setting, three streams—problems, politics, and policy alternatives—converge to create a window of opportunity that allows an issue to move onto the policy-setting agenda. This framework is applied here to describe a successful experience of problem identification, policy formation, and legislative action in one state.

The Problem Stream

National Perspective

After almost a decade of a national nurse shortage, progress has been made regarding increased enrollment in undergraduate nursing schools, improved work environments, and increased salaries. The concerted efforts of many organizations have dramatically increased interest in nursing as a career. The National League for Nursing (NLN, 2004) reported a 50.3% increase in enrollment in all types of pre-licensure registered nurse programs. However, the American Association of Colleges of Nursing (AACN, 2005) found that 29,425 qualified applicants were turned away from entry-level baccalaureate nursing programs in 2004 because of faculty shortages, limited budgets, restricted availability of clinical sites, and insufficient classroom space.

The main reason for limited capacity in nursing school across the country is a national nursing faculty shortage. The realities cited by the AACN (2005) for this shortage include the retirement of 200–300 doctorally prepared faculties annually from 2004 to 2012, with a 18% decrease in faculty between ages 36 and 45. The AACN acknowledges that the underlying reason for increased employment of doctoral graduates in settings other than schools of nursing is driven by the salary disparity between clinical and academic settings. Contributing factors include a decline in doctoral program enrollees as a result of tuition and loan burden for graduate study and a prolonged "time to degree" for doctoral education (AACN). Workplace environment issues for nursing faculty were also cited by the AACN report, including job dissatisfaction because of workload and role expectation issues, student population challenges, and an expectation to "do it all"—teach, practice, and research.

A disturbing conclusion from a longitudinal study in North Carolina was that nurses who are initially prepared at the associate degree level are much less likely to continue their education to graduate studies (Bevill, Cleary, Lacey, & Nooney, 2007). Based on these findings, the North Carolina Center for Nursing proposes that the most immediate way to increase the potential nursing faculty pool is to increase the number of graduates with a bachelor of science in nursing degree, especially men or members of a racial or ethnic minority (Cleary, Bevill, Lacey, & Nooney, 2007).

Vermont Perspective

Progress in combating Vermont's nursing shortage has been made since the 2001 Blue Ribbon Commission on Nursing convened and issued recommendations (Cohen, Palumbo, & Rambur, 2003). The data from the Vermont Office of Nursing Workforce (ONW) reveal increases in the numbers of enrolled students at all levels, nurse graduates, and male nurses. There also appears to be some positive progress since 2003 in terms of reducing the likeliness of nurses to leave their jobs because of dissatisfaction with their salaries (ONW, 2005a). Decreased vacancy rates in hospital and home health agencies were found in 2005 in comparison with 2003 data (ONW, 2005b, 2005c). These gains can be credited, in part, to several initiatives undertaken in the state. Expansion of nursing educational offerings to Vermont students in rural locations have been made by Castleton State College, Vermont Technical College, and the University of Vermont. The Nursing Educational Loan Repayment Program for pre-licensure nursing students was first funded in fiscal year 2001 by the state of Vermont, through the Department of Health, with an appropriation of $148,000 for loan repayment and forgiveness. New graduates (LPN, ADN, BSN) must commit to working at least 20 hours per week in a hospital, nursing home, or home health agency in Vermont. One year of service is required for each year of receiving the award. In 2001, 57 new graduates of RN/LPN programs applied, and 22 received funds. In 2002 there were 85 eligible candidates for $180,000. All 85 were considered, and 24 students received awards ranging from $3,000 to $6,000, depending on their total educational debt.

Despite this progress, the number of baccalaureate-prepared nurses in Vermont remains roughly half (32%) of the recommendation of the National Advisory Council on Nursing Education and Practice (Division of Nursing, 1996), which is to have 60% of the RN workforce prepared at the bachelor's degree level by 2010. Realizing that more should be done, Vermont nurse leaders and other stakeholders gathered in June 2004. The results of this meeting were summarized in a report titled *Next Steps for Vermont Nurse Workforce Planning: Increasing Educational Capacity* (ONW, 2004). The next course of action was collaborating to write a white paper titled *Nurses' Educational Advancement Is Necessary to Increasing Educational Capacity* (ONW, 2006), which suggested that Vermont nurse leaders must actively encourage nurses to further their education so that all nurse faculty roles can be filled. Yet in 2005 home health agencies were the only health care setting in which the majority of employers (70%) offered differentiated pay based on educational preparation (ONW, 2005c). According to the 2005 Vermont Health Workforce Assessment Survey pay was not differentiated for nurses with BSN or other credentials in the majority of hospitals and nursing homes in Vermont (ONW, 2005b, 2005c).

The Vermont RN re-licensure surveys by the ONW are a method by which progress toward nursing workforce goals is tracked and evaluated, thus providing an evidence base. This survey is included in the re-licensure material mailed to every nurse registered in Vermont every 2 years (up to 11,000). This survey is not mandatory but has a high response rate (greater than 60% for the last four surveys). Only data from nurses who report currently working in the state are used (approximately 5,000).

In a comparison of the years 2003 and 2005 in the Vermont RN re-licensure surveys (ONW, 2003, 2005a), some small progress is noted at the master's level, but there is little change at the doctoral level. Faculty with master's and doctoral degrees in nursing are needed at all Vermont nursing schools. Less than 5% of Vermont nurses have master's degrees or higher, and many of these nurses are in clinical practice or administration. Consequently, the five schools of nursing in the state are hard pressed to accommodate the renewed interest in careers in nursing. This is related directly to resources available for additional faculty positions, not to mention the problems finding appropriately educated faculty to fill existing positions. Student clinical placement sites also are limited by availability. Unfortunately, applications submitted to the only graduate program in nursing in the state did not increase significantly in the past decade.

In 2004 the nurse leaders were able to provide data that led to the establishment of more financial incentives for nursing graduate studies, which opened up graduates' choices for taking a nurse educator position. With graduate nursing education costs between $15,000 and $40,000, the following Vermont-based scholarships were developed:

- Freeman's Scholarship extended to graduate students
- Vermont Nurse Foundation Light the Lamp Scholarship
- Vermont Organization of Nurse Leaders' Advanced Degree Nurse Leadership Scholarship

The ONW data were essential to provide the evidence support to create these policy changes, which helped to address the problem—a shortage of nurse faculty.

THE POLITICAL STREAM

Understanding Vermont's "citizen legislature" is an important part of this account of a successful nursing policy initiative. The Vermont legislature meets part-time (from January to late spring every year). Legislators may be teachers, farmers, lawyers, or real estate agents or even nurses who take leave from these jobs during the legislative session. One hundred fifty members of the House of Representatives and 30 senators are elected every 2 years. The governor and lieutenant governor of Vermont also are elected every 2 years. Vermont legislators pride themselves in being accessible to their constituents. It is not uncommon to chat with the Senate Chair of Appropriations at the grocery store or to see the Speaker of the House of Representatives selling snacks at a basketball game.

In 2004 the voters elected a new governor, who established a mandate for creating jobs. The political stream was also primed because of the previous success of the Blue Ribbon Commission on Nursing, loan repayment programs, and a newly legislated requirement for the state health plan to address human resources (i.e., nurses). One key advisory group to the governor and the legislature was the Workforce Development Partnership (WDP) subcommittee of the Vermont Department of Labor's Human Resource Investment council. The WDP was established on the advice of the Workforce Investment Boards from every region of Vermont, who collectively identified the health care sector as a top employment priority. Multidisciplinary committee members were selected from labor, education, health care settings, and government. Approximately 10 members of a 20-member roster meet monthly for the purpose of creating regional and statewide solutions for recruitment and retention of qualified health care workers at all levels. The WDP was involved in every step of converging the problem with the political opportunities and in the preparation of an acceptable policy solution.

THE POLICY STREAM

Ideas were generated from the WDP meeting, statewide health care workforce conferences, and work sessions involving the following groups: Academics, Department of Labor, Hospital Association, Health Department, Area Health Education Center, Human Resources Investment

Council, Vermont State Nurse Association, legislative members, and the Office of Nursing Workforce.

Information was also gathered from the several states that have enacted legislation to address the nurse faculty shortage and that, consequently, have been able to increase student capacity at their schools of nursing. For example, New Mexico has legislation to mandate improved interactions between health care facilities and higher education and to supplement faculty salaries (Bailey, 2003). The Kentucky state legislature has created a board to do the following: Establish and administer an application process, criteria and procedures for awarding scholarships or loan repayment assistance to registered nurses pursuing advanced degrees to become nursing faculty; and establish and administer an application process, criteria and procedures for hospitals that provide nursing scholarships to receive matching funds (Nursing Workforce Foundation Act, 2002).

During this period, New Hampshire's governor announced a financial incentive of $65,000 for 15 nurses to become nurse educators (Haberman, 2003). State mandates are in place to increase or double nursing school enrollments in Nevada, Oregon, South Dakota, and Arizona. Some of these mandates, however, lack appropriations to support faculty development, and others carry quite generous appropriations (e.g., Illinois and Virginia) In addition, small and large foundations have developed faculty initiatives to increase the supply of faculty and, hence, RNs. A major health foundation, the Robert Wood Johnson Foundation, is implementing a faculty initiative in its home state of New Jersey.

When proposing new policy, it is important to consider all possible solutions, explore the technical feasibility of each, consider the value acceptability for all stakeholders, recognize any future constraints, and estimate the actual cost. The view of the public must also be considered, given that perceived public support will be important to any elected representative who may carry forward a policy initiative.

Five possible solutions to the nursing faculty shortage policy solutions were considered for implementation in Vermont. In Table 17.1, the five possible solutions are compared and contrasted. The most feasible program for Vermont was determined to be loan repayment for new faculty at the five schools of nursing as of September 2004. Because a nurse loan repayment program was already in place, the faculty program would fit into the existing structure of application review and award allocation. Taking this one step further, the addition of incentives for health care facilities to support educational progression and create

Table 17.1

ALL OPTIONS CONSIDERED

SOLUTIONS	TECHNICAL FEASIBILITY	VALUE ACCEPTABILITY	FUTURE CONSTRAINTS	COST	PUBLIC ACQUIESCENCE
Faculty loan repayment	Model already in place for nurse loan repayment, easy to replicate.	Data on Vermont faculty must be made available to legislators/others.	Sustainability of funding	$100,000	Debate over allocation of limited state resources could impact outcome.
Scholarships for nursing faculty	Merit scholarships are available currently through an in-state private foundation; the extension to faculty might be possible, and this would not need legislation.	Very acceptable	Sustainability of funding	None to taxpayer, Freeman Scholarship program to be approached	Public is supportive of private means of funding worthwhile initiatives.
Joint clinical appointment incentives	Barriers exist for joint clinical appointments, and few currently exist between the 5 nursing schools and practice sites.	The creation of "teaching" clinical sites around Vermont needs some positive PR.	Rise in fringe benefit costs	Minimal cost for awards of "Nursing Education Advocate"	Administrators of hospitals and health systems may or may not value these incentives.
Support of educational progression to doctoral level	With more online options and one in-state master's program, it is becoming more feasible for RNs to progress to the doctoral level.	Many Vermonters do not place a high value on doctoral education.	Innovative and no-cost ways to reward support of continuing nursing education need to be developed.	Unknown (research of tuition reimbursement paid by hospitals for graduate studies is needed)	Nurse educators and researchers need some positive PR to increase support for and value of doctoral education.
Mandate increased capacity of nursing schools	Not feasible without support for faculty development. Exact projections on ideal capacity are needed.	Turning away potential nursing students will be unacceptable in the years to come.	Upgrade of facilities at all nursing schools will be necessary; clinical sites are limited.	2,000,000 or more	Unfunded mandates will not be popular with the state college system.

joint appointments with schools of nursing also were encouraged. For example, a formal designation and award from the governor as a "Nursing Education Advocate" was suggested to highlight the creation of joint clinical appointment by hospitals and schools of nursing.

Windows of Opportunity

Clear identification of the problem, supported by national and local evidence, provided the incentive for the opening of a window of opportunity for the nurse leaders, as well as the earlier political successes regarding a nurse faculty shortage. The following bullets (Anderson, 2003) demonstrate how a "window of opportunity briefly opens for an issue, as it did for the Vermont nurses leaders, who were poised to act.

- Streams converge effort around "salient issues"
- Changes in other policies increase public interest
- Events increase public interest (natural, staged, planned, cyclic)
- Agenda setting relies on timing and luck (p. 89)

Looking back on the 4-year effort to get legislation and funding to support nurse faculty loan replacement in Vermont provides a good example of an open window of opportunity. It is now clear how the convergence of interest in job creation and concerns about a health care workforce shortage created an atmosphere that was ripe to accept a new policy solution. The nurse leaders planned events that highlighted the problem and helped move the solution closer to acceptance by the policy makers. The agenda moved slowly, so patience was required by stakeholders as their agenda moved slowly through the ups and downs of the political process. The following description of the strategic plan and timeline illustrates the need for stakeholders' patience.

Strategic Plan/Timeline

Getting the Bill Written

November 11, 2003—The WDP reviewed a draft of a proposed nurse faculty loan forgiveness program developed by the Office of Nursing Workforce. The leadership group agreed to support it, and Representative Vincent, the legislator member of the group, volunteered to request a slot for pending legislation for this proposal.

November 14, 2003—Proposed legislation went to Senators Kittell and Bartlett, Representative Vincent, the Vermont State Nurses Association, and the Vermont Organization of Nurse Leaders. The advice at the time was to have it introduced in both the House (with two sponsors) and the Senate (with seven sponsors).

November 19, 2003—Senator Sara Kittell wrote,

Hi Mary, Thanks for the note and information about loan repayment and incentives to expand the number of nurse educators. I will send this info to our legislative council and draft a bill for you to look at. Let me know if this is the direction we should be going in. Regards, Sara

January–May 2004—The director of the Office of Nursing Workforce provided testimony or information as requested to legislators for both House Bill 538 and Senate Bill 268. House Bill 538 proposed to establish a program of education loan forgiveness for nursing faculty who serve in Vermont and an incentive for health care faculty and schools of nursing to establish joint clinical appointments. Senate Bill 268 proposed to establish a program of education loan forgiveness for nursing faculty who serve in Vermont. The testimony focused on the following five points:

1 Jobs—Vermont currently has a nursing shortage (eased in part by expensive traveling nurses), and the Department of Labor predicts a 34% increase in RN positions in the next 10 years.
2 Vermont's ability to educate nurses—In order to meet projected health care needs in 2010, investments were needed to increase the educational capacity of Vermont's nursing schools. In 2004 three out of the five schools of nursing reported that they had turned away qualified applicants.
3 Faculty shortage—The number one barrier to expanding educational capacity was, and remains, the shortage of adequately prepared nursing faculty because clinical nurse positions offer graduate-prepared nurses much higher salaries than do faculty positions. Moreover, the mean age of the current faculty is 50 years, and there are few younger nurses available to replace them when the current faculty retire.
4 The need to build a pipeline—With a required 8:1 student-to-faculty ratio, building a pipeline of qualified nursing faculty is an essential part of addressing Vermont's nursing shortage.

5   Loan repayment and joint clinical appointments—Loan repayments are an effective strategy to encourage nurses to pursue advanced education and then move from high-paying clinical jobs into faculty roles. A joint clinical appointment is a collaborative agreement between facilities and schools of nursing to share expert nurses. H583 would take the necessary first steps to address nursing faculty shortages.

During the legislative session of 2004, the WDP worked to advance the legislation through lobbyists connected to their organizations (University of Vermont, Vermont State Nurse Association, Vermont Association of Hospitals and Health Systems, and the Area Health Education Center). By June of 2004, the legislative year ended, and there had been no movement on the legislation in either House or Senate.

Outcomes: 2005 Legislative Session

- June–December 2005—Plan for reintroduction of nursing loan repayment legislation (House Bill 058) that proposed to direct the Commissioner of Health to establish an education loan forgiveness program for expenses related to an advanced nursing degree for nurses serving on the faculty of certain Vermont postsecondary institutions, to establish a nurse educator advocate award, and to appropriate $200,000.00 for the nursing loan forgiveness program. This bill had 26 sponsors. In addition, Nurses' Week Celebration planning began for a celebration on the State House lawn.
- Nurse's Week Celebration in May 2005 included a tent on the State House lawn and the creation of a giant puzzle, which stated, "In puzzling times, nurses put the healthcare pieces together." The lieutenant governor invited the nurses to put the puzzle together again for a press conference including the governor. A "treasure box" of nurses' stories was also presented to the governor at this press conference and was later summarized and posted on the lieutenant governor's Web site.
- H058 was left "on the wall" in the House Appropriations committee with no action taken.
- Senator Bartlett, chair of Senate Appropriations, included funding ($50,000) for nurse faculty loan repayment in "waterfall funds" for fiscal year 2006. This was a one-time appropriation.

- In 2006, 10 applications were received, and 5 were awarded, with an average award of $10,000. The range of debt was $10,117 to $91,290 (mean $39,325).

General Eligibility Requirements for Nurse Faculty Educational Loan Repayment

- Applicant must be employed as a Vermont academic nurse educator/faculty.
- Applicant must be a nurse with outstanding educational debt acquired in pursuit of an advanced nursing degree *and* must either have incurred nursing program educational debt *after* July 1, 2005 *or* have been *first* employed on the nursing faculty after July 1, 2005.
- Applicant must work a minimum of part-time as nurse educator/faculty during the academic year.

Strategy for 2006

Securing ongoing funding for nursing faculty loan repayment at greater than $50,000 per year was the next step. An opportunity to include this goal in an initiative to keep more young adults in Vermont arose with the recommendations of the Next Generation Commission. The collaborating partners made the issue visible with the launching of Health Care Career Awareness Month in October 2006. A kick-off event held at a local high school included speeches by the governor and the secretaries of health, labor, and economic development. A Plinkit game was unveiled that gave the high school students prizes and information about health care careers in a fast-paced and fun format. This whole event brought more attention to the need for a future health care workforce and an endorsement from the executive branch of the Vermont state government.

Legislation was finally passed in May 2007 that included nurse faculty loan repayment on an ongoing basis and that increased funding for scholarships for young adults who receive their education in Vermont or return to Vermont to work. Act 46 was signed by Governor James Douglas and provided the funding for $75,000 of loan repayment specifically for nursing faculty each fiscal year. A total of $500,000 was appropriated for health care loan repayment for nurses, dentists, and primary care providers, and these funds are administered by the Area Health Education

Table 17.2

A SUMMARY OF ALL THE LEGISLATION THAT WAS INTRODUCED FOR NURSING FACULTY LOAN REPAYMENT IN VERMONT

2004 H-583 (introduced)
http://www.leg.state.vt.us/docs/legdoc.cfm?URL=/docs/2004/bills/intro/H-583.HTM

2004 S268 (introduced)
http://www.leg.state.vt.us/docs/legdoc.cfm?URL=/docs/2004/bills/intro/S-268.HTM

2005 H-058 (introduced)
http://www.leg.state.vt.us/docs/legdoc.cfm?URL=/docs/2006/bills/intro/H-058.HTM

2006 Act 46 (passed)
http://www.leg.state.vt.us/docs/legdoc.cfm?URL=/docs/2008/acts/ACT046.HTM

Center with a service requirement as part of each award. See Table 17.2 for a summary of all the legislation that was introduced for nursing faculty loan repayment and the Web site where the legislative language can be retrieved.

CONCLUSIONS

It is important to be prepared for windows of opportunity or at least to recognize when the window may be cracking open, and it is time to pull together to take advantage of this. Applying the Kingdon theory to this situation, the three streams did converge around the salient issue of creating jobs to keep young adults in Vermont. The formation of the Next Generation Commission was the catalyst that energized nurse leaders and other stakeholders to push for permanent funding for nurse faculty educational loan repayment. Public interest was heightened around this issue because the governor made keeping young adults in Vermont a campaign priority, and the legislature (dominated by the opposite political party) favored loan repayment over scholarships. Therefore, the issue was constantly being debated and covered by the press. This afforded the opportunity to create a venue to highlight health care careers and push for funding for loan repayment.

However, it was the analytical work produced by the ONW through surveys that provided the strong evidence base for a new policy. The reports generated by the ONW clearly demonstrated the need for a policy designed to increase the number of graduate-prepared faculty in order to create a steady stream of new recruits into Vermont nursing.

In addition, all along the way, opportunities to have fun and make nursing more visible were employed. The large white tent on the State House lawn, the giant jigsaw puzzle, the treasure box of nurses' stories, and finally the Plinkit game and declaration of Health Care Career Awareness month made enjoyable moments to reward all the hard work. The 4 years that it took to accomplish permanent funding for nurse faculty loan repayment in Vermont will be looked back on as time well spent.

REFERENCES

American Association of Colleges of Nursing. (2005). *Faculty shortages in baccalaureate and graduate nursing programs: Scope of the problem and strategies for expanding the supply.* Retrieved April 23, 2008, from http://www.aacn.nche.edu/publications/pdf/05FacShortage.pdf

Anderson, J. (2003). *Public policymaking* (5th ed.). Boston: Houghton Mifflin.

Bailey, S. (2003). *Registered nurse shortages: Public policy and higher education in western states.* Retrieved September 30, 2003, from https://www.wiche.edu/Policy/Policy Insights/Nursing2003/Nursing.pdf

Bevill, J. W., Cleary, B. L., Lacey, L. M., & Nooney, J. G. (2007). Educational mobility of RNs in North Carolina: Who will teach tomorrow's nurses? A report on the first study to longitudinally examine educational mobility among nurses. *American Journal of Nursing, 107*(5), 60–70.

Cleary, B. L., Bevill, J. W., Lacey, L. M., & Nooney, J. G. (2007). Evidence and root causes for an inadequate pipeline of nursing faculty. *Nursing Administration Quarterly, 31*(2), 124–128.

Cohen, J., Palumbo, M. V., & Rambur, B. (2003). Combating the nursing shortage: Vermont's call to action. In H. Feldman (Ed.), *The nursing shortage: Strategies for recruitment and retention in clinical practice and education* (pp. 3–24). New York: Springer Publishing.

Division of Nursing. (1996). *National Advisory Council on Nurse Education and Practice: Report to the Secretary of the Department of Health and Human Services on the basic registered nurse workforce.* Washington, DC: U.S. Government Printing Office.

Haberman, S. (2003, October 1). Benson seeks to help nursing shortage. *Portsmouth Herald.* Retrieved April 24, 2008, from http://archive.seacoastonline.com/2003news/10012003/news/52962.htm

Kingdon, J. W. (1995). *Agendas, alternatives, and public policies* (2nd ed.). New York: HarperCollins.

National League for Nursing. (2004). *Startling data from the NLN's comprehensive survey of all nursing programs evokes wake-up call.* Retrieved December 15, 2004, from http://www.nln.org/newsreleases/datarelease05.pdf

Nursing Workforce Foundation Act. 2002 Ky. Acts ch. 272, sec. 7. Retrieved April 24, 2008, from http://www.lrc.state.ky.us/Statrev/ACTS2002/0272.pdf

Office of Nursing Workforce Research, Planning, and Development. (2003). *Registered nurses in Vermont.* Retrieved April 22, 2008, from http://www.choosenursingvemont.org/reports/rptRN_2003.html

Office of Nursing Workforce Research, Planning, and Development. (2004). *Next steps for Vermont nurse workforce planning: Increasing educational capacity.* Retrieved June 2, 2007, from http://choosenursingvermont.org/reports/pdfs/next_steps_2004.pdf

Office of Nursing Workforce Research, Planning, and Development. (2005a). *Registered nurses in Vermont.* Retrieved April 22, 2008, from www.choosenursingvermont.org/reports/pdfs/rn2005.pdf

Office of Nursing Workforce Research, Planning, and Development. (2005b). *Vermont Health Workforce Assessment Survey Hospital Nursing Study 2005.* Retrieved April 23, 2008, from http://www.choosenursingvermont.org/reports/pdfs/hosp2005.pdf

Office of Nursing Workforce Research, Planning, and Development. (2005c). *Vermont Health Workforce Assessment Survey Home Health Nursing Study 2005.* Retrieved April 23, 2008, from http://www.choosenursingvermont.org/reports/pdfs/home2005.pdf

Office of Nursing Workforce Research, Planning, and Development. (2006). *Nurses' educational advancement is necessary to increasing educational capacity.* Retrieved April 23, 2008, from http://www.choosenursingvermont.org/reports/PDFs/inc_ed_cap.pdf

18

Using Research to Influence Federal Policy: The Nephrology Nurses' Experience

LINDA FLYNN, CHARLOTTE THOMAS-HAWKINS, AND SANDRA M. BODIN

Nurses make up the largest sector of health care professionals in the nation and are, therefore, at the core of health care delivery services. As a result, nurses occupy a front-row seat at the point where health care policies impact patients, making nurses visible experts in the myriad issues influencing the safe delivery of health care services. Consequently, nurses, many of whom may not recognize their potential role in policy development, have a solemn responsibility to use their expertise to advocate for policies and decisions that will protect the health and safety of the many patients who place their trust in them.

Although not necessarily at the bedside, nurses educated at the doctoral level are certainly not exempt from this professional responsibility to shape organizational and public policies in ways that maximize patient safety and positive outcomes. Rather, doctoral-prepared nurses are uniquely positioned to identify and utilize research findings as credible evidence on which to base necessary, appropriate, and effective health care initiatives. The purpose of this discussion is to describe the research–policy connection and to present a real-life example of how nursing research can influence policy development.

THE RESEARCH–POLICY CONNECTION

According to Kingdon's model of policy development, health care advocates must lie in wait for a window of opportunity if they are to be successful in getting their proposed initiatives translated into health care policy (Kingdon, 2003). Just as the surfer who waits for the perfect wave must be ready to paddle when the big one comes along, so must advocates be ready to push their policy initiative when the political window opens. Kingdon explains, however, that to be ready fully for the window of opportunity, or perfect wave, there are three streams that must be joined: (a) an important problem must be recognized; (b) a viable solution to the problem must be proposed; and (c) the solution must have political support.

The coalescence of these three streams is challenging to say the least, and most well-intentioned policy initiatives fail because one or more of these important prerequisites is lacking. Although this is not specifically mentioned in Kingdon's model, we are proposing that nursing research can merge these three streams into a powerful political force. Dating back to when Florence Nightingale first used a pie chart to illustrate the impact of nursing services on soldier mortality, nursing research, when utilized, has been effective in influencing health policy. Through nursing research, the magnitude of the problem can be quantified, the efficacy of the proposed solution can be tested, and political support can be more easily garnered when the problem and solution are supported by evidence. Therefore, we are proposing a slight modification to Kingdon's model to specifically include nursing research as a mechanism by which the three requisite streams of problem identification, solution, and political support can be joined.

THE REVISED MODEL IN ACTION

Recently, the leaders of the American Nephrology Nurses Association (ANNA) saw their window of opportunity open when the existing federal regulations regarding the provision of renal dialysis services, as delineated in the Medicare Conditions of Coverage, were up for review and possible revision by the Centers for Medicare and Medicaid Services (CMS). As they were currently written, the regulations required the presence of a nurse during dialysis treatment; the nurse," however, could be either a registered nurse (RN) *or* a licensed practical nurse (LPN). This latitude in staffing was a source of concern among nephrology nurses represented by the ANNA. They recognized that patients suffering from end-stage renal disease were at risk for a variety of adverse events that might occur during dialysis treatments, including hypotensive episodes, unexpected bleeding, vascular access occlusion or infection, and prematurely terminated treatments. Consequently, the expert assessment and surveillance that is best provided by an RN during hemodialysis was considered essential by ANNA members to preventing or reducing the likelihood of adverse patient events. Therefore, to ensure the safety of patients and quality of care, the ANNA was advocating for a change in the regulation that would require the presence of at least one RN in the dialysis facility during hemodialysis treatments.

In keeping with Kingdon's criteria for readiness, the ANNA was, in many ways, prepared to seize the political opportunity and bring about a policy change. As a respected professional organization, it represented a large and visible membership that spoke with one voice in favor of the RN staffing requirement. The ANNA had also been very active in encouraging states to enact an RN staffing regulation requiring the availability of RNs during dialysis treatments. Through state initiatives, political support was mounting for a change in the federal policy. What was lacking, however, was evidence to support the policy change. Although there was a large body of research supporting the link between RN staffing and patient outcomes in hospitals, little research at the time had investigated the association between RN staffing and adverse patient events in chronic dialysis centers.

Consequently, the elected leaders of the ANNA voted to fund a research proposal, submitted by two researchers from Rutgers College of Nursing, designed to quantify the association between RN staffing levels and adverse patient events as reported by nurses practicing in hemodialysis centers. The sampling frame for the study consisted of members of the ANNA who identified themselves as RNs working as staff nurses in hemodialysis centers in the United States. Staff RNs were selected because they have demonstrated in previous research to be reliable informants regarding staffing levels and patient outcomes because of their close proximity to patients and knowledge of their working conditions and workload (Aiken, Clarke, Sloane, Sochalski, & Silber, 2002).

In all, a total of 2,000 RNs were randomly selected from the membership list to receive a survey packet mailed to their home address. To protect the rights of survey participants, the study was approved by the university's institutional review board prior to data collection. Using a modified Dillman (2006) survey method, reminder postcards and follow-up survey packets were mailed to nonrespondents. A 52% response rate produced a final sample of 1,015 RNs practicing in hemodialysis centers.

Nurse staffing and patient adverse events were measured by survey items that had previously been developed and tested at the Center for Health Outcomes and Policy Research, University of Pennsylvania (Aiken, Clarke, & Sloane, 2002; Aiken, Clarke, Sloane, Sochalski, & Silber, 2002; Aiken et al., 2001). Items describing adverse patient events were modified to reflect those adverse events that are known to occur during hemodialysis. Findings indicated a significant correlation between RN staffing and the frequency of reported adverse patient events. The higher the patient-to-nurse ratio, reflecting lower levels of RN staffing, the higher the frequency of reported negative outcomes during hemodialysis, including hypotension, skipped treatments, missed treatments, and patient complaints. Similar significant associations were found when the analyses were delimited to nurses' reports on chronic hemodialysis settings (Thomas-Hawkins, Flynn, & Clarke, 2007).

Armed with findings from this study, as well as another concurrent nursing study that also had found an association between RN staffing levels in dialysis centers and adverse patient events (Gardner, Thomas-Hawkins, Fogg, & Latham, 2007), the leadership team from the ANNA met with regulatory experts at CMS to discuss a proposed change in the Medicare regulations that would require dialysis facilities to ensure the presence of at least one RN in the treatment center during dialysis treatments. In keeping with Kingdon's policy development model, the three core streams necessary to influence policy were now coming together: (a) a significant problem was identified in that research evidence indicated adverse patient events frequently occurred during dialysis treatments; (b) a viable, evidence-based solution was proposed in that research findings indicated higher RN staffing levels were linked to fewer adverse patient events; and (c) political support for RN staffing in dialysis units was garnered from professional associations as well as several state governments. In total, the amalgamation of evidence-based problem identification, an evidence-based solution, and political support for the solution from professional organizations and state legislators provided a potent influence.

As a result, when a draft of the interpretive guidelines for the revised federal regulations was released by CMS for public comment, they contained a proposed regulation requiring the presence of at least one RN in the dialysis facility during dialysis treatment. In explanation of the proposed regulation, the draft guidelines noted that "recent data in the nursing literature demonstrate an evidence-based correlation between the availability of professional nursing service and patient outcomes" (CMS, 2007). Happily, the proposed regulation was adopted and at least one RN is now required during dialysis treatment.

CONCLUSION

The evidence produced from nursing research can be instrumental in the development and adoption of evidence-based health policy initiatives. Consistent with Kingdon's policy development model, research findings can be invaluable in identifying a problem, proposing a solution, and securing political support for the solution. Nurses prepared at a doctoral level, whether it is via a Doctorate of Nursing Practice (DNP) or a research doctorate such as the Doctorate of Philosophy (PhD), have an important role in creating this research–policy connection. Doctorally prepared nurses are uniquely qualified to identify or produce valid research findings that can inform health policy decisions. Professional nursing organizations are also an invaluable mechanism for influencing health policy. Through professional nursing organizations, nurses at all levels of practice and education can collectively channel their knowledge, skills, energy, and financial resources to bring about policy initiatives that protect patients and maximize positive outcomes.

As Florence Nightingale so aptly demonstrated, nurses have the ability as well as the responsibility to advocate successfully for policy initiatives that will improve patient care and safety. Working together, nurse clinicians, nurse researchers, and nurse leaders can and should propose meaningful, evidence-based solutions to the many challenges that threaten the delivery of high-quality patient care.

REFERENCES

Aiken, L. H., Clarke, S. P., & Sloane, D. M. (2002). Hospital staffing, organization, and quality of care: Cross-national findings. *International Journal for Quality in Health Care, 14*(1), 5–13.

Aiken, L. H., Clarke, S. P., Sloane, D. M., Sochalski, J. A., Busse, R., Clarke, H., et al. (2001). Nurses' reports on hospital care in five countries. *Health Affairs, 20*(3), 43–53.

Aiken, L. H., Clarke, S. P., Sloane, D. M., Sochalski, J., & Silber, J. H. (2002). Hospital nurse staffing and patient mortality, nurse burnout, and job dissatisfaction. *Journal of the American Medical Association, 288*(16), 1987–1993.

Centers for Medicare and Medicaid Services (2007). *Draft interpretive guidelines for end stage renal disease.* Retrieved November 27, 2007, from http://www.cms.hhs.gov/GuidanceforLawsAndRegulations/05_Dialysis.asp

Dillman, D. A. (2006). *Mail and Internet surveys: The tailored design method* (2nd ed.). New York: Wiley.

Gardner, J., Thomas-Hawkins, C., Fogg, L., & Latham, C. E. (2007). The relationships between nurses' perceptions of the hemodialysis unit work environment and nurse turnover, patient satisfaction and hospitalizations. *Nephrology Nursing Journal, 34*(3), 271–281.

Kingdon, J. W. (2003). *Agendas, alternatives, and public policies.* New York: Longman.

Thomas-Hawkins, C., Flynn, L., & Clarke, S. (2007). *Relationships between registered nurse staffing, processes of care, and nurse-reported patient outcomes in chronic hemodialysis units.* Manuscript in preparation.

SECTION VI. MAKING THE RESEARCH TO POLICY CONNECTION: LESSONS LEARNED

Linda Flynn

The responsibility to influence policy decisions by making the research to policy connection has been an essential and legitimate aspect of nursing practice since Florence Nightingale established the profession. By influencing policy initiatives at the organizational, professional, and governmental levels, we are working to ensure the health and safety of the public, our patients, and ourselves. Yet, as Lucille Joel so eloquently reminded us in chapter 16, it is easier to become a complacent *inhabitant* of the profession, allowing others to develop plans and make decisions for us, than to be fully engaged as true citizens. Whether we are practicing as clinicians, administrators, educators, or researchers, it is tempting to let the challenges of our day-to-day activities keep us from developing the ideas and decisions that will shape our collective future. It is no longer acceptable to be distracted from the important issues of our place and time; Joel warns us that such distraction and complacency are dangerous.

LESSON 1. HOW WE CAN INFLUENCE POLICY

From Joel, we learned some practical and specific ways through which we can influence policy development. It may be more efficient, for example, to impact federal policy at the point of regulation or rule making as opposed to legislative action. Or it may be that a focus on state policy is a more appropriate approach given that state law prevails whenever the state shares the cost for a program or initiative. Whether the focus is a policy initiative at the organizational, local, state, or federal level, we learned specific techniques, related to coalition building, lobbying, and relationships with elected representatives.

Perhaps most importantly, we learned that our profession, like the world in which we work and live, has moved to a new level of sophistication. Policy makers at all levels now look to evidence to inform their plans and decisions. Fortunately, the profession of nursing has (a) the capacity for the science to produce the evidence, (b) the political savvy to use the evidence, and (c) the numbers to ensure our perspective is heard. To create the research to policy connection we need only to act as citizens instead of inhabitants—a lesson crucial to successful policy formation.

LESSON 2. EVIDENCE-BASED POLICY CAN ADDRESS A STATE FACULTY SHORTAGE

In chapter 17, Mary Val Palumbo exemplified the lessons learned in chapter 16, sharing her experiences as a citizen-researcher who used scientific evidence, political savvy, and coalition building to advance a policy agenda in her home state. Using Kingdon's (2003) political action theory as a framework, she and the nurse leadership in Vermont, leveraging research-based evidence, took advantage of an open window of policy opportunity by (a) identifying a problem, (b) jumping into the political stream, and (c) developing a plan aimed at addressing the nurse faculty shortage in Vermont.

Describing their experiences at each phase of the process, Palumbo explained how research findings produced by the Office of Nursing Workforce (ONW) were, indeed, invaluable in establishing the problem—a shortage of nurses and nurse faculty in the state. Having the political savvy to recognize that a new governor with a new emphasis on workforce development provided an opportunity to advance solutions to the problem, they engaged in coalition building, bringing together representatives from academia, the Department of Labor, hospital associations, health departments, the state nurses association, and members of the legislature. The coalition reviewed approaches implemented in other states to address the faculty shortage and considered all possible solutions before selecting a solution that was acceptable to all stakeholders. Before advancing the proposed solution, however, the coalition evaluated any future constraints of the initiative, the cost, and public support. Last, an elected representative who would introduce and support the initiative was identified. Although the road to success was long and sometimes rocky, this process resulted in legislation and funding to create a nurse faculty loan forgiveness program—an exemplar of the research to policy connection.

LESSON 3. EVIDENCE CAN INFLUENCE NATIONAL POLICY

Finally, in chapter 18, Charlotte Thomas-Hawkins and Sandra Bodin joined me in sharing successfully our approach to influence the federal regulation or rule-making activities of the Centers for Medicare and Medicaid Services (CMS). Congruent with Kingdon's (2003) model, we also recognized a window of opportunity when the existing Medicare

Conditions of Coverage for provision of services in dialysis centers were opened for review and possible revision by the CMS. We sought to have the conditions revised to require the presence of at least one RN on-site during dialysis treatments. We also recognized, however, the power of empirical evidence, so we slightly revised Kingdon's model to incorporate research at each phase of the policy process. As researchers, Charlotte and I joined forces with Sandra, who was the current president of the American Nephrology Nurses Association. With the power of empirics and a large association of nurses supporting us, we met with the staff at CMS and presented our research findings, as well as the findings of others, which indicated significant associations between higher RN staffing levels and fewer adverse patient events in dialysis centers. This blend of evidence and association support proved to be powerful in that the RN requirement was adopted into federal regulation. This was a perfect example of the use of evidence, numbers, and knowledge to effect policy change.

In summary, nurses have a responsibility as citizens of the profession to participate in the decisions that affect our practice, our patients, and our communities. To be effective, however, we need to marry our clinical and research skills with political skills. In this section, contributors have shared their insights, experiences, and advice with respect to that marriage. Will we be inhabitants or citizens? There really is no choice.

Epilogue

19

From Research to Policy—The Ultimate Translation

LINDA FLYNN AND GERI L. DICKSON

Throughout this book contributors have shared their knowledge and experiences regarding the use of research findings in the development of evidence-based health policy. They have discussed everything from methods to politics in hopes of encouraging and equipping other nurse colleagues in this important endeavor. But our work here is not quite done. We conclude by discussing a final prerequisite for creating the research to policy connection—the translation of findings into usable and actionable information.

There may have been a time in the world of researchers and evaluators when their project responsibilities were complete with the dissemination of findings through peer-reviewed journals and oral presentations. That time, however, has come to a close. In the last several years, a major shift has occurred in the endgame. The goal of research has been expanded to include not only the generation of new knowledge, but also the *translation* of that knowledge into constructive information that is (a) practical, (b) accessible, (c) actionable, (d) solution oriented, and (e) actively used by decision makers at clinical, organizational, or public policy levels (Clancy, Slutsky, & Patton, 2004). Such translation is absolutely essential in creating the research to policy connection, whether the venue is the public or the private sector or the focus of the research is system-oriented or clinically oriented. Translation, in contradistinction to dissemination,

355

requires that researchers and evaluators adopt new frameworks to ensure that their "products" are understandable and useable.

The Promoting Action on Research Implementation in Health Services (PARIHS) framework suggests that to enhance successful translation of findings into useable information, researchers should consider (a) the nature of their evidence, (b) the contextual characteristics surrounding its intended end-use, and (c) the type of facilitation that will be needed for translation to occur (Rycroft-Malone, 2004). The following discourse considers each of these factors more closely.

With respect to the nature of evidence, findings from randomized controlled studies remain the gold standard for credibility, compared with evidence produced from a single, nonexperimental investigation (Melnyk & Fineout-Overhold, 2005). Yet regardless of the level of evidence, few policy makers will be able to interpret findings amid the statistical language required in peer-reviewed research journals. Such language and format act as barriers, effectively limiting the access of potential end-users to the valuable information embedded in the findings.

This is not to say that peer-reviewed dissemination is unnecessary—it is necessary to ensure adequate scrutiny and critique of the research by the scientific community. But although necessary, peer-reviewed dissemination of findings is not sufficient. Moreover, dissemination is not translation. In order to begin the translation process, researchers must convert their findings to a message—a message that is clear, concise, short, and compelling, such as "high nurse workloads throughout the state are jeopardizing patient safety, as nurses teeter on the brink of exhaustion!" It is your message that will capture the attention of policy makers and engage them in the translation process.

Now, let us include a word of caution. Although excited about the policy implications of our findings, we must avoid *prematurely* promoting the application of those findings to real-world problem solving and avoid generalizing the applicability of the findings beyond what is valid. Is a follow-up study or evaluation really needed before findings can appropriately inform decision making? Does the study or evaluation need to be replicated in a larger or more diverse sample? The level of existing evidence, the internal and external validity of the study, and the critique of the scientific community will guide the answers to these questions and help us find that sometimes-elusive line between paralyses of analyses and appropriate translation.

Also according to the PARIHS framework, the context or environment in which evidence will be used is a factor to consider when translating research into actionable information. Toward this end, ongoing interaction and collaboration between researchers and policy makers is required to ensure that researchers are investigating questions that are relevant to policy makers; that studies focus on priority problems, settings, or situations; that policy makers receive the evidence they need to inform their initiatives; and that researchers respond to their questions and queries in timely fashion (Clancy, Slutsky, & Patton, 2004; Estabrooks, 2007; Lavis, 2006). Although the *message* may initially engage policy makers in the translation process, it is the ongoing *collaboration* that keeps them engaged for the long haul. As in any collaboration, however, mutual trust, reciprocity, and negotiation are key ingredients to sustaining successful partnerships between researchers as the producers of evidence and policy makers as the users of evidence (McDonald & Viehbeck, 2007).

Facilitation of the translation process is the third consideration when translating research into informed action. Facilitation refers to the identification and engagement of those persons, organizations, or other entities that can assist the researchers in getting their message to decision makers, establishing researcher to end-user collaboratives, and ultimately, using evidence to influence policy. In previous chapters, we learned that funding sources can be excellent facilitators of the translation process. Foundations such as the Robert Wood Johnson Foundation and the Northwest Health Foundation invest millions of dollars to connect researchers with decision makers and other potential consumers of evidence. Likewise, one of the core missions of the federally funded Agency for Healthcare Research and Policy (AHRQ) is to facilitate the visibility and usability of research findings to all levels of decision makers. Consequently, it has established an array of programs and activities to achieve this aim, including evidence-based practice centers, evidence clearinghouses, Web page announcements, and Web access to findings. Moreover, there are a plethora of other people and organizations that can serve as invaluable translation facilitators, including chief nursing officers, advanced practice nurses, professional organizations, consumer organizations, professional lobbyists, and union leaders.

Last, it is important to note that policy decisions are, by no means, determined solely on the bases of empirics. As Kingdon (2003) describes, many factors influence policy decisions, including personal and societal values, economics, politics, historical events, and the general mood of the public or organization. Our goal as researchers and evaluators—as citizens of our profession and advocates for our patients—is to effectively *inform* those decisions by ensuring that valid, rigorously produced, actionable, and understandable evidence is in the hands of the policy makers when decisions are made.

In conclusion, we are reminded that policy is a purposeful plan of action that is frequently codified in the form of standing rules, principles, or protocols within an organization or system. Over time, policy can become embedded in culture—it becomes "the way we have always done things." Consequently, we cannot afford, as members of the nation's largest health profession, to underestimate our responsibility to inform and influence clinical, organizational, and public policy. As trustees of the pubic good, our voice, carrying the message of our evidence, needs to be heard. By informing and influencing policy, we achieve Nightingale's vision for the profession—in short, we achieve the ultimate translation.

REFERENCES

Clancy, C. M., Slutsky, J. R., & Patton, L. T. (2004). Evidence-based health care 2004: AHRQ moves research to translation and implementation. *Health Services Research, 39*(5), xv–xxiii.

Estabrooks, C. A. (2007). Prologue: A program of research in knowledge translation. *Nursing Research, 56*(4 Suppl), S4–S6.

Kingdon, J. (2003). *Agendas, alternatives, and public policies* (2nd ed.). New York: Longman.

Lavis, J. N. (2006). Research, public policymaking, and knowledge-translation processes: Canadian efforts to build bridges. *Journal of Continuing Education in the Health Professions, 26*(1), 37–45.

McDonald, P. W., & Viehbeck, S. (2007). Circle of research and practice: From evidence-based practice making to practice-based evidence making: Creating communities of research and practice. *Health Promotion Practice, 8*(2), 140–144.

Melnyk, B. M., & Fineout-Overholt, E. (2005). *Evidence-based practice in nursing and healthcare.* Philadelphia: Lippincott Williams & Wilkins.

Rycroft-Malone, J. (2004). The PARIHS framework: A framework for guiding the implementation of evidence-based practice: Promoting Action on Research Implementation in Health Services. *Journal of Nursing Care Quality, 19,* 297–304.

Index

AACN. *See* American Association of Colleges of Nursing

AARP. *See* American Association of Retires Persons

Access®, 72, 77, 86, 90

Advanced practice nurses (APNs), 259, 318

Advanced practice, 324–325

Agency contacts, 243–246

Agency for Health Care Research and Quality (AHRQ), 253–269
  areas of emphasis and, 255–257
  career development awards, 265
  dissertation grants, 264–265
  implications for researchers and clinicians and, 254–255
  Initial Review Group (IRG), 261
  mission of, 254
  priorities of, 255
  research infrastructure support programs, 265–266
  See also Research funding opportunities (AHRQ); Research grants (AHRQ), obtaining; Training (AHRQ)

Agenda setting theory. *See* Kingdon, John

Aggregate, state-level supply and demand, 81–83
  with replacement data from the state, 84

AHA. *See* American Hospital Association

AHRQ. *See* Agency for Health Care Research and Quality

AIDS inpatient care, models of specialty care and, 28

Aiken, Linda, 27–28, 44

Allen, Kyle, 262

The Alliance, 323

American Academy of Nursing, 327

American Association of Colleges of Nursing (AACN), 184, 227–228, 323, 330

American Association of Retires Persons (AARP), 289

American Board of Emergency Medicine, 227

American Council on Graduate Medical Education for Graduate Medical Education in Surgery, 226–227

American Hospital Association (AHA), 72
  Organization of Nurse Executives, 275

American Nephrology Nurses Association (ANNA), 344–347

American Nurses Association (ANA), 45, 322–323
  advanced practice groups and, 324–325
  position paper on nursing education and, 188
  staffing survey, 157, 158, 159–160

American Nurses Credentialing Center (ANCC), 180, 327

American Organization of Nurse Executives (AONE)
  Acute Care Hospital Survey of RN Vacancy and Turnover Rates, 45, 158
  NurseWeek and, 45

American Statistical Association, 44

ANA. *See* American Nurses Association

ANCC. *See* American Nurses Credentialing Center

359

ANNA. *See* American Nephrology
  Nurses Association
AONE. *See* American Organization of
  Nurse Executives
APNs. *See* Advanced practice nurses
Area Health Education Center, 333,
  339–340
Area Resource File (ARF), 72, 83, 84,
  86, 87, 108
ARF. *See* Area Resource File
Army Nurse Corps, 8
Associate degree (AD) nurse, 91–92, 94,
  95, 183–184
Associate degree program in nursing
  (ADNs), 213–214
Association of Nurse Executives, 323

Bachelor's of science in nursing (BSN),
  28, 92, 94, 95, 188, 213–214, 216,
  217
Balanced Budget Act of 1997, 10, 12
Barcode Medication, 279
Bartlett, Andrew, 337, 338
Baseline data, FCN
  comparing, 91–94
  differences in, 95–97
Bingham, Ray, 155
BJBC. *See* Oregon Better Jobs Better
  Care program
Black boxes, 72
Block grants, 321–322
BLS. *See* Bureau of Labor Statistics
Blue Ribbon Commission
  on Nursing, 333
Bodin, Sandra, 318, 350
BON. *See* Florida Board of Nursing
Brewer, Carol S., 40, 122–123
BRIC. *See* Building Research
  Infrastructure and Capacity
Building Research Infrastructure and
  Capacity (BRIC), 265–266
Bureau of Health Professions, 72
Bureau of Labor Statistics (BLS), 72,
  83, 87
Burnout
  agitated emotions and, 164
  control variables and, 168

deep acting emotions and, 165, 166
emotional foundations of, 158–161
emotional labor and, 165, 171–172
emotional mentors and, 173–174
influencing factors of, 170–172
MBI and, 164
negative emotions and, 164–165
operationalization of feeling rules and,
  167–168
policy and practice implications and,
  172–175
positive emotions and, 165
surface acting and, 165–166
understanding of, 170–172
workload and, 173

CAARE Project, 161, 164, 173, 174
Cadet Nurse Corps, 8–9
Campaign for Nursing's Future, 157
Career development awards (AHRQ),
  265
Caring for Our Future: Strengthening
  the Long Term Care Workforce
  and, 304–305
Carnegie Foundation, 6, 7
Casewise deletion, 111
Castleton State College, 331
CathSim™, 225
Center for Health Outcomes and Policy
  Research, 27–29, 44, 346
Center for Nursing Research, 11
Center for Rural Health (University of
  North Dakota), 185, 190
Centers for Medicare and Medicaid
  Services (CMS), 258–259, 314,
  318, 344
Centre of Excellence for Surgical
  Education and Innovation, 226
Changing Attitudes About Retention and
  Emotion. *See* CAARE Project
Chemeketa Community Colleg, 300
Civil War, 5
Clackamas Community College, 300, 303
Cleary, Brenda, 185, 235, 236, 260
*Clinical Instruction in Prelicensure
  Nursing Programs*
  (NCSBN), 228

Clinical simulation
  benefits of, 219
  computer screen simulation, 224–225
  defining simulation and, 220
  high-fidelity patient simulators,
    221–224
  incorporating in health care
    professions, impetuses for, 220
  standardized patients and, 225–226
  types of, 221–222
  See also Evidence-based policy
CMS. *See* Centers for Medicare and
    Medicaid Services
Colleagues in Caring minimum
    data set, 45
College of Nursing, Washington
    University Vancouver, 301
Columbia University, 7
Community Based Care Nurses
    Association, 306–307
Community Health Leaders program, 288
Computerized Physician Order Entry, 279
Computer screen simulation, 224–225
Conditional mean imputation, 113–117
Congdon, Joann, 258, 314
Congressional earmark legislation,
    239–252
  federal budget process and, 246–252
  getting involved in, 239–241
  initiatives, limiting number of,
    242–243
  MCs, lobbyists, and agency contacts
    and, 243–246
  plus-up and, 240
  questions, philosophical and practical,
    241–242
Cover letter, 61
Coxcomb diagrams, 3
Crimean war, 3–4
Cunningham, Regina, 259
CyberPatient, 226

Dall, Timothy, 90
Danesh, Valerie, 123
Data
  Colleagues in Caring minimum
    data set, 45

emotional demands of nursing study
    and, 163
  NSM and NDM, comparisons of, 82,
    83
  nursing demand and supply models
    and, 84
  sub-state, FCN, 84
  See also Baseline data, FCN;
    Missing data
Data collection
  FCN, 86
  North Dakota Nursing Needs Study,
    195–196
  survey research and, 62–66
Data replacement, FCN, 86, 90
Data substitution, 72
Data validity, FCN, 96–97
Dear, Brian, 224
Decision making in high school,
    192–193
  diversity of people and, 193
  factors influencing choice and, 193
  informed decisions and, 193
  three-stage model of decision making
    and, 192–193
Deep acting, 165, 166
Demand-side comparisons, 91, 92
Democracy, 319–320
DFS. *See* Division of Facility Services
DHHS. *See* U.S. Department of Health
    and Human Services
DIANA (Digital Animated Avatar), 226
Digital Animated Avatar, 226
Digital virtual human actors, 226
Dillman, Donald, 59, 122
Dillman Tailored Design Method of
    survey methodology, 40
Diploma nurse, 91–92, 94
Dissertation grants (AHRQ), 264–265
Division of Facility Services (DFS), 108
DNP. *See* Doctorate of Nursing
    Practice
Doctorate of Nursing Practice (DNP),
    347
Doctorate of Philosophy (PhD), 347
Donaldson, Nancy, 261
Douglas, James, 339

EBP. *See* Evidence-based practice
ECLEPs. *See* Enriching Clinical
    Learning Environments Through
    Partnerships in Long-Term Care
Econometric forecasting approach, 73
Educational policy. *See* Research and
    educational policy
*Educational Preparation for Nurse
    Practitioners and Assistants to
    Nurses: A Position Paper* (ANA),
    188
Emotional demands of nursing study,
    155–175
    data and sample used in, 163
    emotional measures used in, 164–168
        (*See also* Burnout)
    field evidence and, 161–162
    on nurse staffing crisis, 156–157
    results of, 168–170
    on why nurses leave direct patient
        care, 157–158
Emotional labor, 160, 165, 171–172
Employment projections, 110
Enriching Clinical Learning
    Environments Through
    Partnerships in Long-Term Care
    (ECLEPs), 305
Entry-into-practice mandate, 188
*The Essentials of Baccalaureate Nursing
    Education* (AACN), 227–228
Evidence-based policy, 219–229
    See also Clinical simulation
Evidence-based practice (EBP), 260
Excel®, 72, 80–81, 84, 86, 90
Executive Nurse Fellows program, 288
Expanding Capacity to Prepare Entry-
    Level Nurses, 300–301

FCN. *See* Florida Center for Nursing
    (FCN), HRSA models and
FDA, See U.S. Food and Drug
    Administration
Federal Information Processing
    Standards (FIPS), 107
Federal policy, using research to
    influence, 343–347
    research-policy connection and, 344

revised model and, 344–347
Federal Register, 327
Federation of Nurses and Health
    Professionals (FNHP), 158
FIPS. *See* Federal Information
    Processing Standards
Flexner, Abraham, 6
Flexner Report, 6–7, 8
Florida Agency for Workforce
    Innovation, 86, 87
Florida Board of Nursing (BON), 86,
    95, 96
    Licensure Database, 86, 88
Florida Center for Nursing (FCN),
    HRSA models and, 85–100
    data collection and, 86
    data replacement and, 86, 90
    data validity and, 96–97
    decision to use, 72–73
    experiences in using, 85, 98–100
    running, further testing and, 97
    sub-state data and, 84
    Workforce Florida partnerships and,
        86
    See also Baseline data, FCN
Florida Center for Nursing License
    Renewal Survey, 86, 88, 96
Florida Department of Health, 88
Flynn, Linda, 40, 318
FNHP. *See* Federation of Nurses and
    Health Professionals
Focus groups, 45–50
Foley, Mary, 157
Forecasting
    econometric approach to, 73
    in individual states, 81–85
    nursing needs-based approach to, 73
    nursing personnel-to-population
        utilization approach, 73–74
    supply and demand of RNs (*See*
        Health Resources and Services
        Administration (HRSA))
Fragmentation of a policy system, 189
Freeman's Scholarship, 332
FTE. *See* Full-time-equivalent
Full-time-equivalent (FTE), 74–76, 91,
    96, 116–117

Funding research to policy
  Agency for Health Care Research and
    Quality (AHRQ) and, 253–269
  congressional earmark legislation and,
    239–252
  Robert Wood Johnson Foundation
    (RWJF) policy influences and,
    271–290
  See also individual headings
Future of nursing profession. *See* High
  school student survey

Gap estimates, 82
Gelmon, Sherril, 299
Gladwell, Malcolm, 14–17, 311
  policy change and, applying theories,
    16–17
  stickyness of ideas and, 14–17
  The Tipping Point and, 12–13,
    14, 311
Goldmark, Josephine, 188
Goldmark Report, 8, 188
Gordon, Suzanne, 33
Graduate programs, 10
Grady, Mary, 314
Grafting, 303
Grandfathered nurses, 188
Grassroots activities, 326

Hassmiller, Susan B., 314
Hatfield, Mark O., 297
Health Care Career Awareness Month,
  339
Health Professional Shortage Area
  (HPSA), 108
Health Resources and Services
  Administration (HRSA), 72–73
  See also Nursing demand and supply
    models, HRSA
Health System Change Study, 129
Higher Education Act, 241
High-fidelity patient simulators, 221–224
High school student survey
  early age-related perceptions of
    nursing and, 191
  middle school students and, career
    considerations of, 191–192

nursing as a career vision in high
    school and, 193–194
  See also Decision making in high
    school; North Dakota Nursing
    Needs Study
Hill-Burton Act of 1946, 9, 11–12
Hispanic nurses, 307
Home health nurses (workload, quality
    of care, and job satisfaction),
    143–152
  background and significance of,
    144–145
  findings of, 147–150
  method of, 146–147
  policy implications and, 150–152
  recruitment and retention difficulties
    and, 144–145
Hospital restructuring, impacts of, 28
House Bill 058, 338
House Bill 538, 337
HPSA. *See* Health Professional
    Shortage Area
HRSA. *See* Health Resources and
    Services Administration
Human Capital Portfolio, 288–289
Human Resources Investment Council,
    333–334

Information technology, 279
Informed consent, 61
In-house law, 323–324
Initial Review Group (IRG), 261
INQRI. *See* Interdisciplinary Nursing
    Quality Research Initiative
Institute for Healthcare Improvement, 274
Institute for the Future of Aging
    Services, 200
Institute of Medicine, 219
Institutional Research Review Board
    (University of North Dakota),
    195, 196
Interdisciplinary Nursing Quality
    Research Initiative (INQRI), 279,
    286, 288
International Council of Nurses, 323
International Pharmaceutical
    Federation, 323

Investigator in Health Policy Research
Award, 279, 282
"Investing in a Healthy Future:
Strategies to Address the Nursing
Shortage," 298

Jargon, 51
JCAHO. *See* Joint Commission on
Accreditation of Healthcare
Organizations
Job satisfaction. *See* Home health nurses
(workload, quality of care, and
job satisfaction); Workplace
satisfaction, NSSRN and
Joel, Lucille, 317–318, 349
Johns Hopkins University, 6
Johnson & Johnson, 157, 184
Johnson, Mary, 260
Joint Commission on Accreditation
of Healthcare Organizations
(JCAHO), 44

K08 development awards, mentored
clinical scientist, 265
Kendrick, Kathleen, 314
Kingdon, John
agenda setting and, 13–14, 17–17
community of specialists and, 13–14
fragmentation of a policy system and,
189
national perspective and, 330
open window of opportunity concept
and, 12, 13
policy change and, applying theories,
16–17
policy stream and, 13, 333–336
political stream and, 13, 333
problem stream and, 13, 330–332
Vermont perspective and, 331–332
Kittell, Sara Branon, 337
Kovner, Christine Tassone, 40, 122–123,
262
K02 awards, independent investor, 265

Lacey, Linda M., 40, 122
Laerdal, Asmund, 221, 222
Lashley, Felissa R., 185, 236

Leadership at the Point of Care: Moving
into Action, 309
Lewin Group, 90
Licensed practical nurse (LPN)
demand for, NDM projections and,
73, 74–76
NDBON rules for entry into nursing
parctice and, 188
Linfield College Good Samaritan School
of Nursing, 305–306
Listwise deletion, 111
Loan forgiveness, education, 337–338
Loan repayment, state funding for,
329–341
education loan forgiveness and, 337–338
eligibility requirements, 339
opportunity and, windows of, 336
outcomes (2005 legislative session),
338–339
strategic plan/timeline and, 336–340
Lobbying/lobbyists, 243–246, 324–326

Magnet hospitals, 25, 28, 327
Magnet Recognition Program, 25
Magnet status, 180
Mail survey methods, 58–62
cover letter and, 61
envelope appearance and, 60
multiple follow-up contacts and, 62
personal connections with recipients
and, 61
population representation and, 58–59
postage and, 60–61
response rate and, 59
sampling frame and, 63
Making Oregon Vital for Elders
(MOVE), 306
Makulowich, Gail, 314
Mannequin simulators, 221
MAR. *See* Missing at random
Marquis Health Services Companies,
305–306
Maslach Burnout Inventory (MBI), 164
Master's of science in nursing (MSN),
214, 215
Maximum likelihood estimation (ML),
115–116

Mazzocco, Gail, 260
MCAR. *See* Missing completely at
    random
McDonald, Claudia L., 313
M. Chase doll, 221
Mean imputation, simple and
    conditional, 113–117
Medicaid, 247, 258–259, 320–321
Medical Education Technologies, Inc.,
    222
Medicare, 247, 320–321, 323
    Conditions of Coverage, 344
    nursing home reforms and, 325
Medicare Enactment of 1965, 10
Melichar, Lori, 314
Members of Congress (MCs), 243–246
METI, the human patient simulator™
    (HPS), 222
Metropolitan Life Insurance Company, 5
Metropolitan Statistical Area (MSA), 81,
    83, 128–129
MI. *See* Multiple imputation
Middle school students, career
    considerations of, 191–192
Migration, 97
Minority Research Infrastructure
    Support Program (M-RISP), 265
Missing at random (MAR), 110–111, 112
Missing completely at random (MCAR),
    110, 111
Missing data, 103–118
    casewise deletion and, 111
    employment projections and, 110
    listwise deletion and, 111
    MAR and, 110–111
    maximum likelihood estimation and,
        115–116
    MCAR and, 110
    mean imputation and, simple and
        conditional, 113–117
    the missing item and, 105
    missingness and, analyzing and
        classifying, 107–111
    multiple imputation and, 116
    in multivariate analyses, 112
    reasons for, suspect, 106–107
    sources and causes of, 104–107

survey nonresponse and, 104–105,
    108–109
techniques, recent developments in,
    115–116
in univariate analyses, 112
zip codes and, 107–108
Missing item, The, 105
Missingness, analyzing and classifying,
    107–111
M. J. Chase doll company, 221
ML. *See* Maximum likelihood estimation
Montag, Mildred, 9, 183–184
Moulton, Patricia, 39–40, 121, 234, 235
MOVE. *See* Making Oregon Vital for
    Elders
M-RISP. *See* Minority Research
    Infrastructure Support Program
Mrs. Chase models, 221
MSA. *See* Metropolitan Statistical Area
Multiple imputation (MI), 116
Multivariate analyses, 112
Multnomah County Health
    Department, 300

NAHN. *See* National Association of
    Hispanic Nurses
National Advisory Council on Nursing
    Education and Practice, 331
National Association for Home Care and
    Hospice, 148
National Association of Hispanic Nurses
    (NAHN), 307
National Center for Health Workforce
    Analysis, 72
National Council of State Boards of
    Nursing, Inc. (NCSBN), 89, 228
    Practice, Regulation and Education
        Committee, 228
National Home and Hospice Care
    Survey (NHHCS), 72
National Institute of Nursing Research,
    11, 12
National Institutes of Health, 11
National League for Nursing (NLN), 34,
    45, 184, 323, 330
National Nurse Funders
    Collaborative, 287

National Organization for Public Health Nursing, 5

National Research Service Award (NRSA), 264

National Sample Survey of Registered Nurses (NSSRN), 45, 89
job satisfaction and, 159
limitations of, 127
NSM data and, 82
See also Workplace satisfaction, NSSRN and

National Sample Survey of RNs (NSSRN), 72

NCCN. *See* North Carolina Center for Nursing

NCIOM. *See* North Carolina Institute of Medicine

NCLEX-RN National Council of State Boards of Nursing, 96–97

NCLEX-RN Pass Rates, 88

NCSBN. *See* National Council of State Boards of Nursing, Inc.

NDBON. *See* North Dakota Board of Nursing

NDCC Nurse Practices Act, 189

NDNA. *See* North Dakota Nurses Association

Nehring, Wendy, 185, 236

New Jersey Board of Nursing (NJBON), 40, 60

New Jersey Collaborating Center for Nursing, 40, 60, 61, 62

New York University, 262

Next Generation Commission, 339

Next Steps for Vermont Nurse Workforce Planning: Increasing Educational Capacity (ONW), 331–332

NHHCS. *See* National Home and Hospice Care Survey

Nightingale, Florence, 3–5, 167, 344, 349

Nightingale Training School for Nurses, 4–5

NIH Guide for Grants and Contracts, 257, 262

NJBON. *See* New Jersey Board of Nursing

NLN. *See* National League for Nursing

Nooney, Jennifer, 123–124

North Carolina Board of Nursing, 211, 260

North Carolina Center for Nursing, 260

North Carolina Center for Nursing (NCCN), 104, 185
NSM and NDM data comparisons and, 82, 83
See also Nursing faculty crisis, NCCN study on

North Carolina Institute of Medicine (NCIOM), 210–211, 235

North Dakota Board of Nursing (NDBON), 188, 189–190

North Dakota Healthcare Association, 196

North Dakota Health Workforce Summit, 201

North Dakota High School Student Study, 185, 190

North Dakota Nurse Practices Act, 185, 188–189

North Dakota Nurses Association (NDNA), 189

North Dakota Nursing Needs Study, 194–204
data collection and, 195–196
discussion on, 200–201
nursing education history of North Dakota and, 188–189
policy impact of, 201–202
policy recommendations of, 202–204
procedure and participants of, 195
results of, 196–199
sample of, 195

North Dakota State Board of Higher Education, 189

North Dakota State Legislative Council Interim Healthcare Budget Committee, 201

Northwest Health Foundation (NWHF), 287, 294–295
Caring for Our Future: Strengthening the Long Term Care Workforce and, 304–305
Community Based Care Nurses Association and, 306–307

ECLEPs and, 305
Expanding Capacity to Prepare
Entry-Level Nurses and,
300–301
Linfield College Good Samaritan
School of Nursing and Marquis
Health Services Companies
partnership and, 305–306
long-term investment in programs
to ensure sustainability and,
301–302
MOVE and, 306
National Association of Hispanic
Nurses (NAHN) and, 307
OCN and, 309
Oregon Better Jobs Better Care
program (BJBC) and, 305
Oregon Model and, 302
*Oregon's Nursing Shortage:
A Public Health Crisis in the
Making*, 297
Partners Investing in Nursing's Future
and, 302
Strengthening Capacity to Prepare
Entry-Level Nurses and, 301
See also Oregon nurse shortage
Northwest Organization of Nurse
Executives, 297
NPs. *See* Nurse practitioners
NRSA. *See* National Research Service
Award
NSSRN. *See* National Sample Survey of
Registered Nurses
Nurse Faculty Scholars program, 288
Nurse Practices Act (North Dakota),
185, 188–189, 326
Nurse practitioners (NPs), 272–273
Nurse Reinvestment Act, 157
Nurse Scientist Training Grant, 11
Nurse's Week Celebration, 338
Nursing Against the Odds (Gordon), 33
Nursing assistant (NA), demand for
(NDM projections), 73, 74–76
Nursing demand and supply models,
HRSA
aggregate, state-level supply and
demand, 81–83

aggregate, state-level supply and
demand with replacement data
from the state, 84
changing model assumptions and, 84–85
forecasting in individual states, 81–85
NDM, 72, 73, 74–77
NSM, 72, 73, 77–81
overview of, 73–74
supply and demand at disaggregated
sub-state level, 83–84
See also Florida Center for Nursing
(FCN), HRSA models and
Nursing demand model (NDM), 72, 73,
74–77
Nursing Educational Loan Repayment
Program, 331
Nursing faculty crisis, NCCN study on,
209–217
discussion on, 214–216
findings of, 213–214
issues related to, examining, 213
policy implications of, 216–217
roles of faculty and, 212–213
supply and demand of faculty and,
210–212
Nursing needs-based forecasting
approach, 73
Nursing Organizations Alliance, 323
Nursing outcomes research, 19–30
at Center for Health Outcomes and
Policy Research, 27–29
challenges in, 22–23
future and role of, 29–30
health services research and, 20–22
on staffing, work environments, and
hospital outcomes, 23–25
trends in health care system and
workforce and, 25–27
Nursing personnel-to-population
utilization forecasting approach,
73–74
Nursing Research, 11
Nursing shortage
education loan forgiveness and,
337–338
emotional demands of nursing and,
156–157

GAO report on, 158
Healthcare Research and Services Administration's forecasting report and, 34
national perspective on, 330
nursing outcomes research addressing, 25–26
post World War II, 183–184
public and provider anxieties and, 26–27
reasons why nurses leave direct patient care and, 157–158
Vermont perspective on, 331
See also Emotional demands of nursing study; Nursing faculty crisis, NCCN study on; Oregon nurse shortage
Nursing supply model (NSM), 72, 73, 77–81
Nursing Work Index, 28
Nutting, M. Adelaide, 3, 7, 183
NWHF. *See* Northwest Health Foundation

Occupational Employment Statistics (OES), 72
Occupational Outlook Handbook (U.S. Bureau of Labor Statistic), 187
OCN. *See* Oregon Center for Nursing
OCNE. *See* Oregon Consortium for Nursing Education
OEDR. *See* Office of Economic and Demographic Research
OES. *See* Occupational Employment Statistics
Office of Economic and Demographic Research (OEDR), 89
Office of Management and Budget (OMB), 240, 241
Office of Nursing Workforce, 336
OLS. *See* Ordinary least squares (OLS) regression
OMB. *See* Office of Management and Budget
O'Neill, Tip, 326
ONLC. *See* Oregon Nursing Leadership Council

ONW. *See* Vermont Office of Nursing Workforce
Open window of opportunity concept, 12, 13
Ordinary least squares (OLS) regression, 168
Oregon Better Jobs Better Care program (BJBC), 305
Oregon Center for Nursing (OCN), 298, 304, 308–310
Oregon Consortium for Nursing Education (OCNE), 185, 217, 300, 303
Oregon Council of Associate Degree Programs, 297
Oregon Council of Deans, 297
Oregon Model, 302
Oregon Nurses Association, 297
Oregon nurse shortage, 293–312
educational programs and, increasing capacity of, 304–306
farming and, relationship to, 295–296
funding efforts and, 306–308
key findings and, 310–312
long-term investment programs and, 301–304
nursing environment and, cultivating, 296–300
nursing policy agenda and, 308–310
NWHF and, 294–295
stimulating new growth and, 300–301
Oregon Nursing Leadership Council (ONLC), 297–298, 299, 300
Oregon's Nursing Shortage: A Public Health Crisis in the Making (NWHF), 297
Oregon State Board of Nursing, 297

PA. *See* Program announcement
Palmer, Sir Geoffrey, 240–241
Palumbo, Mary Val, 318, 350
PARIHS. *See* Promoting Action on Research Implementation in Health Services
Partners Investing in Nursing's Future (PIN), 287–288, 302

Pass-through legislation, 321
Patient encounters, 225–226
Patient-to-nurse ratios, 28
Peace Harbor Hospital Foundation, 300
Pew Health Professions Commission, 202
PhD. *See* Doctorate of Philosophy
PIN. *See* Partners Investing in Nursing's
    Future
PLATO (Programmed Logic for
    Automated Teaching Operations),
    224
Pluralism, 322
Plus-up, 240
Policy changes, past, 4–12
    applying theories to, 16–17
    higher education for nurses and, start
        of, 7–8
    for nurses and hospitals, 8–10
    nursing schools and, formation of, 4–5
    public health movement and, 5–6
    scientific base for nursing and, moving
        towards, 10–12
    in scientific medicine, impact on
        nursing, 6–7
Policy development and nursing, 319–327
    citizenship in a democracy and,
        319–320
    democratic community and, nurses as
        participants in, 320–322
    numbers and, power of, 322–323
    politics and, 323–327
Policy making, theoretical framework of.
    See Kingdon, John
Policy stream, 13, 333–336
Political action theory. *See* Kingdon, John
Political stream, 13, 333
Politics and policy, 12–17
    Gladwell's stickyness of ideas and, 14–17
    grassroots activities and, 326
    in-house law and, 323–324
    Kingdon's agenda setting and, 13–14,
        16–17
    lobbying/lobbyists and, 243–246,
        324–326
    nursing and, 323–327
    politics defined, 323
    rule making process and, 326–327

Portland State University, 299
Postage stamps, 60–61
Practice Environment Scales, 28
Problem stream, 13, 330–332
PROC MI, 116
PROC MIANALYZE, 116
Program announcement (PA), 260, 261
Project Connect, 284
Promoting Action on Research
    Implementation in Health
    Services (PARIHS), 356–357
Promotoras, 301, 303
Public health movement, 5–6
Public Health Service, 8

Registered nurse (RN)
    AD, 91–92, 94, 95, 183–184
    BSN, 28, 92, 94, 95, 188, 213–214,
        216, 217
    demand for, NDM projections, 73,
        74–76
    diploma, 91–92, 94
    FTEs, 74–76, 91, 96, 116–117
    supply of, NSM projections, 77–81
R18 grants, research demonstration and
    dissemination, 258–259
Report cards, 258–259
Request for applications (RFAs), 260, 261
Research and educational policy
    evidence-based policy, 219–229
    high school student survey and,
        187–204
    nursing faculty crisis, NCCN study on,
        209–217
    simulation in health care professions,
        incorporating, 220
    See also individual headings
Research and workplace policy
    emotional demands of nursing study
        and, 155–175
    workload, quality of care, and job
        satisfaction study, 143–152
    work satisfaction, NSSRN and,
        127–140
    See also individual headings
Research funding opportunities (AHRQ)
    conference (R13) grants, 259–260

examples of AHRQ funded research
projects, 261–262
investigator-initiated, 257–258
large research (R01) grants, 257–258
notices of special emphasis, 262–263
program announcements, 261
requests for applications (RFAs), 260
research demonstration and
dissemination (R18) grants,
258–259
small research (R03) grants, 259
solicited research funding, 260
Research grants (AHRQ), obtaining,
266–268
application submission, review, and
ward process, 267–268
application, tips for completing, 267
common problems, 268
proposal, developing, 266
technical assistance, 268
Research to policy connection
federal policy and, using research to
influence, 343–347
loan repayment and, state funding for,
329–341
policy development and nursing and,
319–327
translation and, 355–358
See also individual headings
ResusciAnne, 221
RFAs. *See* Request for applications
Robert Wood Johnson Foundation
(RWJF) policies, 271–290
building capacity of individuals and
institutions and, 288–289
Community Health Leaders program
and, 288
creating evidence to convince policy
makers, 279–281
Executive Nurse Fellows program
and, 288
governmental policy and, 272–273
Human Capital Portfolio and,
288–289
improving health policy through
strategic communications and,
283–285

Interdisciplinary Nursing Quality
Research Initiative (INQRI) and,
279, 286, 288
Investigator in Health Policy Research
Award and, 279, 282
lobbying restrictions, 285–286
National Advisory Committees of, 290
National Nurse Funders Collaborative
and, 287
Nurse Faculty Scholars program
and, 288
organizational policy and, 273–275
Partners Investing in Nursing's Future
and, 302
priorities, identifying, 275–278
Project Connect, 284
solutions, identifying, 278–279
strategic effort to retain experienced
nurses and, 157
strategic partners and, engaging,
286–288
Teaching Nursing Home Project
and, 327
translating and synthesizing
information to influence policy
makers, 281–283
Rockefeller Foundation, 8
R13 grants, conference, 259–260
Rudel, Rebecca, 234, 235
Rule making process, 326–327
Rutgers College of Nursing, 345
RWJF. *See* Robert Wood Johnson
Foundation (RWJF) policies
R01 grants, large research, 257–258
R03 grants, small research, 259

Safety in the workplace, 139
St. Thomas Hospital, 4–5
Sampling frame, 63
SAS statistical software, 107–108,
114, 116
School of Nursing, Oregon Health and
Science University, 301
School of Nursing, University of North
Carolina–Chapel Hill, 260
Scott, Jill, 261–262
Senate Bill 268, 337

SF 424 application, 266
Shaw, George Bernard, 62
Sheppard-Towner Act of 1921, 7
Sim Man, 222
Sim One, 221
Simple mean imputation, 113–117
Simulation. *See* Clinical simulation
SMG Foundation, 301, 303
Social Security, 247, 320
Southern Illinois University School of
    Nursing, 222
Specialty care, AIDS inpatient care used
    as a model for, 28
Staking, 302
Standardized patients, 225–226
Stevens, Kathleen, 259–260
Stickyness of ideas, 14–17
Strengthening Capacity to Prepare
    Entry-Level Nurses, 301
StudentMax, 308–309
Summa Health System, 262
Supply and demand at disaggregated
    sub-state level, 83–84
Supply and demand of RNs, forecasting.
    See Health Resources and
    Services Administration
Supply-side comparisons, 91–92
Surface acting, 165–166
Survey methodology, 40
Survey nonresponse, 104
Survey questions, 50–58
    focus groups and, 45–50
    inadequate categories of, 54
    language barriers and, 51–52
    multiple-choice, 47–49
    open-ended, 45–47
    order of, 57
    research, 44–45
    respondents to, screening, 50–51
    scale measures and, 55–56
    shared reference point and, 56–57
    stopping, 57–58
    unanswerable (double-barreled), 52–53
    vague and ambiguous, 53–54
Survey research
    data collection and, 62–66
    individual interviews and, 45

    specialized groups of people and, 43
    topic of, determining, 44–50
    See also Mail survey methods; Survey
        questions
Survey research, complexities of, 43–66
Susannah Maria Gurule (SMG)
    Foundation, 301, 303

Tailored Design Method (TDM), 59, 60,
    61, 62
Tanner, Christine, 297
Task Force on the North Carolina
    Nursing Workforce, 210–211
TCAB. *See* Transforming Care at the
    Bedside
Teacher's College (Columbia University),
    7, 183
Teaching Nursing Home Project, 327
Texas A&M University, 262
    Corpus Christi for Pulse!!, 240,
        242–243
Thomas-Hawkins, Charlotte, 318, 350
The Tipping Point (Gladwell), 12–13,
    14, 311
Tocqueville, 319–320
To Err Is Human (Institute of Medicine),
    219
Training (AHRQ)
    and career development programs,
        263
    goals and opportunities, 263–264
    grants, pre/postdoctoral, 264
    Nightingale Training School for
        Nurses, 4–5
    Nurse Scientist Training Grant, 11
    U.S. Nurse Training Act of 1964, 10
Transforming Care at the Bedside
    (TCAB), 274–275
Translation, 355–358
Tri-Council for Nursing, 323

UCF. *See* University of Central Florida
    (UCF) School of Nursing
U.S. Bureau of Health Professions, 273
U.S. Bureau of Labor Statistic, 187
U.S. Census Bureau, 83, 84, 86, 89
U.S. Children's Bureau, 7

U.S. Congress. *See* Congressional earmark legislation
U.S. Department of Health and Human Services (DHHS), 143, 326, 331
See also Agency for Health Care Research and Quality
U.S. Food and Drug Administration (FDA), 227
U.S. House of Representatives, 246
U.S. Nurse Training Act of 1964, 10
U.S. Senate, 246
Univariate analyses, 112
University of California, San Francisco, 261
University of Central Florida (UCF) School of Nursing, 95
University of Colorado, 258, 262
University of Florida, 226
University of North Dakota
Center for Rural Health, 185, 190
Institutional Research Review Board, 195, 196
University of Pennsylvania, 259, 346
University of Texas Health Science Center, 259
University of Vermont, 331
Unruh, Lynn, 123

Vermont Department of Labor's Human Resource Investment council, 333
Vermont experience. *See* Loan repayment, state funding for
Vermont Nurse Foundation Light the Lamp Scholarship, 332
Vermont Office of Nursing Workforce (ONW), 318, 331, 332
Vermont Organization of Nurse Leaders, 337
Advanced Degree Nurse Leadership Scholarship, 332
Vermont State Nurses Association, 334, 337
Vermont Technical College, 331
Vincent, Val, 337
Virtual operations, 225
Virtual reality software, 225
Virtual world, 225

Wald, Lillian, 5, 12
WDP. *See* Workforce Development Partnership
When, Not If… A Report on Oregon's Registered Nurse Workforce (OCN), 308
Williams, Josie, 262
Windows®, 72, 77
Woodruff, Judith, 315
Workforce analysis and projections. *See* Missing data
Workforce Development Partnership (WDP), 333–334, 336–338
Workforce Florida, 86
Workforce information sources, 45
Workforce issues and policy decisions. *See* Nursing outcomes research
Workload. *See* Home health nurses (workload, quality of care, and job satisfaction)
Workplace satisfaction, NSSRN and, 127–140
demographic characteristics and, personal, 131
emotional labor and, 160
findings of, 130–131
job opportunities and, perceived, 133–136
job market indicators and, objective, 134
variable and, analyses of relationships among, 134–136
methods of, 129–130
policy implications and, 138–140
safety in the workplace and, 139
sample of, 128–129
work attitudes and, 133
work characteristics and, 131–133
World Dental Federation, 323
World Health Professions Alliance, 323
World Medical Association, 323
World War II, 8–9, 183–184

Zip codes, 107–108
ZipList5 CBSA, 107

CPSIA information can be obtained
at www.ICGtesting.com
Printed in the USA
FSOW04n2224090617
35113FS